COMBAT
SURGEONS

By the same author

MILITARY

*Brassey's Battles: 3,500 Years of Conflict,
Campaigns and Wars from A–Z*
War Annual 1
War Annual 2
War Annual 3
War Annual 4
War Annual 5
War Annual 6
War Annual 7
War Annual 8
Middle East Journey
Return to Glory
One Man's War
The Walking Wounded
Digger: The Story of the Australian Soldier
*Scotland the Brave: The Story of the
Scottish Soldier*
Jackboot: The Story of the German Soldier
*Tommy Atkins: The Story of the English
Soldier*
Jack Tar: The Story of the English Seaman
*Swifter than Eagles: Biography of Marshal
of the RAF Sir John Salmond*
The Face of War
British Campaign Medals
Codes and Ciphers
Boys in Battle
Women in Battle
Anzacs at War
*Links of Leadership: Thirty Centuries of
Command*
Surgeons in the Field
Americans in Battle
Letters from the Front 1914–18
The French Foreign Legion
*Damn the Dardanelles: The Agony of
Gallipoli*
The Australian Army at War 1899–1974
*The Israeli Army in the Middle East Wars
1948–1973*
Fight for the Falklands!
*On the Western Front: Soldiers' Stories
1914–1918*
The Man the Nazis Couldn't Catch
*The War of Desperation: Lebanon
1982–85*
Battlefield Archaeology

*The Western Front 1917–17: The Price of
Honour*
*The Western Front 1917–18: The Cost of
Victory*
Greece, Crete and Syria 1941
Secret and Special (Australian Operations)
Holy War: Islam Fights
World War I in Postcards
Soldiers of Scotland (with John Baynes)
British Butchers and Bunglers of World War I
The Western Front Illustrated
*Guide to Battlefields of the Western Front
1916–1918*
Digging Up the Diggers' War
Panorama of the Western Front
Western Front Companion
*We Will Remember Them: AIF Epitaphs of
World War I*
Brassey's Book of Espionage
Gallipolii and the Anzacs
Australians on the Somme
British VCs of World War Two
Raiders
*The Battle of Hamel: The Australians'
Finest Victory*

GENERAL

*The Hunger to Come (Food and Population
Crises)*
New Geography 1966–67
New Geography 1968–69
New Geography 1970–71
Anatomy of Captivity (Political Prisoners)
Devil's Goad
Fedayeen (The Arab–Israeli Dilemma)
The Arab Mind
The Israeli Mind
The Dagger of Islam
The PLO Connections
The Arabs as Master Slavers
Know the Middle East
Fontana Dictionary of Africa since 1960
  (with John Grace)
Hitler Warned Us
Aussie Guide to Britain
*The Spirit and the Source: A Poet and his
Inspiration*
and other titles, including novels

COMBAT
SURGEONS

JOHN LAFFIN

SUTTON PUBLISHING

First published in 1970 by J.M. Dent & Sons Limited

Revised and updated version first published in 1999 by
Sutton Publishing Limited · Phoenix Mill
Thrupp · Stroud · Gloucestershire · GL5 2BU

British Library Cataloguing in Publication Data
A catalogue record for this book is available from the British Library

ISBN 0 7509 2173 0

For my grandchildren Luka, Dimian,
Kirstie, Owen, Erin

 ^{TM} ALAN SUTTON^{TM} and SUTTON^{TM} are the
trade marks of Sutton Publishing Limited

Typeset in 10/12 pt Plantin Light.
Typesetting and origination by
Sutton Publishing Limited.
Printed in Great Britain by
Redwood Books, Trowbridge, Wiltshire.

CONTENTS

Acknowledgements

A book such as this must depend on the general assistance and professional authority of various people. I thanked them in the edition of 1970, which was published under the title of *Surgeons in the Field*, and I do so again now.

Major-General N.G.G. Talbot OBE, TD, QHS, MD, FRCOG, Director-General Royal Army Medical Corps, for permission to study the unique collection of books, pamphlets, documents, manuals, letters and diaries in the Muniments Room of the Royal Army Medical College and for permission to reproduce the graphic Waterloo sketches of Sir Charles Bell.

Mr Malcolm Davies, librarian of the RAM College for his suggestions on primary sources and his unfailing assistance.

Major-General R.E. Barnsley, CB, MC, MB, B.Ch., a former director of the RAMC and later curator of the RAMC Museum, Keogh Barracks, Ash Vale.

Lieutenant Colonel John Moore, for lending me certain rare books.

Mr Tomlinson, photographer of the RAM College and Mr L.M. Payne, librarian, Royal College of Physicians.

Librarians of the Royal United Services Institution, Ministry of Defence, Admiralty and RAF, the Library of Congress and United States Army HQ, the US Signal Corps, the Imperial War Museum, especially Mr C. Brennan of the Photographic Section, and the Australian War Memorial. I am grateful to Dr Felix Abner for reading and approving my observations concerning French military medical practice.

My late wife, Hazelle, was an enormous help in the preparation of the original edition, as she was with all my books.

The 1970 version of this book, published by Dent, became a collector's item and nearly thirty years after its publication I was still receiving letters asking me where a copy could be found. I was unable to help. It says much for the enterprise of Sutton Publishing, one of the leading history publishers, and especially their editorial director, Peter Clifford, and military editor, Jonathan Falconer, that they have produced an enlarged and updated edition for new generations of readers.

I have always believed that research is part of authorship. I do not employ researchers, therefore I have nobody but myself to blame for any errors in the book. *Combat Surgeons* is not a technical book for medical professionals but the British Medical Association's *Journal* and *The Lancet* both highly praised the earlier edition.

'In battle you will live dangerously and you will feel the grip of stark fear; you will be unarmed amid violent, indiscriminate lethality; to you the hurt and the frightened will turn for easement and comfort; through your devoted service the profession of medicine will gain added dignity. The work that you do, under conditions which will range from the merely inconvenient to the utterly impossible, will be of the very greatest importance, for it is upon the quality of this initial treatment that all the rest depends.'

A Royal Army Medical Corps officer, in 1941, to young doctors about to join the Army.

'Throw away, in the first place, all ambition beyond that of doing a day's work.'

Sir William Osler, at the graduation of the first class of the US Army Medical School, 28 February 1894.

'Le bien le plus précieux est le sang du Soldat.'

Marshall Turenne, 1666.

CHAPTER ONE

'Glorious Dead' and 'Gallant Wounded'

A remarkable thing about the Great Captains is that they rarely write, in their often voluminous memoirs, about the men who bled and died for them in battle, though they may refer to 'casualties' being light or heavy or 'not disproportionate' to the gain of ground. The word 'casualties', when referring to the human cost of a battle or campaign, has been used so frequently that it is now invested with a strange abstract quality, almost as if it does not refer to human beings but to some aspect of logistics. The greater the number of casualties the more abstract and the more unreal the term becomes, so that half a million casualties at Ypres or a million at Verdun somehow do not shock. The figures are too great to be comprehensible and they are unmoving in the abstract collective.

Newspaper lists of casualties shock only those people whose close relationship to the soldiers concerned renders them shockable. *Killed in Action, Died of Wounds, Died of Illness, Missing, Wounded* – all are merely convenient labels for various classifications, and modern man is accustomed to dealing in classifications. This is something he understands intelligently. But they have no emotional context for him.

Neither he nor the Great Captains look beneath the labels, and if the impulse occurred to them their built-in defence mechanism of non-involvement would reject it. This is understandable, for should the general allow himself to consider subjectively the quantity of blood, bone and flesh he necessarily expends he might easily cease to be effective as a commander. The citizen, following the same impulse, might not be able to speak with so much admiration of his own gallant boys and with so much hatred for the beastly enemy.

Another conveniently glossy phrase, much used by some politicians, poets, preachers and pressmen, is 'our glorious dead', followed by 'our gallant wounded'. Two of the great clichés of war literature and war propaganda, they have survived thousands of years of battlefield carnage, and in nearly all cases the users have never seen any glorious dead and rarely any gallant wounded. A special mentality is required to *see* the human wreckage of a battlefield and *then* to refer to it as glorious dead. No mentality at all is required to mouth the phrase if one has never been near a military action. Military doctors and nurses see many dead and wounded, but see no glory in the dead or quivering flesh they tend.

Georges Blond saw no glory in the bombardment of Verdun in February 1916:

> . . . nothing existed but a roaring, thundering monster that lashed and ripped the earth, tossing huge chunks of it up into the cloud of smoke, dust and debris which had replaced the breathable air. A rain of branches, stones, fragments of metal, cloth, and human bodies fell uninterruptedly from the yellowish sky. No other movement was possible; the human presence was reduced to flattened terror. In every man not yet smashed to bits the violence of the shock produced a constriction of the blood vessels that wiped out every feeling but sheer animal fear and the desire to hide underground the palpitation that still persisted in the centre of his body, just above the diaphragm. Men's eyes were not closed but wide open, their pupils dilated: they did not blink when, a few yards away or even within reach, the bodies of their fellows were transformed into a flat spot beside them or torn to pieces or erased from their sight. Unable to move, the soldiers stared at the rain pouring around them. They were not divided into the living and the dead; there were also wounded men, whose shrieks and groans had even less chance of being heard than the crackling of an uprooted tree.[1]

There *is* glory in the bravery of soldiers, sailors and airmen, but not one of them would see anything glorious in being dead, even if in the dying he were helping to make his country a better place to live in, which, history proves, is doubtful. Dying on a battlefield – which is often not a field at all but a ditch or a patch of mud – is very unpleasant; being badly wounded but managing to survive for a long time until help arrives can be even more unpleasant; being patched up in hospital can be protracted and painful. And so many servicemen are not even granted the luxury of death on the battlefield at the hands of the enemy – the 'perfect soldier's death' – they die of typhoid or cholera or malaria or scrub typhus or dysentery or scurvy or frostbite or one of the many other afflictions which have cursed generations of soldiers. It is rather disconcerting to note how few balladeers or poets have sung the praises of heroes who had died of illness far from home. Perhaps they have seen nothing heroic in such a death. It is, in truth, rather a shabby death and an aesthetically unsatisfying one for a soldier. Yet many more soldiers throughout history have died of illness rather than of wounds and in the cold ignominy of bed and not in the heat of battle. Smollett, in a sober account of Admiral Vernon's expedition against Cartagena, 1741, has drawn a dreadful picture of the sufferings of the seamen:

NB: The note numbers that appear in the text refer to sources which can be found on pp. 235–8.

They were destitute of surgeons, nurses, cooks, and proper provisions; they were pent between decks in small vessels, where they had not room to sit upright; they wallowed in filth, myriads of maggots were hatched in the putrefaction of their sores, which had no other dressing than that of being washed by themselves with their own allowance of brandy; and nothing was heard but groans, lamentations, and the language of despair invoking death to deliver them from their misery.

During the Seven Years War – 1756–63 – of the 185,000 men raised for service in the Royal Navy no fewer than 135,000 died of disease, with scurvy as the principal cause.

There is another form of death too. Insanity. Many men have gone mad under the stress of continual shellfire or from living too long in a muddy, bloody, corpse-strewn trench or through having so much pride and will as to remain on duty to the point where protesting nature covers the havoc with a crazy quilt. All too euphemistically, insanity is known as 'the silent wound'.

Only a very honest poet such as Wilfred Owen, or an honest observer such as Henry Dunant or Philip Gibbs, will write of soldiers gone mad, but then they saw no glory in war. Nor do the photographers, who can hardly help but report war honestly. The great majority of war artists of all nationalities and all ages have been content to illustrate the heroics of a cavalry charge, the capture of a fort or a besieged stand at bay against fearful odds. Their corpses are always so carefully and artistically posed – and they rarely bleed. Not for them the offence to the eye of a leg detached from its trunk or entrails torn from a stomach. Indeed they are very guilty men, the war artists, with their steady line of archers, their crimson-coated, sabre-waving horsemen, the magnificent line of lancers, the toiling gunners, the unshakable infantry standing serene in square, the wave of impetuous boarders foaming onto the deck of an enemy ship. . . .

But what happens when the arrow bites, when the sabre slashes down and the lance thrusts through and the shell bursts amid flesh and the infantry are struck by showers of shrapnel and the boarders lay around them with cutlass and musket barrel and belaying pin? One end product is victory or defeat. This is what the politician sees. Another is blood. This is what the surgeon sees.

Casualties are men. There is no such thing as 'fifty thousand casualties', but fifty thousand separate and individual tragedies. It would be better if the conventional labels gave way to newer ones, such as:

Blown to pieces by a high explosive shell
Thomas Carter, thirty, married with three children . . .

Burnt alive in a tank
William Dyson, nineteen, only son of . . .

Paralysed by bullet through spine
Joseph Cash, twenty-three, recent university graduate . . .

Suffocated in sinking submarine
William Carter, twenty-one, next-of-kin Mrs V. Carter, widow . . .

Severely wounded, cheek and nose torn off
Robert Gray . . .

Severely wounded, emasculated
Aiden Croft . . .

Severely wounded, both legs crushed
Alistair Duke . . .

Gravely ill, exposure, exhaustion and meningitis
John Harrow . . .

But in war truth dies before a shot is fired, and such revealing details would perhaps not induce men to volunteer for service. Further, they might prevent women from inducing men to volunteer.

No race of people is prepared to publish in its newspapers the intimate details of its casualties. If critical of the government a paper may refer to battle 'slaughter' or 'massive casualties' or 'scenes of carnage', but these, too, are phony phrases, mere abstractions. Sometimes we encounter 'rivers of blood', but the hyperbole defeats any intent to startle. Readers *know* the reporter is not serious – though rivers have been known to take on a reddish colour from the slaughter committed on their banks, as at the Boyne. And gutters have run red after severe street fighting, as at Blenheim.

Military surgeons and physicians, nurses, stretcher-bearers and medics – the people, with the padres, who know most about the human and inhuman side of casualties – are strangely inarticulate. Relatively few have recorded their experiences, and many of those who have done so write clinically; since their records are intended for other doctors to read they speak of anonymous 'cases'. This is reasonable; one could not ask a physician* or surgeon to become subjectively involved to the point where his own reason is in jeopardy. Considering what they have seen and heard and smelled military doctors have managed to remain astonishingly sane, sober and sanguine. Their professionalism has been their armour. Their skills, which have grown in range and sophistication in the twentieth century and the competent complexity of the entire military medical system, have given the serviceman greater confidence in his survival.

Hygiene, diet, preventive medicine, antibiotics, anaesthetics, transfusions and surgical techniques, including plastic surgery, have vastly improved the soldier's prospects. He gives very little thought to the commensurate increase in the sophistication of death-dealing wound-inflicting and disease-

---

* The word *physician*, in old Ionian dialect, meant 'extractor of arrows'.

inducing techniques. And no matter how medicine and surgery develop they can do little to mitigate the immediate effects of battle wounds, burns, concussion and crushings.

Still, throughout the ages doctors and surgeons have experimented and innovated and improved, often having to fight apathy, ignorance and conservatism to gain their legitimate end – better conditions and treatment for the fighting man. Their humanity is equalled in intensity only by the sufferings and fortitude of their soldier patients.

CHAPTER TWO

Early Military Doctors

To take part in battle is the logical fulfilment of a military life; wounds and sickness and the possibility of a premature death are the natural concomitants of the fighting man's trade. He will spend his life believing that neither enemy weapon nor infection will get him – though he concedes that they may get his comrades – but by virtue of the weapon he holds in his hand he must accept the risk of personal disaster.

The chances of his being *exposed* to the risk have always depended on the machinations of politics, the skill or ineptitude of his commanders and the attitude of society. A fighting man of the First World War had every chance of suffering, for politics were vicious, generals inept, and society, demanding in the name of humanity that humanity be saved, encouraged inhumanity on the battlefield.

The chances of a man *surviving* his wounds or illness have improved with each war, since medicine and surgery somehow manage to keep ahead of the technological efficiency of killing.

It is true to say that in no two fields of human activity has so much ingenuity been displayed as in the martial infliction of death and wounds and in the treatment of these wounds. But it is wrong to assume that life is held more precious now than it was in ages past. Only those peoples with a population so small as to make security precarious have valued life highly, hence the interest of the numerically weak Byzantine armies in restoring their casualties to health.

Since earliest times the fighting man has been at the mercy of his society, his politicians, his leaders and his surgeons. Giving service, he has not always been given service, though he has at least a natural right to expect somebody to try to cure his illness and patch up his wounds according to the standards of the times.

The armies of ancient Egypt had surgeons and physicians, and though we do not know their duties we do know that they were prohibited from receiving rewards from the soldiers they treated. The practice of healing was restricted to priests and in time became fused with the mythology of the country, while incantations and astrology were freely used in the treatment of disease. According to the priest-surgeons no fewer than thirty-six demons presided over the human body, each demon having authority over a particular region. The duty of the doctor was to invoke the deity capable of giving relief. The treatment was not wholly confined to forms and ceremonies; the squill – a diuretic (urine-producing), purgative bulb – was administered for dropsy and oxide of iron was used for various ailments. The Egyptians also knew about trepanning – removing part of the skull to relieve the brain.

The ancient Greeks probably drew their knowledge of surgery and medicine from the Egyptians, and Greek surgeons became highly honoured; Greek history sings the praises of army surgeons almost as loudly as it does those of the army commanders. The greatest of them all was the mythological Aesculapius, the 'father of medicine', who is said to have been the son of Apollo by Coronis, daughter of Phlegyas, king of Orchomenus. His birth was posthumous and he was placed in the care of Chiron. He became a naval surgeon, accompanying Castor and Pollux on the Argonautic expedition – variously said to have taken place in 1263 BC or 937 BC. Aesculapius set up in private practice but was killed by a thunderbolt loosed by Zeus because, tradition says, Aesculapius was poaching on the preserves of the gods. The names of four of his daughters and two of his sons are known. The girls were Hygiea (health), Panakeia (universal remedy), Iaso (healing) and Aigle (splendour). The two sons, Machaeon and Podalirius, were the earliest army surgeons whose names have survived. Both accompanied the expedition against Troy, 1192 BC, and not only attended the wounded but fought in the ranks. When Machaeon was wounded by Paris, Achilles himself asked anxiously after the 'wounded offspring of the gods'. The whole army was interested in his recovery, for as they said 'a leech* who like him knows how to cut out darts and relieve the smarting of wounds by soothing unguents is to armies more in value than many other heroes'.[2]

However, it seems that Machaeon and his brother did little more than dress the men's wounds. 'If the men are sound,' they said, 'wine and cheese will not hurt them; if not, let them die and make room for better men.' Neither father nor sons had any knowledge of preventive medicine or hygiene, for whenever disease struck the Greek camp their only action was to deliver incantations to Apollo and other deities.

Other Greek military doctors, however, soon learned about hygiene. Temperance, cleanliness, air and exercise became their great resources, and they highly recommended sound diet and exercise on horseback.

Pythagoras, who about 500 BC was the first to bring psychology into medicine, must be claimed as an army physician. He was captured by the Persians, but, having successfully treated King Darius's dislocated ankle and a breast cancer for Queen Atossa, he was royally rewarded.

In the fourth century BC Alexander, in his Indian campaigns, took medical men with him, but had little confidence in them; he was unattended by a doctor in his last illness at Babylon 324 BC after he had

---

* Leechdom or the art of healing was derived from the Saxon word *laece*, meaning physician.

contracted a fever, partly from exposure and partly from debauchery. Nevertheless Alexander throughout his expeditions bestowed much attention on the sick and wounded of his armies and personally visited those men wounded in battle, and conferred privileges and exemptions on the families of the fallen.

The armies of ancient Persia had medical men, and Cyrus, 530 BC, was careful to appoint the most competent physicians and surgeons, to attend his troops in the field and at sieges. After capturing Babylon he formed a depot there for military medical supplies. Still, much of the medical practice was astrology and magic, and regular army hospitals were unknown.

Hannibal is said to have studied medicine in his youth, and this may be responsible for his including able doctors in his armies. After an engagement during his crossing of the Alps, 219 BC, he had litters made to carry the wounded. But the Huns, at least until the death of Attila, AD 452, had no means of treating or transporting sick and wounded and after an action they left their casualties in the field, where they were destroyed by the camp women.

In Rome curative medicine appears not to have been practised earlier than the first century BC, although hygienic principles had been followed for at least three centuries, as can be seen from the Roman sewers, aqueducts, baths and cisterns. At some time during the first century BC medical men accompanied or followed the imperial armies, and apparently they superintended the food, clothing, encampment and general hygienic conditions of the troops. In all weathers the men were compelled to take part in gymnastic exercises, in sheds if the weather was severe.

During Caesar's time medical administration had at least reached the point where Caesar thought of establishing military hospitals. The night before an engagement was contemplated Caesar had all sick and wounded sent into the nearest town. When static, a part of the camp – the valetudinarium – was set apart for the unfit men. The surgical appliances and instruments were simple, but they always accompanied the army. The Romans introduced the British to military medical organization. When Claudius invaded Britain in AD 43, each of his cohorts included a surgeon or physician, and in each legion, the senior formation, was a higher grade of medical man. The greatest contribution of Rome to medicine, however, was the hospital system, which was closely linked to the army. Each military camp had its valetudinarium to accommodate the sick and wounded. When they withdrew from Britain 400 years later, most Roman customs and organization were stamped out by Teutonic invaders, though the army surgeon of Roman times did survive in Wales – there is mention of 'medici' attached to the forces of Welsh kings.*

---

* The Welsh 'medici' were not necessarily in the Roman army tradition; the chronicler would use the only Latin word he knew for 'doctors' to suggest any sort of medical attendants.

In seventh-century Britain the Anglo-Saxons studied and practised medicine as a science. We do not know much of the treatment of the sick and wounded of the *fyrd* – the name of the first attempt at militia in the time of the Saxons – but considering the very small differences that existed between the military and civil classes it is likely that no special arrangements were required. Religious houses were open to both.

A contemporary prescription for gout advised:

> Take the heads of tuberose isis [probably iris] and dry them very much and take thereof a pennyweight and a half, and the pear tree and roman [rowan?] bark and cummin, and a fourth part of laurel berries and of the other herbs half a pennyweight of each, and six peppercorns and grind all to dust and put two egg shells full of wine. . . . Give it to the man to drink till he be well.

The armies of the Byzantine emperor, Leo VI, in the ninth century, had surgeons, and field hospitals – the first of their kind – were established for the wounded. The cavalry had a form of ambulance operated by men known as *deputati*, whose duty it was to carry wounded men in leather straps on the left side of a horse.

History is accustomed to tracing the origin of military hospitals and systematic treatment of sick and wounded to the period of the Crusades. During these times many a knight who had survived the dangers of the battlefield fell victim to disease while nursing his plague-stricken comrades. But the standards of surgery and medicine were low, and the assistance given to wounded men was often unsystematic and not particularly sympathetic. The common soldier was bought to be sacrificed; he was used while in health and when sick or wounded left to die. The most interesting exception to this barbarous, but, by the standards of the times, logical, practice was in the Byzantine armies of the tenth century. They had an ambulance corps that had no modern equivalent until the seventeenth century. A surgeon served each company of 250 men and had under him six or eight stretcher-bearers, who were rewarded for saving severely wounded men. It is not merely coincidental that the Byzantine army was such a formidable one.

In England it was not until the Norman Conquest (1066) and the introduction of the feudal system that some rudimentary form of medical attention returned. Each Norman lord had an armed force of retainers, and to many of these households 'leeches' – the usual term for a doctor – were attached. In the twelfth century medicine and surgery, up till now practised simultaneously, were separated by the Edict of Tours, 1163, though monks continued in the dual role until 1216, when Pope Honorius III directed that not only should no priest practise surgery – because in doing so he shed blood – but that all priests should refuse their benediction to those who professed surgery. They continued to be responsible for the teaching and administration of medicine, but barbers took over the surgeon's knife, and surgery became a trade.

A number of leeches accompanied Richard Cœur de Lion to the Crusades in Palestine (1190), but they lacked the knowledge and the skill of Saladin's surgeons. Richard's armies were plagued by dysentery and typhus, and suffered just as severely from disease as the two earlier Crusades. But along the lines of communications a great medical organization appeared, set up on a military basis by the Knights of St John of Jerusalem, who wore a black mantle with an eight-pointed white cross, and whose vows required them to protect and care for pilgrims on the way to the Holy Sepulchre. Expelled from Palestine after the Crusades, they occupied Rhodes for two centuries and Malta for nearly three. The order survives today and includes the familiar St John Ambulance Association.

Saladin's medical officers included Abd-Allatif, a physician from Baghdad, who wrote a description of the sultan's camp. It had in its midst 'a large square containing a hundred and forty farriers' shops; in a single kitchen were twenty-eight coppers, each one capable of containing a sheep entire'. The camp had more than a thousand baths and a bath cost a piece of silver.

The death of King Richard at the siege of Châlus, 1199, was due to the unskilful extraction of an arrow from his shoulder, but Edward I, while in Palestine, was luckier. He had in his army a surgeon, name unknown, whose reputation survives. In 1272 Edward was attacked and severely wounded by a member of an assassin band; his surgeon, by making deep incisions and cutting away the mortified parts, restored him to health within a fortnight. Edward's rank was his fortune. Treatment of most wounds from arrows, sword, lance, dagger or club was confined to salves, ointments, powders and decoctions of herbs, to some of which magical properties were attributed. It was considered that suppuration was the natural physiological sequel of every wound, that a wound could not heal properly without suppuration, and if it did not occur it was made to do so.

About 1260 an Italian surgeon, Theodoric, began to modify the usual suppurative treatment of wounds by substituting dressings soaked in arnica – an antiseptic method. A pupil of Theodoric, Henri de Mondeville, surpassed his tutor and reached a state of knowledge far ahead of his time. He became surgeon to Philip-le-Bel, King of France, and wrote, between 1306 and 1320, a treatise on surgery. In this he advocated a new treatment for wounds, but his methods had to wait 600 years for general acceptance.

Mondeville's treatment of wounds to the large intestine was very much as is practised now. He advised that if the large intestine were wounded it should be sutured – 'as furriers sew a skin'. The wounded intestine should then be replaced in the abdominal cavity and the abdominal wall sutured. He saw wounds of this sort, sutured and closed immediately, heal in a short time with a single dressing.

Describing the treatment for fresh wounds which had penetrated the cavity of the chest, he wrote:

From whichever side the wound may be, one treats it in just the same way as wounds penetrating the skull, that is to say, removing foreign bodies, closing the edges of the wound, and giving powder with the pigment. One need only add that these wounds and those of the abdomen should be closed more quickly, should be joined more strongly, and should be sutured by stitches closer and tighter even though they may be smaller than wounds of other parts. . . . One must act so for three reasons: so the vital heat should not be exhaled through the wounds; and in order that the surrounding cold should not annihilate this heat; and in order that the entry of circulating air should not cause suppuration of the wound. . . . Bandages must be broad and sewn together so that they do not slip.

The fact of St Louis having witnessed the work of army surgeons in the field led to the founding of a college of surgeons in Paris in 1268 and the promulgation of an order that wounds and sores would be treated gratis on the first Monday of each month – though by 'barbers' who had received no professional education. Imperfect though this step was it counted as progress.

As England had no standing army until the middle of the seventeenth century surgeons and physicians were engaged, as were the troops, 'for the duration only' in the wars of the Middle Ages. They were generally part of the king's retinue and acted as personal medical attendants to the sovereign and his staff. Wounded troops were sent to monasteries or billeted with the civil population for treatment, or discharged on the spot with a small sum of money sufficient to get them home; in some cases the severely wounded were put out of their misery by their own comrades. Arrangements varied with each campaign, and there are some instances of attempts to organize the evacuation of the sick.

The lordly and knightly combatants were treated by their ladies, many of whom could competently treat flesh wounds; the historians of the fourteenth century extol the surgical knowledge of the ladies. It was believed that professors of medicine had access to worlds unknown to ordinary mortals, so that 'the possession of more than mortal knowledge was readily ascribed to a pure unearthly being like woman and the knight who felt to his heart of hearts the charm of her beauty was not slow in believing that she could fascinate the very elements of nature to aid him'.

Henry III included in his expeditionary force to France in 1253 Master Thomas Weseman, 'who knew how to cure wounds, a science particularly useful in the siege of castles', but he was probably the king's personal surgeon, and it was not until the following reign that paid medical officers attending an army are mentioned in the king's accounts. To Edward I, in fact, is given the credit of making the first attempt to set up a military medical service during his campaigns against Scotland, 1298–1300, while Edward II's ordinary 'chirurgeons' received fourpence a day, and also shaved the men, receiving another twopence from each soldier on pay day as 'regards' – a custom which lasted for over 200 years.

Of the five campaigns against Scotland, those of 1298 and 1300 are especially interesting for the earliest indications of anything like an organized army medical service. The accounts for the 1300 campaign have been preserved, giving particulars of disbursements. These include interesting details concerning the medical men who were present, their pay, the clothing they received and the horses they had. The king had in his train his physician, de Kenleye, with two servants, or juniors, also his surgeon, Master Philip de Beauveys; in addition there was Master Peter, who had served in the campaign of 1298. The king's physician and surgeon each received a knight's pay, two shillings a day, and the others, who ranked as esquires, half that sum. In addition to their pay, the king's physician and surgeon each received four marks for clothes for winter wear, and while they were with the court they received their board and lodging free. Master Philip, the surgeon, was allowed the sum of forty shillings annually for supplying medical stores for men injured, and Master Peter was allowed half that sum.

The expedition to Scotland in 1322 deserves mention; there is a record of the medical stores which were sent for use of the troops by Master Stephen of Paris, the king's surgeon. This document, the earliest of its kind, proves that there was at this time some sort of organization to provide for the medical needs of the army, and that somebody was entrusted with the preparation and dispatch of the material, probably Master Stephen. The drugs were packed in two great 'paniers' – the first mention of the containers which were to become ubiquitous. They cost 6*d* each and were sent from London to Newcastle by ship, then to Edinburgh and from there back again to Hayleland. The total cost of the goods, including carriage from London, was £91 3*s* 9*d*. The stores themselves, called 'drogueries and implastra', are specified minutely, and include 3 lb. of oxerocrosin, 3 lb of dyataroscoe, 6 lb of apostolicon, 2 lb of Saunguys Draconis and various other forms of ointment.

Little is known of medical arrangements for the English forces at the battle of Crécy (1436) or the siege of Calais (1347), but a large number of the sick and wounded – after treatment in monasteries – were shipped home from the French port for discharge. Some attention was paid to the wounded on the battlefield at Poitiers (1356), which the English nearly lost through being vigorously counter-attacked when engaged in getting their unfortunate comrades out of the fighting line to the rear. The leading English surgeon of the period was John of Arderne, who wrote the first English book on surgery.

There is an illuminating passage in Froissart which is probably a correct picture of the times. It concerns the famous knight, Sir John Audley, who fought at Poitiers. He suffered several wounds, and when overcome by them he was carried out of the press by his four squires, who laid him under a hedge, took off his armour to examine his wounds, dress them and sew up the most dangerous. The châtelaines – wives of the knights – probably taught these squires how to bandage and treat wounds. Part of the duty of the squire was to carry dressings and salves.

During the fourteenth century France had a great surgeon, Guy de Chauliac, who was so advanced that he did not employ astrology and resisted most superstitions. He favoured healing wounds by first intention, that is, a once-and-for-all treatment rather than in stages, and recommended dry dressings and treatment by desiccators and balsams. To prove that a wound had penetrated he closed the patient's mouth and nose and held a lighted candle near the wound or held a piece of cotton close to it, watching for escaping air to move the thread. De Chauliac recommended that there should be no delay in opening, dilating and draining the wound and that the patient should be rolled on the side to allow the fluids to run out. If the patient was very ill, de Chauliac practised counter-incision, with a razor, through one of the lower spaces, the best space being that between the fourth and fifth ribs counting from below.

In 1363 de Chauliac, in probably the first book of its kind, gave advice on the treatment of wounds and advocated methods followed by some German knights – the employment of exorcism, oil, wool and cabbage leaves. According to de Chauliac German surgeons were divided into five sects – the first applied poultices indiscriminately in every description of ulcer or wound; the second in similar cases applied wine only; the third used emollient ointments and plasters; the fourth, chiefly military surgeons, promiscuously employed oils, wool, potions and charms; the fifth consisted of ignorant practitioners and silly women who exploited the saints and praised one another's writings constantly.

Illness was given less attention than wounds, since many diseases were thought to be a sign of the Almighty's displeasure and therefore not to be tampered with, or unclean and therefore to be avoided. In any case, most remedies were useless or dangerous concoctions. Society's attitude to illness among fighting men also saw to it that men received meagre treatment; a battle wound was held to be honourable, while a disease, lacking the heroic connotations of a wound, was almost dishonourable. In much the same way, doctors were more interested in the tangible realities of a wound than in a disease with which they could not come to grips. Preventive medicine, even in the form of elementary hygiene, had to wait a long time for its exponents.

CHAPTER THREE

Weapons and Diseases

Until the introduction of gunpowder in the fourteenth century (in Europe) the arrow was the main missile weapon – in sea as well as in land warfare – in the Middle Ages in Western Europe. The crossbow was so devastating that in 1139 the Second Lateran Council outlawed it, describing it as 'a weapon hateful to God and unfit for Christians'. The Council held, in fact, that long-distance or missile warfare was unchristian. This was one of many futile attempts to limit something not subject to limit – the method of inflicting death in war. The English longbow was more deadly than the crossbow and the archers were the backbone of any English force at the time of Crécy or Agincourt. The bows, mostly of yew and 6 ft 4 in long, shot cloth-yard shafts fitted with a barb of iron and fledged with goose or peacock feathers. They could pierce oak to a depth of two or more inches and cases were reported of one arrow killing three men in file and of driving clean through a horse and killing a man on the other side. Another formidable English weapon was the bill – evolved from an agricultural implement – a staff weapon with a hook, spike and blade. A foot-soldier could drag a horseman from his saddle with the hook, then kill him with the spike, which could be poked through a chink in the armour, or with the blade. The pole-axe and mace were dangerous smashing weapons, and the morning-star – a heavy spiked ball on the end of a length of chain – could inflict terrible injuries. Razor-sharp swords and axes could decapitate or maim at a blow. There was constant danger of being ridden down by cavalry, and many a soldier escaped lance or spear only to die under the hooves of a heavily laden charger. The horsed soldier ran less risk of wounding, but being clad in armour carried its own hazards. A knight could well be wearing gear his own weight, at the time of the Crusades, and if he fell he was helpless; many a fallen knight was burnt to death by Greek fire inside his armour. If a lance pierced armour and broke off, the difficulty of extracting it and getting the victim out of his casing usually resulted in his death. In attacking a castle or town a soldier could be scalded by boiling water or oil or crushed by rocks dropped from the walls. The doctors called upon to treat wounds knew how to amputate and bandage, but they could neither mitigate pain nor prevent infection. Standard treatment for centuries was to pour boiling oil on a bleeding stump or into a gaping wound. That so many men survived not only their wounds and illness but also endured their treatment is a tribute to the resilience of the human body and the spirit which drives it.

Surgeons became part of the British military establishment following the introduction of gunpowder, the manufacture of which Henry V tried unsuccessfully in 1414 to prohibit in England. The following year he had twenty surgeons and a physician in the army of 32,000 with which he invaded France. Thomas Morstede and William Bredewerdyn (or Bradwardyn) as principal medical officers, were entitled to receive prisoners and take plunder.

Preparations for the expedition were started a year ahead, and soldiers were enlisted under contract or 'indenture'. In this way, 2,500 men-at-arms and 8,000 archers were enrolled, and in addition numbers of non-combatants, such as carpenters, smiths, miners, armourers, yeomen of the pavilions, saddlers, physicians, surgeons and chaplains. Thomas Morstede of London, as chief surgeon, was to be ready to attend muster in May 1415 and was to bring with him fifteen persons, of whom three should be archers and the other men of his own craft. His wages for the whole year were to be forty 'marcs' for himself and twenty each for the other fifteen persons, to be paid in advance for the first quarter. Morstede applied for money to purchase medical stores, as well as one cart and two horses to carry them. Here is the germ of a medical service. The provision of one cart and two horses seems ridiculously inadequate to carry all the medical stores for an army preparing for a year's campaign,* but Henry's army was most carefully planned and the best organized and equipped expeditionary force that had ever sailed from England. Henry V was not a devil-may-care adventurer, ready to risk his crown and kingdom on a mad expedition, but a general who took pains to leave as little as possible to chance.

Though the two leading surgeons occupied distinguished positions in London their staff were obviously not much esteemed, for they ranked after shoemakers and tailors – but at least before washer-women – in Henry V's military code. At the siege of Harfleur the surgeons had to deal with an outbreak of dysentery – *cours de ventre* – in which 2,000 men died and 5,000 more had to be invalided home. The disease was epidemic, and affected both knight and common soldier. It ran an acute course, often being fatal in a few days. There is no evidence to show whether it was due to the amoeba of dysentery, which caused such trouble to British troops in Mesopotamia during the 1914–18 war, or to the bacillary form. It seems to have been a common type in northern France, for at the siege of Arras in 1414, when defended by the Duke of Burgundy, 11,000 men died of the flux.† Considering the conditions under which Henry's men fought, the outbreak

---

* As late as 1808, at the beginning of the Peninsular War when Wellesley landed in Mondego Bay, the medical stores for the whole army were loaded into two bullock carts.
† During the 1914–18 war in the Somme area the British and the Germans suffered severely from dysentery of a rather mild and non-fatal type.

of bowel complaints was inevitable. They were short of food, and much they had bought with them had been spoilt at sea. The men drank inordinately after working in the sweltering heat and too freely ate unripe grapes and other fruit. On fish days they wolfed the cockles and mussels that swarmed that year in the muddy creeks, and when chilly nights ended the hot autumn days they lay down where the offal of slaughtered beasts lay rotting in the surrounding swamps. Flies did the rest of the damage. The men endured great hardships in their march up the valley of the Somme, past Abbeville, Pont St Rémy, Hangest, Corbie, Boves, Nesle and Harbonnières towards battle at Arras and Harfleur.

The doctors must have watched the battle with anxious eyes. They were probably stationed during the fight with the baggage animals, and alongside the chaplain, who described the action. Their most notable patient would have been the Duke of Gloucester, dagger-wounded in the abdomen. He made a successful recovery. No provision existed for taking the wounded from the field, but on the following morning the English troops, in marching off, killed all the hopelessly wounded 'for the humane purpose of putting them out of pain'.[3] Each slightly wounded man was given some money and told to find his way home. Useless prisoners were also killed.

The wounded and chronically ill men of any nationality who managed to struggle home after a battle could expect no treatment there. They could only plead for charity, as did Thomas Hollstede, wounded at Harfleur while fighting for Henry V. His petition for royal favour supplies interesting details of wounds suffered.

> To the king our sovereign lord,
> Beseecheth meekly your povere [poor] liegeman and humble horatour [petitioner], Thomas Hollstede, that, in consideration of his service done to your noble progenitors of full blessed memory, king Henry the iiijth and king Henry the fifth, (whose souls God assoile!) being at the siege of Harfleur there smittin with a springbolt through the head, losing his one yee and his cheek bone broken; also at the battle of Agincourt, and afore at the taking of the carracks on the sea, there with a gadde of yrene [iron] his plates smitten in to his body and his hand smitten in sunder, and sore hurt, maimed and wounded, by mean whereof he being sore feebled and debrused, now falle to great age and poverty, greatly endetted, and may not help him self, having not wherewith to be sustained ne relieved, but of men's gracious almesse [alms], and being for his said service never yet recompensed ne rewarded, it please your high and excellent grace, the premises tenderly considered, of your benign pity and grace to relieve and refresh your said povere oratour as it shall please you with your most gracious almesse, at the reverence of God and in work of charity, and he shall devoutly pray for the souls of your said noble progenitors and for your most noble and high estate.[4]

Henry granted the soldier a pension.

Spanish soldiers in service at the end of Hollstede's century were more fortunate than he, for Queen Isabella, a competent military leader in her own right and one of the most efficient quartermasters in military history, placed field hospitals on something like the footing we now recognize. In 1484, during the War of Grenada, 1483–7, Isabella had an army of 18,000 at Antequara, where she had a large six-tent hospital, well equipped, for sick and wounded. 'Isabella, solicitous for everything that concerned the soldiers, sometimes visited the camp in person, encouraging the soldiers to endure the hardships of war, and relieving their necessities by liberal donations of clothes and money.'[5]

Use of gunpowder had led to a great change in tactics, but in military surgery no great change was discernible in the fifteenth century. Not until some time after the introduction of the arquebus in 1450 did gunshot wounds become common. The first authors to write of these were Pfolsprundt in 1460; Braunschweig, whose *Buch der Cirirgia* was printed in Strasbourg in 1497; and Hans von Gersdorf, who published *Feldbuch der Wundarsney* in 1517.

Gunshot wounds of that time were caused by large missiles of low velocity, producing ragged wounds aggravated by indriven pieces of clothing. They were severe and dangerous and they often turned septic. Nearly all surgeons of the time believed that gunpowder was venomous and poisoned the flesh; to neutralize the poison they cauterized the wound by injecting boiling oil, the old standby. Special instruments were made to dilate wounds so that the oil could be poured in.

In the last decade of the fifteenth century fighting men were hit by a sinister disease new to Europe – syphilis. Ironically, Isabella was indirectly responsible for it, since she, with her husband Ferdinand, had encouraged Columbus to sail to America, where the disease originated. At this time King Charles VIII of France laid claim to the two Sicilies; in order to gain the crowns of these two lands he raised an army of 18,000 horsemen and 20,000 infantry in Lyons. The cavalry were Frenchmen, the foot-soldiers mercenaries from every country, including a contingent of 3,000 Swiss, famed for their bravery and their 25-ft pikes.

This army crossed the Alps, reaching the Italian frontier in September 1494. Protected by neutrality treaties, they advanced unhindered through Upper and Central Italy. Milan, Florence and Rome were the scenes of their wild carousing. On 22nd February 1494 Charles VIII and his troops appeared at the gates of Naples, which surrendered without a struggle. A single citadel in which the few of those who had resisted and feared reprisals had taken refuge stoutly resisted. It was defended by Italians aided by Spanish troops whom Ferdinand, flouting the neutrality pact, had sent to the aid of hard-pressed Naples. The Spaniards had not only brought their weapons but also syphilis, which since Columbus's triumphant home-coming had slowly spread in the taverns and the poorer districts of the towns. In this castle during the course of the siege defensive methods were used by the besieged in their distress that proved fatal for both sides and eventually for the whole of Europe.

The anatomist Falloppia (1523–62), whose father was in the fortress, tells how the defenders used every method to save their skins:

> Since they were but a small band, vastly outnumbered by the French, they stole out of the fortress, leaving behind an adequate garrison, and poisoned the wells. Not satisfied with this, they bribed the Italian millers who delivered the corn to the enemy to mix plaster in the meal, and finally, under the pretext that food was short, they expelled from the fortress the whores and women, especially the attractive ones whom they knew were infected with the disease. The French, seized with compassion for the women and attracted by their beauty, gave them asylum.

The French soldiers revelled in the delights of love. While their commander, the king, enjoyed the mild climate of Naples, abandoning himself to *dolce far niente*, his army was busied with the captured whores instead of with weapons. Once before in history an army together with its great leader very nearly succumbed to the charm of its Neapolitan landscape and its women: Hannibal's army, which had gone into winter quarters at Capula during the Second Punic War, retired demoralized and with no stomach for battle. This seductive *genius loci* had persisted down the ages, and Queen Joanna I of Naples (1326–82) found herself forced to issue a decree for the benefit of the women which limited conjugal intercourse in her kingdom – 'Ne quis uxorem suam cogeat plus guam exxies pro die coire') that no man must force his wife to have sexual intercourse more than six times a day).

In the rear of the lascivious conquerors trouble was brewing. Milan, Florence and Venice entered the war on the side of Naples; Germany and Spain revoked their dearly bought neutrality. After a month Charles realized that his lines of retreat had been cut. He broke off the siege and prepared to fight his way back to France, leaving Naples for the north. But near Palma he met an Italian army of 40,000. The French managed to fight their way through the frontier with heavy losses, where the demoralized mercenaries were disbanded to disperse and make their own way home. They were in a lamentable condition.

> Some of the soldiers were covered from head to foot with an appalling type of itch which looked so alarming that, abandoned by their comrades, their only wish was to be left alone to die. Others had the same itch only in certain places, on the forehead and neck, throat, chest, buttocks, etc., but the scabs were harder than treebark and they tore them with their nails, because they were so painful. The bodies of others were covered with innumerable warts and pimples. Some of these broke out on the face, in the ears, and on the nose. This strange rash was also due to scabies from which the mercenaries, like all soldiers of the period, suffered. Some laughed and joked over their troubles instead of complaining.[6]

The survivors of this lost army looked as revolting as lepers and were more dangerous. They shivered with hunger and pain and writhed in agony in the gutters, but they were offered neither bread and water, nor pity and sanctuary. In ragged clothes, in all weathers, they lived on wild berries and roots, crawling through the thickets and slowly rotting in caves, an offence to themselves and to others. However, many of the disbanded soldiers arrived home proud and carefree, looking healthy enough in their fine uniforms. Underneath it was a different picture, for they had rashes like the measles, small ulcers in the mouth and on the gums, the lips or the tongue. They had their pay and many a looted gold piece and now they were ready to spend. In every small town they roistered in the taverns, and slept the night with whores. After a visit to the public stews to be bled, they went cheerfully on their way. But wherever they tarried, wherever they ate, drank, slept and debauched they left poison behind – on the rim of the tankard, on kissed lips, on bodies enjoyed and on the couches where they had lusted. The poison circulated in their blood and infected anyone who came in contact with it; it took possession of a man's body, exuded from all his pores so that he in turn poisoned everything he touched. The abominable disease was not mortal like the plague but hateful and tragic.

At the outset Italy was most deeply affected. The disease flared once more after the death of Charles VIII (he died of syphilis in 1498, at the age of twenty-eight), when his nephew, Louis XII, renewed his claims on the kingdom of Naples. Once more a French army crossed the Alps and marched the length of Italy to Naples and a Spanish army landed in Calabria. The allies began to quarrel over the frontiers of their conquests and a clash followed during which the French were driven not only from Naples but from the whole of Italy. The Spaniards reigned in Naples. Once more a French and a Spanish army with their foreign mercenaries and countless camp followers came into contact with the centre of syphilitic contagion, Naples. Defeated and sick, retiring troops carried new germs of the disease to their native towns and villages and to their families.

The disease spread rapidly across Switzerland to Germany. Augsburg, Nuremberg and Munich were the first large cities where cases were reported, and within a year hardly a town in Europe was free. From this time for nearly four and a half centuries fighting men had a raging enemy – and medical men faced a problem to which there was no apparent solution.

CHAPTER FOUR

Ambroise Paré – New Principles and Pity

It was easier to treat some wounds than illnesses. An early work on gunshot wounds was published in 1514 by Antonio Ferri, physician to Pope Paul III. The orthodox treatment for gunshot wounds was still to pour boiling oil into them. Amputations should be summarily dealt with, Ferri advised, by chopping off the limb with a hatchet, followed by the application of a red-hot iron to the stump.

On the Continent surgery was given status by the skill of the French barber-surgeon Ambroise Paré. Paré, the son of a barber, was fortunate enough to serve as an apprentice in the Hôtel Dieu, the largest hospital in that age. Here he accumulated knowledge from the stream of patients and had opportunity of learning anatomy by dissecting corpses. At the end of his apprenticeship in 1536 he took part in his first campaign with the French Army as a field surgeon. The object of the campaign was the occupation of Milan, to which Francis I of France and the Emperor Charles V both laid claim. In the bloody battle for Turin, Paré came under fire and was greatly moved by the sufferings of the wounded.

> We thronged into the city and passed over the dead bodies and some that were not yet dead, hearing them cry under the feet of our horses which made a great pity in my heart, and truly I repented that I had gone forth from Paris to see so pitiful a spectacle. Being in the city, I entered a stable thinking to lodge my horse and that of my man, where I found four dead soldiers and three who were propped against the wall, their faces wholly disfigured, and they neither saw, nor heard, nor spoke, and their clothing yet flaming from the gunpowder which had burnt them. Beholding them with pity there came an old soldier who asked me if there was any means of curing them. I told him no. At once he approached them and cut their throats gently and, seeing this great cruelty, I shouted at him that he was a villain. He answered me that he prayed to God that when he should be in such a state he might find someone who would do the same for him, to the end that he might not languish miserably.

During his apprenticeship Paré had seen much suffering and death, but soldiering surpassed all. After the bitter fighting for the Susa pass he had many wounded men on his hands. Paré had no experience of gunshot wounds; he only knew that on account of the gunpowder they were considered septic and according to the theories in vogue were to be cauterized with boiling elder oil. With great reluctance, having seen his superiors do this, he set to work. It was repulsive to him because it caused the wounded incredible suffering; they screamed with pain as he poured the burning oil into the wounds, and their groans continued until at last they fainted or fell silent from sheer exhaustion. When his supply of elder oil ran out Paré, rather than leave them untended, dressed a few of the men's wounds with an ointment composed of egg yolk, rose oil and turpentine.

> That night I could not sleep at my ease, fearing that I should find the wounded on whom I had failed to put the oil dead or poisoned, which made me rise very early to visit them where, beyond my hope, I found those upon whom I had put the digestive medicine feeling little pain, and their wounds without inflammation or swelling having rested well throughout the night; the others to whom I had applied the said boiling oil, I found feverish, with great pain and swelling about their wounds. Then I resolved in my heart never more to burn thus cruelly poor men wounded with gunshots.

And that morning Paré added with relief: 'I dressed and God healed.'

Another of Paré's worries concerned the soldiers whose limbs were shattered by bullet wounds and hung in ribbons. Normally these wounded men were abandoned on the battlefield until they bled to death or succumbed from fever. Only the very few who survived the first few days were given medical attention; the surgeons waited until the inevitable gangrene had become localized and then amputated the limb at the decayed zone. It was possible to operate with knife and saw and to amputate the shattered limb, but often the red-hot iron was inadequate to halt the flow of blood and prevent the wounded man from bleeding to death. Paré devised a crescent-shaped needle with which he pricked the blood vessels, led the needle through a pair of pincers and knotted the ends of the thread tightly. The bleeding was thus arrested, and the end of the artery wasted away.

With this type of ligature Paré showed how shattered limbs could be saved from gangrene and soldiers from bleeding to death by swift amputation. High amputations at the shoulder and thigh joints could now be attempted, and operations performed on healthy tissue. Paré insisted upon this, for he knew by experience that, unless completely isolated, gangrene would spread and necessitate further amputations if the patient had not already died of the serious infection.

With Paré's banishment of the hot iron and boiling oil, the introduction of the ligature and the challenge to amputate a healthy limb, surgery in the field (there existed no other) progressed. A type of surgery evolved which was no longer the butchery of sawing and searing; it was deliberate, avoided inflicting pain unless the cure demanded it.

Not everyone followed Paré's recommendations. To amputate a healthy limb, to endure the screams of pain of the sufferer, demanded perseverance, sound knowledge of anatomy and a cool head to sew the arteries and bind them. Speed was essential for any chance of a successful treatment. The Paris Faculty of Medicine vigorously opposed the new theories. 'An ignorant and misguided person has recently dared, from lack of knowledge, to reject burning the arteries with red-hot irons after the severance of the limbs and, flouting commonsense, to substitute a new treatment, the ligature of the arteries without being aware that this ligature is far more dangerous than cauterization with red-hot irons. . . . In truth, anyone who endures this butchery has every good cause to thank God that he is still alive after the operation.' Surgeons were delighted to be excused by this highest authority from complying with demands which very few of them were capable of carrying out. They continued to amputate at localized gangrenous parts and used the easy method of the red-hot iron to stop the flow of blood. Paré's sane practices were dropped, though he served as surgeon to four successive kings of France, followed their armies from 1536 until 1569 and published the results of his vast experience in 1582.

In 1552, when the Grand Master of the Artillery was returning to his tent with a wound in his shoulder, Paré saw a crowd of wounded soldiers trailing pathetically after him hoping that his doctor would be able to find time to give them some treatment. He tells, too, how the Duke of Alva reported to the Emperor that about 200 soldiers were dying and, when told they were not 'gentlemen or men of mark' but just 'poor soldiers', the latter replied, 'Then it is no great loss if they died.'

When the nobles of France, under the Duke of Guise, were besieged in Metz by a great army led by Charles V, Guise sent to his king asking that Paré be allowed to visit the garrison and that the general feeling was that 'Now we shall not die even though wounded for Paré is among us.' Metz was the bulwark of France at that time and the French have always maintained that the presence of this one man so inspired the garrison that it was able to hold the fortress until the besieging army perished.

Paré reveals something of the way in which wounded were evacuated after the retreat from Metz when carts and wagons were requisitioned to bring out the wounded. 'Our carters, when they returned, told us the roads were all paved with dead bodies, and they never got half the men there, for they died in the cart and the Spaniards, seeing them at the point of death, before they had breathed their last, threw them out of the carts and buried them in the mud and mire, saying they had no orders to bring back dead men.'

The 'English Paré', Thomas Gale, was probably the first British surgeon who wrote especially on injuries caused by gunpowder projectiles. He had served in the army of Henry VIII, was present at the siege of Montreuil in 1544 and, at the time of publication of his two books, was sergeant-surgeon to Elizabeth I. In *Wounds, Fractures and Dislocations* he gives a formula for styptic powder, the ingredients of which were alum, lime, arsenic and strong vinegar, mixed and applied by means of tow covered with white of egg. In later works, published in 1586 and 1596, Gale deplored the inferiority of men employed as medical officers. At Montreuil Gale had found all kinds of men usurping the title and functions of surgeons – sowgelders, tinkers and cobblers. These men were dangerous and usually killed their patients by treating wounds with a concoction of a grease used to lubricate horses' hooves, an ointment compound of shoemaker's wax and the rust of old kettles.

Gale left some clear descriptions of his treatment of chest wounds. If non-penetrating they should be treated as other wounds, with tow dipped in restricting powder. If penetrating, but without wound of the inward viscera, they should be stitched and dressed, but if penetrating with inward bleeding then 'with all haste and expedition put in a tent large and long' and roll the patient on to his side to aid drainage. He insisted that a string should be tied to the tent in case it should slip into the pleural cavity. For a man with a bullet in the chest he advised use of a probe to try to dig out the ball, 'but if you cannot without great pain and searching find the the bullet leave it alone lest the air injure the inward part'. In eleven cases at Montreuil Gale let shots remain in men's bodies and all survived and prospered.

Contemporary with Gale was Felix Wurtz, first a barber in Zurich, who became a military surgeon of great skill. He recommended that surgeons should be very clean, and that they should touch wounds only with freshly cleaned hands and should avoid dragging sleeves over men's wounds.

Partly as a result of Paré's suggestions, in 1597 Henry IV of France instituted field hospitals at the siege of Amiens, a boon which so moved his soldiers that they called the siege the 'velvet campaign'. His son, Louis XIII, built the first fixed hospital at Pignerol and Louis XIV the Hôtel des Invalides at Paris.

Several English surgeons were prominent at this period. One, William Clowes, more naval surgeon than a military one, was sent to the Low Countries to take charge of the wounded of Elizabeth's army then helping the Dutch against the Spaniards. In 1585 he wrote a book on syphilis and advocated its treatment by mercury. He too wrote about gunshot wounds, recommending the application of various forms of gum, an important improvement on the barbaric boiling oil.

The first Scot to attain eminence as an army surgeon was apparently Peter Lowe, who served as chirurgeon-major to the Spanish regiment in Paris towards the end of the sixteenth century. Amputations were his special interest; he taught his assistants to amputate a finger or toe with a pair of pliers, 'by which the part was chopped off at once and with the smallest pain'. Sometimes he used a chisel and mallet, 'laying the member in a block and so cutting it off'. Lowe, on retirement from the army, founded Glasgow's medical school.

In 1505 the surgeons of Edinburgh had been incorporated under the denomination of surgeons and barbers. It was required that they be able to read and write, 'to know anatomie, nature and complexion of every part of the human bodie, and lykeways to know all vayns of the saym that he may make flew bothomie in due time, together with a perfect knowledge of shaving beards'.

Among the changes Queen Mary introduced into the organization of the army was the appointment of additional medical officers. In 1557 one surgeon was attached to each company of 100 to 120 men and the rates of pay were revised. A surgeon drew 2*s* a day, a junior surgeon 1*s* 6*d*. In addition to the surgeon's ordinary pay a deduction from that of the soldiers to the same amount as in the time of Edward III continued to be given to him. These low rates attracted men of low education. Gale pointed out to Queen Elizabeth, early in her reign, that army doctors were treated unfairly, but not until 1603 were the qualifications and thus the status of surgeons raised. They then had to be 'men of sobriety, of good conscience, and skilful in their science; able to heal all sores and wounds, specially to take a pellet out of the same'.[7]

All captains – that is, company commanders – were directed to employ a surgeon and to see that he had with him all his 'oils, balms, salves, instruments and necessary stuffs . . . allowing and sparing them carriage for the same'. On each pay day every soldier was required to 'augment' the surgeon's salary, while for his part the surgeon was expected 'readily to employ his industry upon the sore and wounded soldiers, not intermeddling with any other cures to them noysome'. The meaning of *noysome* is obscure, but probably the injunction meant that a surgeon had to prescribe treatment agreeable to the patient. Treatment was certainly not agreeable to the English seamen of the period. Rupture was treated by hanging the patient up by the heels until the prolapsus was reduced. After an amputation the bleeding stump was dipped in boiling pitch to cauterize it, a practice that pertained until after Trafalgar. Pepys met a seaman who had lost an eye fighting the Dutch; the surgeon had stopped the socket with oakum.

But for centuries illness and not the enemy had been the main killer at sea. Commanders' reports made frequent reference to such trouble, as did that of Lord Howard's to Elizabeth on 22 August 1588:

> My most gracious Lady, with great grief I must write unto you in what state I find your fleet in here. The infection [scurvy] is grown very great and in many ships, and now very dangerous; and those that come in fresh are soonest infected; they sicken the one day and die the next. It is a thing that ever followeth such great services, and I doubt not but with good care and God's goodness, which doth always bless your Majesty and yours, it will quench again.

The Navy Commissioners' occasional burst of enthusiasm to keep English seamen fit was generally inspired by their shortage rather than by their sincere regard for welfare or by the efforts of some humane medical man. One such seems to have been a Dr Cogbourne, who in 1602 sold his patent electuary – a medicinal powder mixed with syrup – to the Commissioners, who ordered it to be distributed to seamen in the West Indies fleet.

A prominent surgeon of the Elizabethan period was John Woodall, who began his service career in in 1589 when he accompanied Elizabeth's forces, under Lord Willoughby, to help Henry IV of France. In 1626 he was given medical control of the Royal Navy and later of the East India Company. Between the years 1612 and 1639 he published masses of advice, but his name deserves to be remembered chiefly because he first advocated lime juice as a treatment for scurvy. Not for more than a century, however, did anybody seriously apply the treatment. Woodall applied ligatures to large arteries – instead of using cautery – for control of haemorrhage and suggested amputation at the ankle joint for certain wounds of the leg.

Army surgery was stagnant if not retrogressive in the seventeenth century, and only one military medical officer in British service, Richard Wiseman, published any notable work. Having served in the armies of James I and Charles II, and in the Navy during the Dutch war of 1665, Wiseman was experienced, and between 1672 and 1676 he urged the carrying out of primary amputation in certain cases of gunshot wounds. On chest wounds, Wiseman wrote:

> In my practice of these wounds of the breast I consider the wound, how it is capable of discharging the extravasated [forced out] blood and matter. If it be inflicted so that the blood and matter may be thereby discharged, then it is to be kept open, the welfare of the patient depending mainly upon the dressing and well governing of it; but if it do not lie well for evacuation of that extravasated blood, then it may do hurt and so ought to be healed up.

For gunshot wounds he advocated the extraction of bullets, foreign bodies and slivers of bone; he did not stitch the wounds but drained them. Only one of several chest-wounded patients after the battle of Dunbar, 1650, died under his hands. In the treatment of syphilis he, like Clowes, advocated the administration of mercury so as to cause profuse salivation.

Wiseman had genuine concern for his patients, urging that when an amputation was necessary it should be performed at once before the patient's physical condition or his spirits deteriorated. At the battle of Worcester, 1651, A Scottish soldier was brought to him with his elbow joint mangled by a musket ball. Wiseman wanted to cut off the arm and encouraged the soldier to endure the ordeal, but the man refused, crying out: 'Give me drink and I will die!'

Wiseman recorded; 'They did give him drink, and he made good his promise and died soon after, yet he had no other wound, by which may be perceived the danger in delaying this work to the next day when the accidents have kept them watching all night and totally debilitated their spirits . . . therefore, while they are surprised, and as it were amazed with the accident, the limb is taken off much easier.'

During a sea fight Wiseman cut off a man's arm, but as the fight grew hotter the patient ran to the deck and helped traverse a gun. He was accustomed to sailors begging to have shattered limbs cut off at the moment of wounding, but if for some reason this could not be done until the following day they would prefer to die. 'Amongst us abroad in that service [the Navy],' Wiseman commented, 'it was counted a great shame to the chirurgeon if the operation was left to be done the next day when the patient . . .was spent with watchings.'

While some progress was being made in English practice the Thirty Years War, 1618–48, swept Europe with its horrors, slaughter and arson. The methods that Paré had advocated a century before were ignored and surgery sank back into barbarity. In France his heritage persisted among a few surgeons and, after a long lapse, was enhanced by a valuable innovation made by the surgeon Morel in 1674 in the battles of Flanders. A rod was placed above the amputation spot against the main artery, and a band secured to the limb and pressed so tightly to the bone that the pulse below the ligature ceased to beat; the amputation was then performed. Since the blood vessels were compressed by the pressure of the band and bled very little, they could be sutured without undue haste. This was the first use of a tourniquet. Now for the first time Paré's methods of amputation and stopping the blood flow were used more frequently.

In the later seventeenth century the study of anatomy and physiology was undertaken with more enthusiasm. The discovery of the circulation of the blood, the structure of the brain and the nervous system aided surgeons, some of whom kept detailed clinical notes. But improvements and discoveries were slow to spread and, generally, soldiers and sailors were still at the mercy of practitioners who wielded their saws and scalpels with much more enthusiasm than skill and applied ancient 'remedies' indiscriminately. The prescription for one concoction for application to wounds was: 'Boil in two pounds of oil of lilies two new-whelped puppies till the flesh fall from their bones; add some earthworms in wine. Then strain and to the strained liquor add . . . turpentine and an ounce of spirit of wine.'

The sucking of wounds to cleanse them was considered efficacious even towards the end of the seventeenth century. The suckers merely washed their mouths with a little wine from time to time, and when they had finished applied chewed paper to the wounds. They did not, however, omit to utter some words, supposed to be cabalistic and which gave offence to the clergy, who would not administer the last sacrament to the wounded so practised on.

CHAPTER FIVE

Leeches, Blisters, Bleedings

For centuries a major obstacle in the way of an efficient military medical service was the difficulty in recruiting first-rate medical men. This was due partly to the parsimony of kings and governments in not recognizing that special skills deserved special rates of pay. Physicians and surgeons could make much more money in civil practice – and they could make it more comfortably. At home military practice tended to be boring and abroad it was hazardous. In general army and navy life seemed to attract doctors incapable of making a living in civil practice, or younger, inexperienced men drawn by the apparent glitter of a martial life. A few were men dedicated to military medical work; these were the outstanding ones, those who were to achieve high reputation. Some of them deserve to be as famous as the generals they served – for example, Wellington's McGrigor and Napoleon's Larrey.

During the early part of the seventeenth century in the reign of James I some attempt was made to organize the army medical staff. Two physicians to the forces were appointed, each paid 6s 8d a day, and two apothecaries at 3s 4d. Every regiment of 1,800 men had one surgeon at 4s and twelve assistants, paid 1s each. In 1620 a 'surgeon-major to the camp' was appointed. At this time too surgeons were ordered to wear their sword belts during action 'whereby they may be known in times of slaughter; it is their charter in the field'. But slightly improved status did not attract sufficient medical men to the army and in 1641, when forces were sent to Ireland to quell rebellion, surgeons were ordered into the army with little more ceremony than that given to rank and file.

The formation of a standing army by Charles II in 1660 offered medical officers a permanent career for the first time. They became regimental officers, buying their commissions – or obtaining them through influence – and some drew double pay as combatant officers as well, a somewhat unethical practice which was not abolished until 1796. Still, the desire for double pay was understandable, for the surgeon remained subordinate with no hope of advancement, except in guards regiments, which had surgeons-major.

For many years the medical profession itself believed that only the dregs of the profession cared to enter the army. Their opinion was given some support by a notice in the *London Gazette* for 1689 concerning the surgeon of what was later the 22nd Regiment.

Run away, out of Captain Soames' Company, in his Grace the Duke of Norfolk's Regiment of Infantry, Roger Curtis, a barber-surgeon; a little man, with short, black hair, a little curled; round visage, fresh-coloured; in a light-coloured cloth coat, with gold and silver buttons, and the loops stitched up with gold and silver; red plush breeches and white hat. Whoever will give notice to Francis Baker, the agent of the same regiment, in Hatton Gardens, so that he may be secured, shall have two guineas reward.

To be fair to the surgeons, their job was made difficult through lack of money with which to buy medical necessities for their respective regiments and by commanding officers who cared little for the well-being of their men. In all armies and navies the surgeons could rarely rely on their status to bring about some improvement; they were persistently overruled by inflexible commanders. The doctors' diaries which have survived are full of bitter complaints about the lack of respect accorded them as doctors, their shortage of money and of their difficulties in making officers see reason. Observers throughout the sixteenth, seventeenth and eighteenth centuries attacked the absence of suitable accommodation for sick soldiers. Landlords demanded exorbitant rents for the foul hovels in which sick soldiers were treated, and the regimental surgeon was in no position to supply anything better. The best of hospitals was hardly comfortable enough even to interest a malingerer. All troops had to contribute some of their pay towards medicines, while the sick practically paid for their subsistence through heavy stoppage of pay. The few larger, non-regimental hospitals, though their staffs included apothecaries, purveyors, dispensers, hospital assistants, clerks and orderlies, were not much better than the hole-in-corner regimental ones.

Prior to the wars during the reign of William and Mary, field hospitals had occasionally existed, as in the army of Henry of Navarre and during the war for the conquest of Granada under Ferdinand and Isabella of Spain. William III appears to have been the first to realize their value as part of the necessary establishment of a British army in the field, and such hospitals, then called Marching Hospitals, accompanied the army during William III's campaign in Ireland. The earliest appointment to these hospitals is that of Francis Smith, MD, 'to be Physician to the Marching Hospital', 28 December 1689, but all hospitals were under the command of directors who were not medical officers.

The soldiers admitted to these Marching Hospitals were fortunate. For the surgeon much depended on the attitude towards the hospitals of the commanding officer of a regiment who, like the naval captain, had the power of a despot. Only a surgeon with great will and tact could hope to be much more than a rubber stamp for the great man's whims. The generals, less personally involved with the ordinary fighting man, hardly spared a thought for his health. Marlborough was a notable exception. He organized collecting posts or regimental aid posts where possibly two or three regimental surgeons may have joined together to render first aid to the

British wounded. Marlborough's march to the Danube, culminating in the victory of Blenheim (1704), ranks as one of the world's great feats of arms. Very little has been written about his arrangements for the treatment of his sick and wounded in that campaign. The constitution of the medical establishment of the British Army at the commencement of Marlborough's campaigns in 1702 was simple enough. The regimental medical personnel consisted of one surgeon and one surgeon's mate. The surgeons were qualified men and commissioned officers; the mates, who had been added to the establishment in 1673, were of warrant rank only. The qualifications for a surgeon's mate were very low, yet many surgeons were promoted from the ranks of the surgeons' mates. The need for medical officers of higher rank to direct army medical practice led to the appointment of a physician-general, surgeon-general and apothecary-general. It was also common when an army took the field for a physician to be appointed to the staff of the general officer commanding.

To our modern ideas little effective help can have been given to the British wounded, though the existence of a hospital with a staff of surgeons was an advance. Facilities for operative treatment were limited, as is obvious from a report by Doctor Hare: 'Lieutenant Colonel Philip Dormer (of the Guards) was wounded in the left thigh about 3 in the afternoon by a muskett [*sic*] ball which broke his great artery and expired in the author's arms a little after six.'

But some amputations were made. Capt Windham of Lieutenant Gen Wyndham's Regiment of Horse wrote from Nordlingen on 23 August 1704: 'I was loth to write very soon after the first account I gave you of my being shot in the leg in the late engagement, because truly my surgeons could not tell what to think of the matter; but upon my arrival at this place – which is the hospital for all our wounded – I have got all the help I can desire, and on Tuesday last fortnight my leg was doomed to be cut off and accordingly was that day.'

Windham continued in service and took part in the battles of Ramillies (1706) and Malplaquet (1709). But at Ramillies the wounded had to be left on the field. After the capture of Lille (1708) the sick and wounded were sent to some form of hospital at Douai. At Malplaquet the more lightly injured were treated in the field by their surgeons, and many men, still shocked and bleeding, were then ordered to the ranks again.

From this point military medical services began to improve slowly, at least in British service, and records are studded with the names of innovators, experimenters and reformers. Some of their ideas were, by hindsight, ludicrous, but the doctors, running their heads against official obstruction and apathy, were at least trying. John Ranby, sergeant-surgeon to King George II and present with him at the battle of Dettingen (1743) introduced the practice of bleeding in cases of gunshot wounds and the less injurious if no more beneficial treatment of applying bark (quinine) to wounds. Ranby described arrangements for the wounded at Dettingen as excellent, though 'arrangements' is too complimentary. A soldier with a wife on service with him was more fortunate than a man admitted to hospital; she could be depended on to nurse him devotedly.

Perhaps the most outstanding contribution to military medicine in the eighteenth century was made by Sir John Pringle, Physician-General to the Forces in 1744, and physician to royalty. His book, *Observations on Diseases of the Army*, published in 1750, republished in 1763 and again in 1768, included advice far in advance of its time, especially in the field of military hygiene, long a Cinderella branch of medicine. Pringle believed that his book would become a handbook for army doctors and, while it did not achieve this status, the more enlightened physicians and surgeons, including John Hunter, used it extensively. Pringle knew that cleanliness and reasonable comfort paid dividends in efficiency. His book is as interesting for its explicit details of bleeding, blistering and leeching as for its common-sense suggestions in maintaining health.

He wanted 'under-waistcoats' issued to each man; he had seen how beneficial they were during the winter conditions of the 1745 Rebellion. At this time all foreign soldiers – and all but the poorest civilians – wore warm waistcoats. Similarly he pressed for the issue of heavy coats the men could wear on sentry duty in the cold, and for strong shoes; lack of both led to many respiratory troubles. He suggested, quite reasonably, that every infantry tent have a blanket; remarkably enough, many English and French infantry survived a winter without blankets, though other nations kept their troops warm. The English cavalry were better off; they had issue cloaks which served as blankets.

In keeping with his time, Pringle strongly advocated bleeding.

> As bleeding is the principal remedy in the cure of inflammatory disorders, delaying it too long, or not repeating it often enough in the beginning of bad colds, is the chief cause of their ending in dangerous inflammatory fevers, in rheumatism, or consumptions; and as a soldier applies first to the surgeon of his regiment, on him it chiefly depends to prevent many deaths, by the timely use of the lancet. In general, young practitioners are too sparing in letting blood, and delay it too long. But the surgeon may be assured that soldiers will seldom complain of a cough, or pains with inflammatory symptoms, wherein immediate bleeding is not proper; and from the continuance of the complaints, he is to judge of the necessity of repeating the evacuation, which, in the case of a stitch or difficult breathing, is never to be omitted in some quantity, even in the advanced state of the fever.

Pringle generally ordered from 12 oz to 16 oz to be let at the first or second bleeding, but less at all the rest. He advocated observation of the colour and consistence of the flowing blood; when it was thickish and dark it should be taken away more freely. When large quantities were necessary, it was best to bleed the patient lying, in order to prevent his fainting before enough be drawn. Otherwise, in all inflammatory complaints, the loss of consciousness, upon the loss of blood, was reckoned 'a favourable circumstance'.

Pringle's first practice in every inflammatory fever was to blister, especially in an advanced condition when he believed that the patient could not bear any further loss of blood. When he found that a fever did not respond to blistering he confined blisters to 'those states of the disease in which I could be the most assured of their efficacy'. Such a state was that of a headache when not cured by the first bleeding and by purgative. In this case he found that a blister between the shoulders 'seldom failed of giving ease'. He also applied a blister to the back when the patient had a cough or any other sign of inflammation of the lungs. A stitch in his side was treated by a blister on the side.

Inflammation of the brain required immediate, large and repeated bleedings; the relief was thought to be more certain if the blood could be taken from the jugular. Pringle never advised cutting the temporal artery, since he could relieve his patient by applying three to six leeches to each temple after bleeding in the arm. 'The benefit thence arising may be compared to the effects of an haemorrhage by the nose.'

Pringle also treated phrenitis (delirium) by opening a vein, but if the soldier's pulse was feeble he used blisters and leeches. It was usual in blistering to begin with the head, but Pringle often left the head to the last because army barbers – barbers performed the bleeding – were careless and in cutting the skin they brought on strangury – a disease in which urine was passed painfully and in drops. Sometimes Pringle found the brain 'sensibly relieved' by shaving the head without producing a blister.*

Phrenitis was often caused or aggravated in army hospitals by lack of perspiration and by chill in the feet and hands. Pringle urged that on admission a soldier's hands and feet should be washed with warm vinegar and water and double-flannel fomentations applied to his legs.

Ophthalmia (inflammation of the eyes) was almost endemic in Pringle's time, caused by winter colds and by sun and dust in summer. Only the slighter cases escaped bleeding; more acute cases could not be cured without heavy bleeding, unless some local treatment could be applied.

For this purpose [Pringle noted] blisters are usefully applied behind the ears, especially if they are continued for two or three days, and if the sores are kept running. This part of the cure is sufficiently known. But what I have observed to be sometimes more efficacious, though less generally practised, is bleeding by leeches. Two or more are applied to the lower part of the orbit or near the external angle of the eye, and the wounds allowed to ooze till they stop of themselves. Therefore in all greater inflammations, after bleeding in the arm or jugular, I have used this method, and repeated it more than once if required. The practice is no less proper in an inflammation of the eyes from a hurt or blow . . . some blood is to be first taken . . . and immediately after . . . a brisk purge. But though these means are proper in the common ophthalmia, they are not to be relied on when the disease arises from a scrofulous or venereal cause.

---

* Dr Whytt, Professor of Medicine at Edinburgh University at the time, prevented strangury by shaving the head at least twelve hours before blistering.

Inflammation of the throat, apparently common and severe among men new to the army, Pringle treated by injecting far back into the throat five or six syringefuls of a mixture of mustard, barley water, mel rofarum and vinegar. 'The bleedings, the laxatives, the blisters and this gargle are all the medicines I find necessary,' Pringle said with some satisfaction, though his patients must have found the process wearing. He used the syringe treatment even in cases of ulcerous sore throat.

Itch was a continual problem. Highly contagious, it was most frequently found in hospitals, introduced by soldiers arriving in a dirty state. Pringle was probably the first the distinguish the common itch from a measle-like eruption; the itch mostly affected the inside of the wrists, between the fingers, the sides of the belly and the hams.

Pringle considered that shortage of sleep was rare among soldiers and that soldiers off duty slept too much, 'which enervates the body and renders it more subject to disease. It is well known how necessary it is to keep up the perspiration; and also, how much the uncleanliness of the person will concur with other things to frustrate that intention. I have observed in the hospitals, that when men were brought in from the camp with fevers, nothing so much promoted a diaphoresis [a sweat] as washing their feet and hands and sometimes their whole body and giving them clean linen'.

Without conscious ambiguity or irony Pringle reflected that in wartime, 'by the smallness of his pay a soldier is secured against excess in eating, the most common error in diet'. Since no orders could restrain soldiers from eating and drinking what they liked, if they had the money, the solution was to insist that they eat in messes so that the better part of their pay was spent on wholesome and properly balanced food.

> The greatest impediments to messing are the wives and children, who must often be maintained on the pay of the men. In such circumstances, it is not improper food, but the want of it that may endanger a soldier's health. . . . Take care that the men be supplied with good bread and that the markets to be so regulated that the traders have encouragement to come to the camp, and the messes have good provisions at a moderate price, vegetables in particular, which during the hot weather ought to make the greatest part of their diet. Though the pay of a British soldier is better than that of other troops abroad, yet his economy is less, so that after giving in his proportion to the mess, there is little danger of his having wherewithal to make a debauch.

Despite Pringle's suggestions many British soldiers never saw a green vegetable on service and the only fruit they ate was what they could steal.

Dr Francis Home served with the army in the 1740s and adopted unusual methods of treating gunshot wounds; he freely sacrificed the neighbouring parts in all cases and is said to have cut all the wounds which he dressed at the battle of Dettingen. Like Wiseman and Ranby, he favoured primary amputation and is believed to be the first man to practise inoculation for measles.

In the Low Countries in 1748 advances were made in hospitals. The Duke of Cumberland's sick and wounded had separate and clean beds, frequent changes of linen and were attended by female nurses. Hospital storekeepers and clerks were on hand to provide equipment and to keep records. The presiding administrator was Cumberland's chief surgeon, Middleton, but the inspiration is thought to have been Cumberland's own, and because it was a personal idea it lapsed before the next campaign.

In 1756 a distinct administrative organization was for the first time introduced into the army medical department. Lord Barrington, then Secretary of War, was directed to establish a hospital board for the medical service. The board functioned, but could do little to solve the problem of transport, always inadequate for the wounded so that frequently they had to be left behind, to be butchered by the enemy or tortured and scalped, as happened to the British wounded taken by Indians attached to the French Army in North America. This happened too during the War of Independence. During the Seven Years War transport was better arranged, usually by contract. A Treasury minute of 1762 shows that a Mr Dundas, then contractor for wagons in Germany, transferred to the government his 500 wagons, with horses and drivers, for £88 10s each.

CHAPTER SIX

Hunter and the Portuguese Campaign

A great reformer and soldiers' friend was Dr Brocklesby, appointed physician to the army in 1758 and doctor in charge of army hospitals in Germany in 1760. The 'hospitals' of the period shocked him, for they were merely of one or two small rooms, each of which was an almost continuous bed without spaces. 'They would quickly destroy those who should be confined in them, even if sent there in perfect health,' Brocklesby said. He drew up a code of instructions to preserve the health of men in barracks, in hospitals and in the transports which took them to foreign stations. He asked merely for cleanliness, good ventilation, sound diet and proper exercise, but his seniors in Whitehall obstructed him. He prescribed wine in liberal doses for treatment of fevers – 'a spoonful or more every half hour or three pints in twenty-four hours'. This had, he wrote in 1764, the most decided benefit. Since it probably made the patient more cheerful the benefit was automatic. Brocklesby, like Francis Home, was a keen advocate of post-mortem examination, and he carried out many such examinations on the bodies of his military patients before the practice had become general in civil medicine. He tried to raise the standard of doctors in the army by proposing that medical commissions, still obtainable by purchase, should be raised in value to at least £600 and that candidates should, in addition, undergo a strict professional examination. His scheme was not taken up; doctors were difficult enough to come by and examinations would only reduce the field.

Brocklesby demanded well-built barracks, strongly criticizing those which were then going up – with low ceilings, no ventilation and damp floors. At this time many soldiers were billeted in ale-houses, and Brocklesby could not see how men could be kept constantly 'wholesome and cleanly' unless in efficient barracks. With humanity and foresight uncommon in his time, Brocklesby wrote in 1764: 'The day of battle is once or twice in a long campaign, when men must be used as they are wanted; but our attention to the well-being of the men and the preservation of their health, ought to be a constant business, and an increasing care of their officers as well as of their doctor.'

Dr Donald Monro was campaigning on similar lines in 1764. Monro had served in Germany from 1761 to 1763 and had seen how little regard was paid to hygiene and to the proper conduct of military hospitals. He set out[8] rules of health and hygiene which became commonplace a century later without anybody giving credit to Monro for having first suggested them. He noted that in winter men were healthier if they wore flannel, that each man while on sentry duty should wear a greatcoat and that his period of sentry duty should be limited, that the soldiers should be quartered in the upper storeys of buildings because the air was healthier, that officers should inspect the men's quarters frequently. He advocated well-aired, cleaned and purified troopships, equipped with ventilators or wind-sails; men should be ordered to bathe frequently on board, and ships should be well stocked with vinegar, sugar, lemons and molasses. The men's hammocks should be brought to the deck every day. To Monro the British Army became indebted for the idea of sending hospital ships with expeditions, though at first they were merely marine germ-carriers.

Before an army went into winter quarters it should, Monro urged, echoing Pringle, be provided with a store of potatoes, onions, cabbages, sour crout [sic], pickled cabbages, apples. He strongly recommended that soldiers dine together in messes, an arrangement that was not generally adopted into the Army until the end of the century.

He urged his objections against standing camps, pointing out the evils to men of exposure to putrid effluvia from dead animals and latrines. Portius, Ramanini and other authors who had written about camp diseases centuries earlier, he noted, attributed most of them to the effluvia from the excrements of men and beasts and from the dead bodies of men, horses and other animals lying unburied. 'When the camp begins to turn unhealthy the only means that will preserve the health of the men is to change the ground and leave behind all the filth and nastiness which gave rise to those putrid disorders.'

Monro evolved methods of filtering water. One was a cask with an open end into which was placed a longer cask without ends; this short cask was filled with sand and the inner longer cask just over half filled. The rest of the inner cask was filled with water which filtered through the sand and rose above the sand in the outer cask.

Monro considered that army hospitals should be neutral and protected by all belligerents.* In 'churches and such places' used as hospitals each man should be allotted thirty-six square feet, but in common hospital wards he should have from forty-two to sixty-four square feet, according to the height of the ceiling and the nature of disease of the patient.

On the subject of scurvy affecting troops he pointed out that among its more common causes were the continued use of salted provisions and lack of fresh vegetables, together with exposure of the men to cold and damp. In 1761 there was no authorized scale of hospital diets, but Monro, aware that many relapses

---

* This was in fact accepted by the Earl of Stair and the Duke of Noailles, who commanded the French, in Germany in 1748.

in cases of fever and dysentery were due to lack of special hospital diet, introduced one into his hospitals. It had three scales – full, middle and low:

> Full diet: Breakfast: one pint of water or rice gruel.* Dinner, 1 lb boiled fresh meat. Supper, as for breakfast.
>
> Middle diet: Breakfast, as for the full diet. Dinner, 1 lb of broth, ½ lb of boiled meat. Supper, as for full diet.
>
> Low diet: Breakfast as for full diet or 'according to the patient's palate', Dinner, 1 pint of broth or half a pint of panada [bread boiled to pulp and flavoured] with 2 spoonfuls of wine and ¼ oz of sugar. Supper, as for the other diets.

At this time the daily allowance of bread was 1 lb per man and patients were allowed barley water with two spoonfuls of brandy per pint and a little sugar, or light beer or wine with water and sugar.

Monro, like other military doctors with foresight, wanted improvements in conditions of service for doctors. Not long before a British commander, Lord Granby, had ordered that surgeons' mates should be permitted a joint of meat roasted or boiled for dinner and a bottle of wine so 'that they might not absent themselves from their duty' in a hunt for food. Monro urged some military rank for every commissioned officer of the hospital on service.

There were signs in the sixth decade of the eighteenth century that the British national conscience was stirring, and that this conscience, embodied in hierarchy of war, was beginning to realize that a soldier and sailor were not merely cannon fodder, but somebody's husband, son or brother. During the campaign in Portugal of 1762–3† the greatest efforts to date were made to establish a first-rate hospital, well-staffed with competent men, with women nurses and equipped with instruments, bedding and various comforts.

By February 1762 careful consideration was being given to the provision of medical arrangements for the Portuguese campaign. Sir William Fordyce was asked to provide a scheme for a hospital for 6,000 men. Supposing each regiment to have a quota of 100 sick, Fordyce suggested 100 palliasses or strong Osnaburg cases to be filled with straw. 'If the hospital is fixed and not a field or flying hospital there must be 100 bedsteads with boarded bottoms of strong work.‡

The first surgeon who went to Portugal was John Hunter, one of the great surgeons of history. In 1748, aged twenty, he had gone to London from Scotland to join his surgeon brother William. Ten years later he became a

---

* Water gruel was made of about 4 oz. of oatmeal, a little salt with or without a little sweet oil and two spoonfuls of wine. Rice gruel consisted of 2 oz. of rice, one spoonful of fine flour, a little salt and sugar.

† Spain, resenting Portugal's friendship with England, invaded Portugal, which appealed to Britain for help. Militarily the campaign was insignificant.

‡ Sir William was a little out of date. The Marching or Field Hospitals had disappeared after Marlborough's campaigns and the only hospitals now were the general hospitals.

staff surgeon in the army, and on 29 March 1761 sailed from Spithead with an expeditionary force under General Hodgson to capture Belle Isle. Hunter reached Lisbon direct from Belle Isle. He had with him an apothecary, Hugh Smith, five mates, two servants, one storekeeper, one matron and four nurses. In one letter he referred to these and other colleagues, or some of them, as 'a damned disagreeable lot'.

The general hospital in Lisbon was quartered in four existing buildings. In a report they are described as:

1st. The House of Lobo's (where at present the two physicians, master apothecary, one surgeon and three mates lodge) is calculated to receive
Patients 100

2nd. The House of Panteas (where one mate lodges), calculated to receive
Patients 196
N.B. There is an old Friar lodges in a little cell belonging to this house.

3rd. The Fort (where three mates lodge), calculated to receive
Patients 150
N.B. This is much the worst hospital, the rooms small and is removed at least a quarter of a mile from the others.

4th. Casa de Almirate (where one surgeon and five mates lodge) calculated to receive
Patients 50

On 6 July the hospitals held 202 patients, with a matron, two head nurses and eighteen other nurses. This ratio of one nurse to ten patients was apparently considered too high, for Colonel Cosnam, the Adjutant-General, noted that: 'Though the hospital is at present rather overstocked with nurses for the number of sick none can be discharged as their places cannot be supplied on any emergency and they expect an increase of sick daily.' This seems to imply that these nurses were professionally trained since untrained women could easily have been recruited from among the camp followers.

Hospital discipline was not all that it might have been, as Standing Orders indicated:

A hospital guard is to be appointed and the officer of the guard is to be responsible for the regularity of the hospital and to have the rolls called before every relief so as to see if any of the patients are out. The officer is to give the doctor all the assistance in his power for such purposes as drawing water, burying the dead and in general all kinds of labour above the strength of the nurses. Refractory and disobedient patients are to be confined on bread and water as long as the Doctor shall direct and a Black Hole and Irons are to be provided.*

---

* Among the crimes for which hospital patients were confined were desertion, drunkenness and robbery; two men were kept for 161 nights in the Black Hole for being involved in the murder of a Portuguese.

The Guard will also send frequent patrols to the Tipling houses in the neighbourhood to prevent any men drinking and quarrelling with the inhabitants. . . . The officer of the guard is to see that these orders are to be kept clean and repaired when defaced.

Medical reports give interesting sidelights on march procedure and discipline. The 3rd Regiment of Foot (The Buffs) were moving up; they made part of their journey up the Tagus by boat as far as Port de Muge and then had to march to Santarem. Starting at 6 a.m., they marched at a rate of about two miles an hour, with the surgeon and his mates at front, centre and rear of the regiment. Whenever a man fell sick the companies had orders to leave a careful man with him. The rearguard officer and twenty-two men had charge of all that dropped behind. Water was scarce, the men were choked with heat and dust as they trudged through defiles of sand and they fell down sick so fast that insufficient well men remained to care for them. The total distance covered was only about twelve miles, but eleven men died, resulting in a report from Peter Barnard, regimental surgeon:

> My opinion is, that it was owing to the extreme heat of the weather; likewise to the imprudence of the men themselves who drank immoderate quantities of water (contrary to all advice given them) whenever they were parched with the excessive heat. The attention paid to preserve them was as follows. As fast as any man dropt, I removed them to a shady place and gave them every physical assistance, such as bleeding, volatile spirits, etc. They were then left under the care of proper persons till such time as the proper carriages could be procured to bring them into Town.

By the middle of August many sick were being brought into Santarem, and since there was no proper hospital their condition was distressing. Master Apothecary Smith, sent to investigate, found the sick 'in want of necessities and very near half of them laying on the ground . . . the disorders are in general fevers and fluxes, some of the putrid kind. . . .'

A great difficulty was still that the medical services had no transport of their own. They were entirely dependent on the exigencies of the army generally and had no priority. Doctors were always pleading for wagons or boats. On 20 September 1762 William Wiseman, surgeon to the 75th Regiment, wrote to General Armstrong:

> Sir, I'm left here [Cabassa] with twenty-nine of your sick, eleven of the 75th, and one of Lord Blaney's. Being in a melancholy state to get provision for them, have took the liberty to detail Nicholas McColly of the Major's company in your regiment to interpret for me, that I may get them to Santarem as soon as possible, otherwise the poor sick must inevitably suffer. . . . This morning I sent a corporal and two men to get sheep for the sick, instead of getting them he was threatened by the peasants and a Portuguese dragoon would have killed him if he had not had a stick to defend himself . . . what a miserable situation we are in. . . .

John Hunter, on the same theme, wrote with some exasperation to the commander-in-chief himself, Lord Loudon:

> My Lord, As there is no provision made for the Flying Hospital as in other countrys, we think it incumbent upon us for the better and more speedy carrying on His Majesty's service to acquaint your Lordship of the necessity of having mules and horses to transport our mates, medicines and instruments, many of them having fallen sick from the fatigue and want of those conveniences and also many of the medicines and instruments have been obliged to be left behind. Therefore we hope your Lordship will see the propriety of this application and allow us for each surgeon two beasts and three more to be in common for mates that attend the Flying Hospital.

It is not clear if this reasonable request was granted or if several other practical suggestions which Hunter made were put into effect.

One requisition sent to London at this time illustrates the requirements of a military hospital: the senior doctor asked for 500 complete sets of bedding (a set comprised one palliasse, one bolster, one pair of sheets, a blanket and coverlet), 20 pewter bedpans, 25 chamber pots, 30 bleed porringers and 24 tin candlesticks and extinguishers, 200 white platters, 150 quart bowls, 5 gross of wooden spoons, large quantities of drugs, 2 sets of amputating instruments, 2 sets of instruments for the trepan, 2 dozen dissecting knives; 20 dozen lancets; 6 dozen bag trusses and 4 dozen spring trusses.

There were no convalescent hospitals or centres in 1762, and men recovered from illness but still not fit to join their regiments were quartered in billets and put under the command of a combatant officer, who arranged them in messes and was responsible for their welfare and discipline.

Hunter's experience in Portugal gave him a taste for active service, and from 1779 to 1783 he served in the West Indies, that great graveyard of British fighting men. The death-rate startled Hunter. His figures[9] show that in the 1st Battalion 40th Regiment two-fifths of the unit were lost in a year; in the 79th Foot, four-ninths; in the 88th, one-third; 85th, a half; the 92nd nearly half; 93rd, nine-elevenths, 94th, six-sevenths. Hunter studied the combination of circumstances that was calculated to cause such loss of life and published a list of rules to preserve health:

1. Troops sent to the West Indies should be trained and well disciplined and not newly raised.

2. They should arrive in the West Indies at the coolest time of year.

3. They should be sent from England in roomy transports and the rules of health and hygiene laid down by Captain Cook and Sir John Pringle should be observed.*

---

* Cook advocated lime juice, fresh-air sleeping, exercise and well-spaced hammocks. For Pringle see previous chapter.

4. On landing the men should be quartered in barracks in healthy situations, that is on dry, sandy peninsulas or islands near the shore or in the mountains.

5. A certain number of negroes should be attached to each regiment to do whatever work was required during the heat of the day.

6. Soldiers should be divided into messes for dining.

7. Parades and drills – which should not be long – should be held in the early mornings. Evening parades, when the men's shorts and jackets became sweat-soaked, produced colds, rheumatism and other complaints.

The notable thing about Hunter's suggestions is that they were hardly notable at all, but common sense in man management was rare in his day and even the most obvious measures were not put into effect.

Hunter detected in the illness known to the troops as 'dry belly-ache' – the colica pictonum – and traced its cause to the lead derived from the tubes through which the rum passed in its process of distillation and introduced with the rum into the human system. He suggested treatments for several painful or distressing infections caused by insects, such as the chiger or jigger (*Pulex penetrans*), mosquitoes (*Culex pipen*) and the itch insect (*Acarus siro*). One painful and horrible disease was caused by a large fly depositing its ova in the soldier's mouth or nostrils while he slept.*

---

* Among the obligations which the medical profession owes John Hunter is the museum of the Royal College of Surgeons. He evolved an operation for aneurism – abnormal enlargement of an artery; he advocated delayed amputations in case of gunshot wounds; he was the first to recommend excision of joints as substitute for removal of the whole limb; he reduced the treatment of injuries to the skull to more definite principles; he advanced the treatment of hernia, and diseases of the spine and joints; and published a work on venereal disease which remained standard for a century. He is described on his tomb in Westminster Abbey as the 'founder of scientific surgery'.

CHAPTER SEVEN

Broken Bodies, Broken Hearts

Towards the end of the eighteenth century several articulate doctors, a little more secure now in their professional status, were pressing for reforms. That they were mostly British and French was because these were the two nations with great forces intermittently at war in Europe and with armies and expeditions in many parts of the world. At a time when the British and French were beginning to see the fighting man as a valuable commodity which could, with care, be used again and again until he wore out through the natural process of time, the Prussians, Austrians, Russians and others were still thinking in terms of discarding wounded and sick as embarrassments. The Americans, during the War of Independence (1776–83), suffered acutely, for trained and experienced doctors were at a premium. In the severe winter of 1776–7 those soldiers on the Canadian border suffered terribly from cold and hunger and the diseases induced by both. In Fort Ticonderoga General Anthony Wayne's force was ravaged by famine and disease; whole companies, racked with fever, lay on the stone floors of the fort with old shreds of blankets wrapped round them. Without medicine or competent medical aid they died by the dozen, clutching their blankets helplessly for more warmth.

Dr Rush, serving with the Americans, noticed that men under twenty were most afflicted by camp diseases and called American hospitals the 'sinks of human life', robbing the United States of more men than enemy action.

Besieged in Valley Forge in the winter of 1777–8, the Americans endured raging pneumonia and smallpox. Dysentery quickly killed soldiers who months before had been hardy farmers. One hospital building, crowded with 250 beds made of filthy straw and covered with foul old blankets, was packed with a thousand or more patients, three or four in the same bed, screaming in pain and delirium. As they died they were thrown out into the snow to make room for those coming in. Washington took 10,000 men into Valley Forge in November 1777; by March 3,000 had deserted to the British in an effort to survive and 1,000 had not survived. No medical administration existed; nobody had had any training in cleaning a wound, applying a bandage, making a stretcher, moving sick and wounded, running an aid post or hospital. It was largely because of the total lack of medical assistance during the War of Independence that the United States armies of the future became so conscious of the need for it and would not embark on any operation until a chain of evacuation and treatment had been established.

The British troops during an advance were sometimes so badly mauled by American irregulars, sniping from the flanks, and so hard pressed in retreat that their state became unspeakable. On 7 October 1777, when General Burgoyne retreated after his defeat at Freeman's Farm, a great many of his wounded were still bleeding, dying by inches, and the able had to carry them on their backs while exhausted from starvation and sleeplessness. When Burgoyne surrendered ten days later the wounded had still had no attention. A few surgeons served the British troops garrisoned in North America, but when the surgeon himself succumbed a replacement could be months arriving.

One of the most versatile and progressive doctors in British service was Dr John Bell, far in advance of his time; for instance, he advocated a change of climate for sickly soldiers. Instead of cooping them up in the West Indies he suggested that Britain copy France and order regiments to take regular spells of duty on board ships of war. He wanted to exchange Gibraltar for the Canary Islands, which he saw as sanatoria for soldiers.

In the late eighteenth century sick soldiers were still given their ordinary allowance of salted meat prepared with unrefined sea salt, with the result that it was 'nauseous, bitter and cathartic', as John Bell described it. With this went the daily ration of half a pint of rum. Bell believed that the rum had a pernicious effect and wanted beer substituted. With salted provisions beer was doubly necessary. 'If malt liquor had been more generally used by the army in the West Indies we should not have had so much reason to lament our ability to act offensively in that quarter, nor should we have had such cause of apprehension for the safety of our own islands from the equal

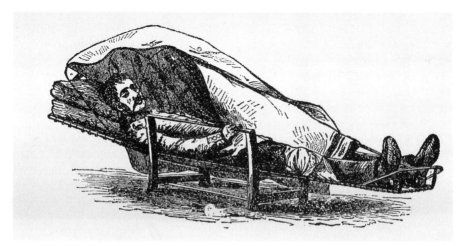

Mule litter used by the American Army during the War of Independence.

inability of the troops to defend them.' Bell advocated the canteen system, which was afterwards introduced into the East Indies and adopted in Britain late in the 1860s. It had taken the government nearly a century to implement Bell's idea.

Bell was really the first to urge an institution in which candidates for medical service in the army or navy would be given special training. In 1798, after experience in the naval hospital at Yarmouth, he wrote to the First Lord of the Admiralty urging 'one great school of military surgery'. It comes as no surprise to learn that half a century had to pass before a similar idea was put into execution. Bell evolved details for the training in this hospital – anatomy, military surgery, medical geography, climates, seasons, coasts of various countries, the manner of conducting soldiers on foreign expeditions, general care of the troops' health, choice of camps, forming of hospitals, carriage of wounded, military economics and so on.

Protesting against the system of recruiting then in force for newly raised regiments, Bell observed that: 'Every art is employed by the lowest and more despicable wretches to entrap the intoxicated, the ignorant and those who, from some silly cause of discontent, have deserted a business to which they embrace the very first opportunity of returning.' He was angry too at a system which would not accept as soldiers men professing to be Roman Catholics; a man aware of this structure was safe from the recruiters.

If a patient were wounded in the belly, head or breast or if he were to keep a limb Bell insisted on bleeding 'almost without bounds'. He considered the French surgeons daring in their bleeding and their successes wonderful. At this time the French were bleeding with an enthusiasm which some British surgeons considered reckless – as much as four times in twenty-four hours and for as long as twenty days.

While complimenting the French surgeons, surgeon Bell castigated the Prussians, for by order of the surgeon-general Bilguer, between about 1762–95, no limbs were cut off. The result was obvious to Bell. 'If all limbs be kept many must gangrene; if no amputation be performed all the shattered stumps must gangrene, then the sloughing stumps and gangrenous limbs, the exfoliating bones, long accompanied by putrid discharge must infect the whole. . . .' Bilguer had admitted just before Bell wrote that Prussian military hospitals were riddled with diarrhoea, dysentery, fever and other diseases. Without a tidying amputation a stump could take six months to heal and a fractured limb nine months, after which time the soldiers were emaciated.

One of the first army doctors to see that health was often sapped by monotony, Bell wrote:

> We cannot too strongly urge the necessity for employment, either of body or mind, especially for newly raised troops, as a powerful means of preserving health, provided that bodily exercise is not carried to fatiguing lengths. . . . Some attention to the morals of soldiers . . . is necessary to preserving health and that the assistance of the chaplain may very frequently render the advice of the surgeon unnecessary.

Perhaps no man had so reasoned an appreciation of the functions of the army medical officer as did Dr Robert Jackson, who served successively in the 60th, 71st and 3rd Regiments.

> The preservation of the health of the soldier is indispensable to the preservation of the conquests which fortune or courage achieves. . . . If genius conquer, prudence preserves. The health of the army, as a preserving instrument ought, therefore, to be a primary condition of the state.

So Jackson wrote in 1791 when soldiers and sailors were still expendable commodities.

> The medical history of armies holds out a dismal picture of human misery. Armies were crippled, almost annihilated by artificial diseases [in the West Indies] that is, by contagious fevers proceeding from ignorance of principles which conduce to the preservation of health or from indifference and negligence in applying them.

He advocated the appointment of sanitation officers, a suggestion not followed for about sixty years.

Dr William Lemprière, who was successively surgeon to the 20th Light Dragoons and Apothecary to the Forces, makes repeated allusions in his writings to the prevailing intemperance among all classes at the time he served – the latter end of the eighteenth century. He saw drunkenness lead to many dangers to health and morals. Soldiers would resort to devious schemes to defeat efforts to keep them sober. The CO of the 20th Light Dragoons confined his men to barracks as a way of keeping them sober, but the women, on the plea of bringing in water or milk for their families, put a cork at the bottom of the spout of a tea kettle, filled up the spout with water or milk – and the body of the kettle with rum. If challenged by a sentry they would merely pour out the water contents of the spout for his inspection. Drunkenness was the perennial, inevitable problem all doctors faced.

It might appear that the greatest hazards to soldiers' health were abroad, but in the British Isles they suffered just as much, though perhaps less exotically. Everything militated against the soldier leading a healthy life. The billets in England and Scotland were always in public houses; the landlord never failed to look on the soldiery not only as a nuisance but as a great obstacle to profit. He treated them coldly and lodged them poorly, generally in some foul-smelling garret or lumber-room. If the landlord had no garret he would erect a few dirty beds in an outhouse fit for no other use.

> The clothes on their beds are frequently so scanty and so worn, as even in summer to be almost unfit to keep them warm, and should it happen to be cold winter weather, altogether insufficient [noted Dr Richard Hamilton, a regimental surgeon for twenty-five years]. This often brings on catarrhal affections and lays the foundation of other more violent diseases of the inflammatory kind, not unfrequently ending in death. The most judicious plans of practice may be laid

down, but it will be next to impossible they can prove successful. That this is a fact many a poor soldier can testify. . . . Many a prisoner in his cell is better lodged than we find many of the soldiery in billets; yet will they seldom complain. . . . Those necessaries which the landlord is obliged by law to furnish the soldier are not only given with reluctance, but are often of the worst quality. Their small beer is what I have chiefly now in view; it is generally vapid and unfit to be drank. Hence it frequently becomes the cause of colics, diarrhoeas, and other complaints of the bowels, that cannot be completely cured till the cause ceases. This is not always in the power of the surgeon to accomplish; he can only attempt a remedy by a complaint to the officer, which often fails. . . .

The surgeon's difficulty in enforcing his professional will was tragically shown in a case of 1780.[10] A strong, well-trained young soldier was sent to the regimental hospital with a small ulcer on a leg. He stayed there for several weeks, the surgeon unable to find a cure for it, until the company officers began to complain that the surgeon might by now have been able to heal such a trifling sore. They brought so much unpleasant pressure to bear that the surgeon had no option but to discharge the man who was 'delivered over to the regiment', as the saying then was. The man's sergeant said that he would soon cure the ulcer even if the surgeon could not and he confined the man to the barrack-room. Once a soldier was struck out of the sick list the surgeon was no longer answerable for him, so he took no further interest in the ulcer case. Two months later a messenger came for him; his former patient was dying. He found the man, once strong, sitting up in bed panting for breath; he had strong palpitations, an oppression of the heart and with all the symptoms of dropsy of the chest. The abdomen was swollen and there were evident marks of general dropsy. The sore leg was swollen and the ulcer much enlarged. He died – a day later – not from the sore on his leg but from close confinement and the sergeant's strict discipline, which included light rations. The officers had noticed the man's deterioration, but having in effect reprimanded the surgeon they were too proud to confess themselves at fault. Thirteen other men lived with the sick man in the room, but none felt able to seek help for him, so great was their fear of the officers and sergeants.

Among fighting men of all races homesickness was an illness with serious physiological effects in an age when families, rural ones particularly, were close-knit and interdependent and men were often of simple nature. Surgeon Hamilton in 1781 at Teignmouth had a soldier patient named Edwards, young, handsome and well built, who complained of universal weakness, giddiness, noises in his ears, insomnia and loss of appetite. Put on a course of medicines and allowed wine, he continued to decline; his pulse became shallow and weak and he developed a fever. Hamilton had almost abandoned the man as lost when the nurse mentioned that Edwards often spoke to her, in a raving way, about home, family and friends. Hamilton took it upon himself to tell the soldier that when he recovered he would have six weeks' home leave. This promise was beyond his power to fulfil, but he importuned the officers and wore them into co-operation. After two months' encouragement along these lines Edwards recovered.

Dr A. Zimmerman, a Swiss military doctor of the same period, noted that his countrymen were extremely subject to homesick-melancholy when in a foreign country. It sometimes quickly proved fatal. 'I believe,' he wrote,[11] 'it will be found among men in every nation, who, in foreign countries, feel the want of those delights and enjoyments they would meet with among their friends at home.'

A French doctor, Barrere, saw it in several Burgundy soldiers, who were forced into the service, or refused discharge. Dr Auenbrucker frequently observed it among Austrian troops enlisted by force. They were 'first silent, languid, pensive, emitted deep sighs, seemed exceedingly sorrowful and gradually became insensible to everything'. Incidence of this condition decreased greatly following a plan for enlisting soldiers for a limited number of years. Dr Auenbrucker found that in several who died of this disease the lungs adhered to the diaphragm, and that part of the lungs was calloused, or had even become more or less purulent (septic). When the disease had not degenerated into phthisis (progressive wasting disease) or insanity, Auenbrucker achieved cures by inspiring patients with the hope of soon seeing their friends and their home.

In 1781 Hamilton assisted at the dissection in Newcastle upon Tyne of a soldier of the South Lincoln militia who, the local surgeon said, had died of love. Before his death he was greatly wasted, with nightly sweats and fever.

> That he died from the effects of this depressing passion, all the corps to which he belonged agreed, some of whom knew his attachment before the regiment marched from their own county. . . . Sometimes the disease acts suddenly and violently; at other times, like intense grief, it gradually undermines the constitution. The more general effects of this tender passion are, a tremulous pulse, deep sighs, an alternate glow and paleness of the cheeks, dejection, loss of appetite, a faltering speech, cold sweats, and watchfulness, which gradually terminate in consumption, or perhaps induce insanity and sometimes suicide.

Hamilton lost a patient from no other cause than the badness of his billet during an attack of typhus. In the bitter March of 1782 the soldier concerned was in one of the worst billets of Hamilton's experience. the room let in wind and rain and the floor around the man's bed was 'a perfect mortar'. Several soldiers were housed in this room. The landlord, fearing contagion, would provide no other billet and nobody in the town would let a house for the regimental sick. Hamilton felt he was fortunate in losing only one patient. He induced his commanding officer to buy a house, but this was no better than the billets and all he would do was to pray for better weather.

The public felt that anything was good enough for a soldier or sailor, and supposed that from a natural hardiness and insensitivity they could bear a surgical operation better than most. Yet surgeons often saw apparently strong men tremble at the sight of a lancet and faint during an operation. Hamilton found only one man in seven calm enough to hold the cup into which his own blood was drained during a blood-letting. That there was some justification for the soldiers' apprehension Hamilton himself confesses by his quotation of a cynical contemporary saying that more men died from the lancet than the lance.

Men died too from the failure of doctors and orderlies to observe the most elementary precautions of hygiene. Yet some survived. 'G.B.',[12] wounded in action in Egypt in 1801, suffered from infection after a musket ball had been extracted. The wound became inflamed and his foot and ankle were swollen. 'I was suspicious that the dirty water with which it was sometimes washed was the cause of the inflammation. An erroneous opinion was entertained that salt water would smart the wounds and as fresh water was short on board [the troopship] only a small quantity of it was available for washing them. A great number of wounds were washed with one basin-full. . . .'

Fighting men of the period were pretty much inured to harsh conditions. Hamilton once opened his door to a former soldier named Watson, a patient of his in the regiment. It was February in London, with hail and sleet, and Watson was bare-armed and shoeless, with torn stockings; he wore neither shirt nor waistcoat and his naked body could be seen through the tears in his coat. He was, however, in perfect health. Hamilton provided him with a complete set of warm clothes, but a week later heard that Watson was walking the streets in his rags. Irritated, the surgeon hunted down the ex-soldier and asked what he had done with the new clothes. 'If your honour obliges me to wear that waistcoat and those thick stockings and breeches I shall be a dead man by tomorrow,' he said. 'Your honour does not know what I suffered the first night and I have been ill ever since.' On examination Hamilton found him feverish, with a severe cough, catarrh, pneumonic inflammation and pains. He was convinced that the difference of temperature between the very warm clothes and almost complete nakedness had induced the man's symptoms.

Army medical zealots produced plenty of sane suggestions, but they ran their heads against solid conservatism. Dr William Blair, practical and experienced, produced in 1798 a book he called *The Soldier's Friend*, perhaps an ill-advised title since it might have appeared to set him on the side of the men against the officers. In fact, Blair was concerned for all soldiers. The uniform of the time struck him as particularly stupid. It was so restricting that soldiers often became exhausted or developed skin rashes. For many years of the eighteenth and nineteenth centuries British soldiers were tortured by the stock worn around the neck – a 'stiff bandage' Blair called it. This leather contraption fitted hard under the chin and was diabolically uncomfortable. Their legs were encased in gaiters – 'tight ligatures that constrain the articulations of the loins and knees'. Blair urged looser, more serviceable and less porous uniforms, but commanding officers like to see their men straight and tight; appearance was more important than utility.

Soldiers rarely exercised or played sports in an organized way; such exercises as they performed were flat and insipid, but again doctors could not persuade the army or navy to introduce gymnastics. Dr Blair, dismayed by the lack of physical training, pointed out that because he kept himself fit he could walk from Edinburgh to London in eleven and a half days. Surely soldiers, who had to march long distances, should be undergoing physical training.

Soldiers' diet was another of Blair's worries. He had noticed that the custom of taking a light and warm breakfast, such as tea or coffee, 'renders men delicate and susceptible of taking cold'. He may have been influenced by the French practice of strictly prohibiting warm breakfasts; every man was allowed half a pint of good wine, which he took with his bread. The French were rarely unfit, even in severe weather. In Britain, Blair suggested, a pint of good porter or sound ale could be substituted for the wine.

As a remedy for the prevailing drunkenness, especially among men who had been tailors, weavers and shoemakers, Blair suggested that instead of liquor the troops be given syrup of vinegar mixed with cream of tartar and sugar with water – 'a very pleasant, wholesome beverage'.* Another drink could be made from ½ lb of bruised raisins in 3 quarts of boiling water, plus liquorice root, figs, prunes and ripe apples.

Biscuit was better than bread for soldiers, Blair advised, because it produced a firmer flesh and gave the soldier more stamina. Officers should eat rusks – presumably because they had more delicate teeth. They should also carry 'portable soup' for eating when fatigued. Every soldier should eat something before exposing himself to the air of low banks, marshes and coasts, should chew a little tobacco or a piece of ginger or drink pure spirits 'infused with Peruvian bark, colombo root, orange peel and tansy'.

Well aware of the great difficulty in keeping soldiers and their quarters clean in winter, Blair had to admit that 'nothing short of punishment is adequate or can create the smallest exertion'. And while he was the soldier's friend he knew that many young men admitted to hospital had no ailments other than laziness and aversion to duty, though they feigned rheumatism or headaches or some other disability difficult to check. 'It is by no means uncommon for a dozen of these men, after a hearty meal, to sit down to cards or even to drinking with the nurses and hospital attendants.' As a further check on hospital excesses Blair would permit neither 'loose women nor visiting females' into an army hospital. Such a ban might reduce the incidence of venereal disease and the secondary infections it led to as soldiers went to quacks, mountebanks, farriers and their own comrades for treatment, which could be as painful as it was dangerous – immersion in acid or scalding water.

---

* The only liquor in ancient armies was vinegar.

Blair at least deserves some recognition for his suggestion, in 1798, of mouth-to-mouth resuscitation – 'blowing strongly into the mouth at the same time stopping the nose'.

While Blair was finding deficiencies among British soldiers, Count Rumford, an American in Bavarian service, was praising the health and husbandry of Bavarian soldiers, whom he saw as the finest, stoutest and strongest men in the world, their countenances showing the 'most evident marks of ruddy health and perfect contentment'. Yet the Bavarian soldier supported himself on less than 2*d* a day, saving another three farthings.

But the Bavarians did not buy medicines out of their own pittance, as did many British soldiers, rather than take the medicines prescribed by their doctor. Most officers and many doctors would have criticized the soldiers as stupid; surgeon Hamilton felt there had to be fault on the doctor's part.[13]

Surgeons could be at fault in more serious ways. One soldier lost both feet from cold in England – and while in a regimental hospital. He reported that his feet were numb and swollen and after several days they were found to be black and gangrenous and were amputated.[14]

CHAPTER EIGHT

Guthrie, McGrigor and the Peninsular War

On active service the initial problem of getting the wounded from battlefield to hospital remained insuperable. Ambulances and transport were not always available for an army under pressure and sometimes men were abandoned. The misery of the sick and wounded in the early years of the Peninsular War (1808–14) is difficult for the modern imagination to conceive. The regimental hospitals had no transport and casualties were dumped in filthy depots along the route. During the long, cold, exhausting withdrawals – such as the British retreat to Corunna in the winter of 1808 – the casualties were loaded roughly into crude Spanish ox-wagons which jerked and heaved over primitive roads. They were given little to eat and no attention. Disease, especially lice-caused typhus, was rampant. Most thought no further than amputation, and only 50 per cent of the wounded could expect to survive gangrene, loss of blood or tetanus. Since operations were still performed without anaesthetic surgical shock was severe and often fatal. Vinegar was the only antiseptic, disinfectant and dressing for wounds. Dysentery and malaria were common.

The men inflicted some of their privations on themselves by their excesses; some of the weaker regiments lost all control and looted, smashed and burned in an orgy of destruction. Yet Spain was not an enemy country, but one they had come to save from the French. Some regiments went in search of wine the moment they entered a town and were soon helplessly or violently drunk. In Benavente a large party of men smashed open hundreds of casks, by firing musket balls at them, and then kneeled deeply into the gushing wine and drank it like water. Drunk, they were easy prey for chills and fevers. At Astorga the commander, Lieutenant Gen Sir John Moore, could no longer risk the bulk of his army by slowing it down with the sick, so about 400 were left behind. At Bembibre another 1,000 men were left behind – so drunk that the disciplined men of the rearguard, the 95th, could not even prod them to their feet with bayonets. The wounds suffered by these drunkards when the French cavalry galloped among them are better not described; but Moore, in an effort to restore discipline, drew up those regiments which had behaved badly and paraded past them those hideously mangled survivors who had managed to reach the British lines. The surgeons could do nothing for these unfortunates other than bind the worst of their wounds, but they knew that even this was a waste of time.

A conscientious and responsible surgeon faced enormous difficulties during the Peninsular War. George Guthrie, Principal Medical Officer at the battle of Talavera (1809), had 3,000 wounded on his hands, yet his only equipment was such as regimental surgeons carried in their panniers. An outspoken man, Guthrie protested vehemently against what he termed 'off with his head' surgery – the all too rapid decision to amputate or bleed. He called one hospital a slaughter-house and made himself unpopular by urging more conservative methods, but he got his way and several of his surgical and medical practices became standard.

What Guthrie was fighting is all too vividly shown by the experiences of Richard Cooper who, suffering from dysentery and fever at the end of 1809, was taken to a convent and put in a corridor with 200 others. 'My case was pitiable, my appetite and hearing gone; feet and legs like ice, three blisters on my back and feet unhealed and undressed; my shirt sticking in the wound caused by blisters . . . and worst of all nobody seemed to care a straw for me.' At Elvas he was one of twenty men put into a room with no ventilation; eighteen died. Somehow surviving, Cooper was moved to another hospital, but it was so crowded he was accommodated in the charnel house. At Celerico he was squashed into another crowded room. At no time did he see soap or towel and he existed on biscuit, salt pork and wine.

Guthrie found 300 French sick and wounded crowded into a convent at San Carlos, Salamanca; they had been left behind by their hard-pressed commander, the Duke of Ragusa. Neglected by the Spanish authorities, who hoped they would all die painfully, the French were in a frightful state. Guthrie bullied the Spaniards into a more humane treatment of the prisoners and supervised their nursing. While at Salamanca a French cavalry officer was brought to him severely wounded, and Guthrie operated on the man and saw him restored to health and activity, in due course to be exchanged for a British officer. The following year Guthrie, near Oporto, was taken prisoner by a troop of enemy cavalry commanded by his former patient who, recognizing his surgeon, set him free on the spot.

It should be obvious from these few brief references that Guthrie was an individualist and a man of character. In the opinion of many medical men he remains the greatest of British military surgeons. He was certainly one of the army's most outstanding personalities, though in no way an eccentric. He had a proper regard for soldiers as men and was a dedicated professional in his craft. During his first battle, Rolica, Portugal (1808), when attached to the 29th Regiment, he observed that there is no standard reaction to a wound. Two hundred men were wounded while storming the heights of Rolica and most of them were lying in a line of 200 yards. 'They were all known to me by name as by person: the conflict was soon over, and the difference of expression in begging for assistance, or expressing their sense of suffering, will never be obliterated from my memory.'

All military surgeons have bizarre experiences. One of Guthrie's occurred during the battle of Talavera when Guthrie, about to move the position of his aid post to avoid ricocheting cannon-balls, saw a man running after him waving his hand and shouting to him to stop. He was impatient when the soldier asked him to examine his head, on which he said a cannon-ball had bounced. But when the man pulled off his cap Guthrie was astonished to see that the skull was driven in and that brains and mashed bone were mingled with the hair. He sent the man to the rear and later searched for him in different hospitals but could not find him.

This man was unlucky. Others were badly wounded through sheer ignorance or stupidity. At Castrojon, just before the battle of Salamanca, an Irish boy of the 27th Regiment, seeing a cannon-ball bouncing towards him, shouted 'Stop it, boys!' and put his foot in the way. It was smashed to pieces and Guthrie had to amputate it.

At this time the two men attached to Guthrie to take care of his supply mule were patients whose arms he had amputated when on service in Canada. In an effort to be discharged from the army these two had fired musket-balls through their left hands. In each case the ball destroyed the wrist joint and fractured the radius and ulna. Guthrie had taken off the lower third of each arm, using the flap operation, and in three weeks the men were well enough to become regimental cleaners, a duty ordered as punishment. Guthrie fitted them with a hook fastened to the cuff of the sleeve, but they could support great weight on the end of the stump and could use it to press the girth hard against the belly of the mule while saddling it. Guthrie, understandably, was pleased with his surgery, which he recommended should be copied.

That these men should survive was not surprising, but Guthrie brought others through after multiple surgical treatment. At Badajoz a soldier was unlucky enough to be so close to a bursting shell that Guthrie removed a leg, an arm and a testicle; the soldier had already lost part of his penis and scrotum. He had several flesh wounds, including a severe one in the back of his thigh and buttock, from which the surgeon took a large piece of shell. This soldier recovered and was granted a pension of 2*s* 9*d* a day – then a respectable amount.

Guthrie admitted that many operations, in the field and in hospital, that the military surgeon would avoid were it not for his conscience, were forced upon him. He cited the case of a soldier who, in addition to a bad compound fracture of the thigh above the middle, had considerable haemorrhage from a deep-seated artery. Guthrie asked, was this man to die unaided because amputation near or at the hip-joint was generally unsuccessful, or was he, assuming that he was anxious for operation, to have a chance of life? As Guthrie saw it, a military surgeon under these circumstances had no alternative, 'for a soldier ought never to die without surgical aid where there is a chance of its being successful. This kind of case will very much decrease the surgeon's average of success, but he will have done his duty'.

Dr Hume, surgeon to the Duke of Wellington, was close by when a soldier of the 7th Hussars was struck on the thigh by a cannon-shot and, as the man was suffering very much, Hume asked Guthrie to help him operate. Both were convinced that the man could not live unless given relief. As the leg was sawed off a French cannon-ball, weighing twelve pounds, fell out from between the muscles. But the man died. Such a death puzzled the surgeons, for the soldier had lost little blood and the operation had been quick and efficient. Had the man been wounded in the same place by musket-shot or small grape, making amputation necessary, he would probably have lived. There was always an incalculable difference between the effects of an injury by cannon and musket-shot in the same part.

Some soldiers underwent amputation with astonishing self-control. Young Mr Fitzroy-Somerset, then an aide to Wellington and later to command the unfortunate army in the Crimea, watched phlegmatically while his arm was taken off. As it was being taken away he called: 'Here, bring that arm back! There is a ring my wife gave me on the finger.'

Guthrie insisted that a ball should never be allowed to remain in a bone. Since balls tended to stick tightly in bone, Guthrie usually prised them out with a sharp-pointed instrument, but if the ball was deeply embedded, as often was the case in the bones of the cranium, he had to apply a trephine, an improved form of trepan or skull operation.

Finding the musket-ball was one of the surgeon's greatest difficulties. At the battle of Toulouse a soldier of the 61st Regiment was hit on the leg and, disabled, was taken prisoner. French surgeons – after the fashion set by Paré long before – made three incisions on the inside of the leg but failed to find the ball. He was returned to the British lines where Dr Chermside, assistant surgeon of the 7th Hussars, having ascertained that the ball was fired from above while the man's leg was bent, reasoned that its course must be obliquely downwards and found the ball near the inner ankle and extracted it; it had struck the bone and was jagged and flattened.

Guthrie criticized those military surgeons who neglected the opinions of one another and those who 'feared to deviate from the road marked out for them by their teachers'. A thinking surgeon himself, Guthrie was well read, listened to others and was acutely observant. Aware of the dangers of blood poisoning he removed all foreign bodies, splintered bones and the missile when accessible. He did not hesitate to enlarge a wound after a musket-ball had fractured a rib. He found that the artery between the ribs, although often injured, rarely caused such haemorrhage as to require a special operation for its suppression, but whenever it did occur he enlarged the wound so as to show the 'bleeding orifice'. Surgeons of

Guthrie's period wrote much about intercostal (between the ribs) bleeding. One, Meyer, gives two dozen methods for suppressing it, including a little distensible pouch. This was to be used by an Italian surgeon in 1917.

Guthrie and Larrey, as well as Valentine, rediscovered the efficacy of closing chest wounds by suture – a practice abandoned for centuries. Characteristically, it was forgotten after Guthrie's period and re-used about 1917. Guthrie noted that immediate closure of an open chest wound relieved the distressful difficulty in breathing. He also noticed that the immediate closure prevented the exit of fluids; such wounds were sucked by the mouths of 'irregular practitioners', generally the drum-major of a regiment when the patient was a soldier. In some cases the results were astonishingly good, but in others quite as unfortunate. Guthrie's practice in the case of a large haemothorax was to puncture it and, if necessary, drain it by incision.

Between the battle of Rolica (1808) and that of Toulouse (1814) Guthrie dealt personally with no fewer than 20,000 wounds. Toulouse was the final combat of the Peninsular War and, since stability was now possible, the military hospitals set up in the town were well fitted and well staffed. French and British surgeons visited one another and together investigated every case of outstanding interest. The medical men were numerous, young, eager and efficient, and it is clear from facts elicited or confirmed that the general improvement in British and French surgical practice began during those months in Toulouse.

Two medical returns made for the period 10 April to 28 June 1814 are particularly interesting.[15]

SURGICAL CASES TREATED AND CAPITAL OPERATIONS PERFORMED ON OFFICERS

diseases and wounds	admitted	total treated	discharged	transferred to Bordeaux	died	remaining	proportion of deaths to the number treated
head	6	6	4	1		1	
thorax	10	10	2	2		6	
abdomen	1	1				1	
superior extremities	33	33	9	15		9	
inferior	49	49	12	21	1	15	1 in 49
compound fractures	7	7		1	2	4	1 in 3½
slight wounds gangrene	11	11	7	2		2	
Total	117	117	34	42	3	38	1 in 39

SURGICAL CASES TREATED AND CAPITAL OPERATIONS PERFORMED ON SOLDIERS

(the final proportions listed are not precise but are as given in the official report).

diseases and wounds	total treated	died	discharged to duty	transferred to Bordeaux	proportions of deaths to the number treated
head	95	17	25	53	1 in $5\frac{10}{17}$
thorax	96	35	14	47	1 in $2\frac{35}{96}$
abdomen	104	24	21	59	1 in $4\frac{1}{3}$
superior extremities	304	3	96	205	1 in 101
inferior extremities	498	21	150	327	1 in $23\frac{5}{6}$
compound fractures gangrene	78	29		49	1 in $2\frac{20}{29}$
wounds of spine	3	3			1 in 1
wounds of joints	16	4		12	1 in 4
amputations arm 7 leg and thigh 41 }	48	10		38	1 in $5\frac{1}{3}$
Total	1242	146	306	790	1 in $8\frac{128}{145}$

Wounded officers . . . 117, not included. Among these, 13 cases of tetanus occurred; all proved fatal.

To Guthrie surgery became indebted for a method of treating wounded arteries – securing both extremities in case the artery was opened. He advocated cutting out the joints as a substitute for removal of a limb wounded by gunshot, and after Waterloo demonstrated the advantage of the straight splint in the treatment of fracture of the femur (thigh bone). After Waterloo too he amputated the leg of a French soldier at the hip joint – a fearsome and formidable operation – without any other pressure being made upon the main artery than that given by the fingers. The case was successful and was later exhibited in London to demonstrate the fact that employment of a tourniquet was not indispensable.

Some surgeons, such as Hamilton, though industrious, did not have the opportunity to impose personality and professional skill in any wider field than a regiment. James McGrigor, who joined the Army in 1794,* had to wait fourteen years for the initial opportunity which was to make him one of the figures in military medicine.

After devoted but unspectacular service he was Principal Medical Officer South-Western District, based at Portsmouth, when the remnants of Sir

---

* For £150, in what was then De Burgh's Regiment, soon afterwards renamed the 88th or Connaught Rangers.

John Moore's beaten army arrived from Corunna in 1808. The number of sick was overwhelming, and McGrigor had to find accommodation, medical attendants, nurses and other staff. He took precautions against the returning men spreading infection to the communities, but their fevers and diseases affected most of Sussex and Hampshire. Still, McGrigor's showing as a medical administrator was impressive.

In 1809 he was associated with a great naval doctor, Sir Gilbert Blane, at Walcheren, Holland, in trying to protect the troops from the illnesses to which the incompetence of their commanders exposed them. The expedition was ill-conceived and disastrous. The parliamentary commission which followed it was told that had Lord Castlereagh followed the advice of the senior medical officers the lives of thousands of men would have been saved. With Blane, and assisted by Doctors Borland and Lemprière, McGrigor had drawn up rules for the preservation of health among the Walcheren troops, asking that they be not 'oppressed with duty', that they be given four consecutive nights in bed, an allowance of spirits before going on guard and hot coffee afterwards. Of the 39,000 men who reached Walcheren no fewer than 23,000 died of disease in four months. Only 217 fell to the enemy.

In January 1812 McGrigor arrived in Lisbon and immediately assumed charge of the health of Wellington's army. Undeterred by Wellington's discouragement, McGrigor established a chain of hospitals all along the route to Salamanca and, since Wellington would give him no ambulances, used commissary transport to evacuate the wounded from the battlefields. He arranged for wooden frameworks of huts to be sent out from England – they could have been the first recorded prefabricated buildings – together with carpenters and set up a village of cottages near the Douro River to accommodate 4,000 sick. McGrigor carried out constant inspections to keep medical staff and others on their toes and, short of British staff, engaged French prisoner-of-war doctors and Spaniards. He instituted medical boards whose authority was required to send officers and troops to the rear except during battle or retreat – thus making sure that malingerers did not evade their obligations and that genuinely unfit men were not kept in the line. This board decided which men would convalesce in comfort amid the orange groves of Lisbon.

Some men survived bizarre wounds. John Kinkaid, a lieutenant in the Rifle Brigade, saw a musket accidentally discharged while a soldier was ramming home a ball. The ramrod was fired from the barrel, entered the soldier's stomach, passed through his body and then wounded a second man by sticking into his backbone. It was hammered loose with a stone. The badly wounded soldier recovered and rejoined his regiment only to be drowned while swimming.[16]

Hardy, and expecting little, men remained surprisingly cheerful. A visitor to a hospital in Spain saw a palliasse in a dark corner and noticed a pelisse of the 18th Hussars used as a quilt. A little round head upon the pillow, a vivid eye, with a countenance of a deadly pallid hue, bespoke a wounded Irishman. 'Do you belong to the 18th?' 'Yes, please your honour' (the right hand at the same time carried up to the forelock). 'Are you wounded?' 'Yes, plase your honour' (again the hand to the head). 'Where?' 'Run twice through the body, plase your honour.' 'Are you in pain?' 'Och! plase your honour, I'm tolerably aisy; the Frinch daacter blid me, and tomorrow I shall see the old rigiment.'[17]

One of James McGrigor's talents was in being able to predict how many troops would *not* see the old regiment. A magnificent medical quartermaster, he became noted for the accuracy of his estimates in anticipated casualties of sick and wounded. He was such an outstanding chief of medical services that Wellington was to comment that: 'The medical department is the only one that will obey orders; on them I can rely for doing their duty.' No commander had ever before thanked his surgeons in dispatches. Napier, historian of the Peninsular War, commented that the remarkable work of the medical officers might be said to have saved the day at the battle of Vittoria (1813), for their exertions had added between 4,000 and 5,000 men to Wellington's army and without them Wellington might well have lost.

Most military doctors were struck by the tendency of nearly everybody to ignore the services of medical men, even those who had directly benefited from them. McGrigor put their bravery on record.

> In the proper execution of their duties medical officers are frequently under fire; and the cases of wounded medical officers were numerous. Some were killed and many lost limbs in sieges and battles. Yet it has been ignorantly advanced by some military men that the medical men have no business in exposed situations and they would deny the medical officer a pension for the loss of a limb. Yet it is well known that the cases are numerous wherein the lives of officers and soldiers have been saved by the zealous medical officers of their regiments being on hand to repress haemorrhage.

McGrigor admitted to French medical superiority in one thing only – the ambulance service. The French usually had plenty of comfortable transport for their sick and wounded, and though McGrigor proposed such a service for the British troops Wellington would not consider it.

The surgery of the Peninsular War was, because of the great opportunities it gave doctors, several years in advance of civil surgery. Physicians too were able to observe diseases and experiment with remedies not always available in England.

In 1814, the war over, McGrigor became Director-General of the Army Medical Department, a post he held for thirty-six years. Before McGrigor's reforming hand arrived bunks for soldiers to sleep in were arranged in double tiers along the sides of the barrack-room and occasionally two men were required to sleep together in the one berth. A place just vacated by a man going on duty would be filled by a man coming off duty. McGrigor's protests gave the soldier the luxury of a bed to himself.

McGrigor preferred regimental hospitals supplemented by field hospitals to general hospitals, since in those days of poor transport a sick or wounded man could be treated more rapidly. He saw that each regimental hospital was independent enough to carry out all treatments and operations. Because a general hospital was necessary during the long and frequently static Peninsular War, McGrigor insisted on separate wards for particular diseases, an almost revolutionary step. In addition, he had surgical wards and convalescent wards. Previously a single ward might contain men suffering from different diseases and disabilities as well as soldier convalescents, many of whom succumbed to a further infection while in hospital.

In 1812 one battalion newly arrived from England lost 500 men to dysentery in a few weeks.* Captain Gronow attributed the cause to change of diet and substitution of the 'horrid wine' of Portugal for English porter. Taking advice to drink a small glass of brandy or rum on rising to prevent dysentery, rheumatism and other ailments, Gronow never had a day's illness.[18] The standards McGrigor set were high and sometimes he insisted on too much form-filling, but his precepts were responsible in the long run, and after some black periods, for the efficiency of the treatment given British soldiers. Indicating that the higher the qualifications the better the prospect of promotion, McGrigor ordered every medical officer in the army to draw up and sign a statement of education and service. He exerted himself to gain the confidence of each medical officer, and 'while by every means I showed myself their friend and used the utmost courtesy to the good officer, I was severe and unrelenting to the bad, the negligent and the ignorant who were averse to learn'.[18]

Still, by the time of Waterloo, only a year after the final battle (Toulouse) of the Peninsular War, no great improvements had been permanently affected. A few surgeons were at the front giving first-aid treatment, but most remained at the rear, where they recklessly sacrificed arms and legs. Again wounded men lay for many hours or even days on the battlefield; many were killed out of hand by Belgian civilian looters or by criminals in the British and Prussian armies. Captain Mercer of the Royal Artillery, a notable figure during the battle, wrote a long description of the field the night after the battle. 'I woke about midnight, chilled and cramped. . . . I got up to look around and contemplate a battlefield by the pale moonlight. . . . Here and there some poor wretch, sitting up amidst the countless dead, busied himself in endeavours to stanch the flowing stream with which his life

---

* A Swiss army doctor, Tissot, advocated fruit as a remedy for dysentery. The disease had nearly destroyed a Swiss regiment in the south of France in the 1780s. A captain bought the entire crop of several acres of vineyard, to which he had the sick soldiers carried. All men were put on a grape diet and according to Tissot nobody died after this and the disease petered out.

was fast ebbing away. . . . From time to time a figure would half raise itself and then, with a despairing groan, fall back again. Others . . . would stagger away in search of succour. . . . It was heart-rending. . . .'

The countless casualties *were* counted: British, 15,000; Prussians, 7,000; French, 25,000 estimated. Three hospitals were commandeered in Brussels and tents were put up in the main square after the hospitals had been filled and the wounded men had been lying in the open for some time. Guthrie, called urgently to the scene, tried valiantly to remedy conditions but, as he said: 'Nothing could recall the past irretrievable mischief the insufficient medical care had occasioned in the first few days.'

Surgeon James found medical work 'grim in the extreme', alleviated only by the heroism of the suffering soldiers. 'When one considers the hasty surgery . . . the awful sights the men are witness to, knowing that their turn on that blood-soaked operating table is next, seeing the agony of an amputation, however swiftly performed, the longer torture of a probing, then one realizes fully of what our soldiers are made.'[19]

CHAPTER NINE

Larrey, Percy and French Humanity

Contemporary with McGrigor and Guthrie⋆ in the British Army were Baron Larrey and Baron Percy in the French.

Two of the great military surgeons of history, Percy and Larrey are conspicuous as originators of the modern plan of removing wounded soldiers from the field by trained attendants in specially designed conveyances. Each originated a distinctive feature in ambulance organization. Larrey introduced the use of light ambulance conveyances specially fitted for following the movements of the advanced guard of an army and so built as to be capable of rapidly carrying the wounded from the fighting, once the first dressings were applied, to the hospitals in the rear.

Percy, for his part, was the first to introduce into any army a regularly trained corps of field litter-bearers, whose duty was to pick up the wounded during an action and to carry them on stretchers to an aid post.

The word *ambulance* needs clarification.† It was adopted in English from the French language and is derived from the latin *ambulare*, to walk. Until the end of the nineteenth century, however, the word had a different significance among all continental people from that applied to it by English writers. An ambulance never meant, among foreigners, anything but a *field hospital* attached to an army, and moving with it – *hôpital ambulant* – for the initial reception and care of sick and wounded. The 'ambulance of the Quartier General' is the field hospital at Head Quarters. The *Ambulance*

⋆ Guthrie became known as 'the English Larrey'.

† 'The supply of ambulances', 'the ambulances for the conveyance of the sick were too heavy' – meaning the transport vehicles; 'the French ambulances' meaning the French mule litters and cacolets – these and similar expressions are constantly found in documents dealing with the Crimean War – but at that time they were all misused. Without this explanation it would be difficult for an English student to comprehend the significance of 'Les secours à donner aux blessés, sur le champ de bataille, comprennent trois phases bien distinctes: 1, le premier pansement fait sur le terrain; 2, le transport à l'ambulance; 3, le pansement, ou l'opération nécessaire, à l'ambulance.' (The aid to be given to the wounded on the field of battle comprises three very distinct phases: 1, the primary dressing on the ground; 2, the transport to the ambulance; 3, the dressing, or necessary operation, at the ambulance.)

Volante, conceived by Larrey, was a field hospital designed for rapid movements; *les caissons d'ambulance, les voitures d'ambulance*, are respectively the store transport and sick-transport carriages of a field hospital. In England the term ambulance was often applied to the conveyance itself, by which sick and wounded were carried to or from the field hospitals or elsewhere; this sense was never used in foreign writings.

After some service in the navy, Larrey joined the army in April 1792. In September, when aide-surgeon-major in the army of the Rhine, under General Custine, Larrey conceived his new system. At this time regulations ordered that the ambulances (movable field hospitals) should be posted a league (about three miles) from the rest of the army. The custom was to leave the wounded on the battlefield until the fighting ended, when they were gathered in some suitable place to which the movable hospital was brought. But military exigencies made it impossible for the hospital to reach the scene in less than twenty-four hours, so that many wounded died. After the capture of Spires (1792) Larrey was distressed to see several men die who could easily have been saved. He suggested a system for carrying prompt aid to the wounded on the battlefield itself. The ordinary field hospitals and the heavy hospital carts employed with them would no longer constitute the first line of surgical assistance.

Larrey wrote: 'My proposition was accepted, and I was authorized to organize this movable field hospital, which I named the flying ambulance [*ambulance volante*]. I then conceived the idea of a system of carriages [*voitures d'ambulance*] suspended on springs, which should combine solidity with speed and lightness. This institution created a sensation among the soldiers, and they now felt confident that they would receive succour at whatever moment they might be wounded.'[20]

Larrey's plans did not spread throughout the French Army, but in 1797, while Professor of Anatomy at the Military Hospital of Instruction, he was ordered by Bonaparte to travel to Italy and form a system of flying ambulances. His ambulance establishment then had three divisions, each comprising 12 spring vehicles to transport severely wounded men and 4 store wagons; a personnel of 113 commanded by a surgeon-major, the whole being directed by the principal medical officer in the field. The staff included 14 mounted surgeons, 12 mounted ambulance orderlies and 24 orderlies on foot. All orderlies carried a red woollen waist scarf, which could serve to carry a wounded man, and leather knapsacks with dressings. Of the 12 spring carts, 8 were two-wheeled vehicles drawn by 2 horses, and arranged for carrying 2 men at full length; and 4 were four-wheeled to carry 4 men lying down. The 12 carriages could remove 32 men at one time.

Larrey's *ambulance volante*, then, combined two principles: the first a flying field hospital for instant attention on the field, the second an arrangement for rapid transport to the field hospital. It was, to Napoleon, 'one of the happiest conceptions of the age'. He took Larrey with him to Egypt, where he found methods of treating the ophthalmia which afflicted the French Army.

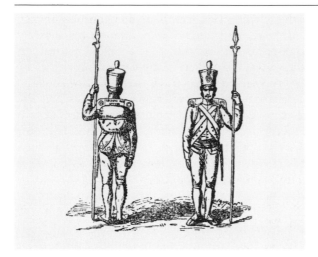

Percy's stretcher-bearers in
marching order.

While Larrey was absent in Egypt, Percy, chief medical officer to the Army of the North, under General Moreau, organized another system of ambulance. In 1799 he devised a light carriage intended to carry surgeons, attendants, hand-litters and surgical dressings. A long carriage on four wheels and drawn by six horses, Percy's conveyance was commonly known as a *wurtz*★ but sometimes as a *char de chirurgie* (surgical cart). Along the body was a long narrow case containing surgical instruments and materials; astride it sat eight surgeons. In front and rear of this carriage were two smaller chests and on each of these sat two hospital corps men; four other attendants sat on the four leading horses. The chests on the *wurtz* held dressings for 1,200 wounded. Stretchers were carried under the long case on the body of the wagon. The purpose of the *wurtz*, said Percy, was to see that 'the art of preserving life should contest in activity and celebrity with the art of destroying life'.

Each *wurtz* was to keep up with its division. When an action began and soldiers were wounded, the attendants ran and picked up the fallen men even though under fire and brought them on stretchers to the *wurtz*, where the surgeons applied the first dressings. If the wounded became numerous and too distant for stretcher-removal then the *wurtz* itself was sent to them. In April 1800 General Lecombe published a general order: 'We all give a tribute of praise to this new institution created by Citizen Percy – the movable corps of surgical aid. The medical officers of these corps have succoured the wounded on the field of battle itself, and have so distinguished themselves by

---

★ The word in French writings is spelled 'wurtz', but is *wurst* in its original German. When used alone in German it signified a thick, short sausage, a cylinder, but when joined to *wagen* signified a long wagon. The French word was therefore an abbreviation as well as corruption of the German *wurst-wagen*.

their zeal and devotion that the soldier reverences them, and consoles himself when he is wounded, because he sees that assistance is given to them with a rapidity hitherto without example.'

Percy's conveyances fell into disuse after the war when the Army of the North was disbanded, and when war broke out a few years later the custom of wounded being carried to the rear by their own comrades was continued. The *soldats d'ambulance* of that period – the first years of the nineteenth century – served only in hospitals.

Percy, as Surgeon-in-Chief with the French Army in Spain, again provided a special corps of stretcher-bearers for removing wounded. This was the beginning of an institution which was to last for a century.

> Tired of the ceaseless disorder [wrote Percy] caused by assemblage of undisciplined hospital attendants; distressed at seeing the deaths of so great a number of soldiers whose lives might have been preserved and limbs saved . . . having seen, moreover, the necessity of having near the line of battle men specially trained to carry off the wounded instead of leaving them to the care of soldiers who too often seized this opportunity for leaving the ranks, I took upon myself to organize a regular corps of army hospital attendants [*soldats infirmiers*] to whom I gave the name of *Compagnies des Brancardiers* [bearers of stretchers]. I selected a hundred soldiers from among the bravest, strongest and most adroit. . . . The service of the sick and wounded soon changed its appearance. Companies of ambulance bearers must be of chosen men uniting courage, strength and address. One cannot too often repeat, the chief consolation and the assistance of first importance to a wounded man is for him to be carried promptly and properly away from the scene of conflict.

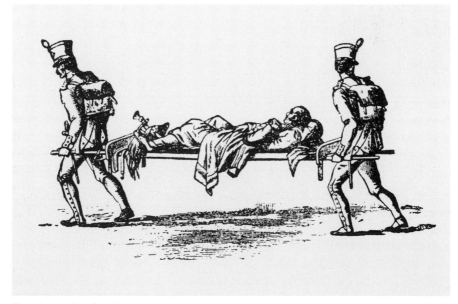

Percy's stretcher fitted for carrying wounded.

An imperial decree established Percy's system throughout the French Army in 1813.

Both these enlightened men, Larrey and Percy, were very much front-line surgeons. Larrey was present during all Napoleon's campaigns and was active at no fewer than 60 battles and 400 minor engagements. A man of professional principle, Larrey, whenever present, saw to it that the sick and wounded British captured during the terrible retreat to Corunna were treated kindly. In April 1808 he had under his charge many wounded on the island of Lobau in the Danube. His patients were starving and, unable to import supplies, Larrey had horses killed to make soup. This was most courageous in an age when horses were less expendable than men, but Napoleon endorsed his surgeon's action. He was so impressed with Larrey that he awarded him the Legion of Honour and created him baron.

At the battle of Wagram (1809) Napoleon further rewarded Larrey with a pension of 5,000 francs annually. During this battle the artillery commander, General Daboville, was seriously wounded when hit on the right shoulder by a cannon-ball, which destroyed the joint and tore away flesh and muscles, making 'an enormous and frightful' wound. Larrey's prompt treatment in amputating at the shoulder joint brought the general from the edge of death.

Larrey was prominent throughout the march to Moscow and the retreat. He performed hip-joint amputations twice during this campaign; on a Russian soldier who bore the operation with great courage, but who died on the twenty-ninth day from dysentery, and on a French dragoon who was believed to have survived. At the Beresina River he crossed and recrossed several times to arrange passage for the sick, until his position was so dangerous that the soldiers, who revered him, had to rescue him from himself.

Larrey's surgical techniques were, like Guthrie's, courageous and definite. In the case of a penetrating wound of the chest with the missile lodging internally Baron Larrey had a six-point pattern of treatment for Napoleon's soldiers:

> To excise the wound as far as the fractured ribs.
> To extract loose splinters of bone.
> To ligature the intercostal vessels if bleeding.
> To cut off jagged ends of ribs if necessary, either with saw or cutting forceps.
> To seek carefully for the ball and remove it if within reach.
> The wound was then sealed with an agglutinative plaster.

Larrey tried to prevent inflammation by local bleeding, by venesection (cutting of a vein) and antiphlogistics (inflammation-reducing agents). He did not like sucking of wounds, though this was common among the French. He thought it might disturb a clot or that the saliva of the sucker or the blood of the sucked might convey a virus. Larrey appreciated the necessity of not leaving large numbers of wounded soldiers in the one place when it could be avoided – congregation spread disease – and only lack of adequate transport prevented him from dispersing them.

Infinitely resourceful, Larrey, after the battle of Bautzen, Saxony, in the summer of 1813, had many wounded on his hands but inadequate transport to get them to Dresden, thirty miles away. He commandeered the country wheelbarrows. The Bautzen barrow was long, well balanced and, as wheelbarrows go, fairly comfortable, but the strain on a wounded man during the ten-hour slog must have been great. Larrey counted as many as 150 barrows, trundled by civilians, on a single stretch of road.[21]

The improvements which Percy and Larrey effected in the French Army attracted more notice among British surgeons than the systems adopted by the other European powers. As late as 1893 Surgeon Sir Thomas Longmore noted that: 'It seems . . . that the observations which were made [by the French] during the Peninsular campaigns have ever since had an influence on the views which have been held by English surgeons on the subject of transport of wounded.'

But neither Larrey nor Percy could be in more than one place at once. The French troops suffered because there were so many of them and so few doctors. Much has been made of the fact that the French performed few amputations compared with the British. The chief reason for this was not one of medical principle but shortage of surgeons; the French doctors were so overworked that they avoided difficult and time-consuming amputations.

Napoleon took 400,000 troops with him on his march to Moscow in 1812, but only 100 surgeons. These few could not cope with the men who fell to the climate or to the Cossacks. No official provision was made for the sick and weak; those who survived did so through luck or through the charity of their comrades; there was little charity in the grim days of the winter retreat. In the advance Russian prisoners existed on the flesh of rotting animals found along the roadside; if they could not keep up they were shot. In the retreat the French and their allies existed on horseflesh, and no sooner did a man collapse from exhaustion than the next man stripped him before he was dead. Many men lost the power of speech and many others went insane from cold and hunger. In this atmosphere the French surgeons who survived did little more than give superficial treatment to senior officers. The many women who accompanied the armies were given no treatment, but most endured their privations better than the men; the greatest loss of women occurred during the return crossing of the Beresina when they fell from the pontoon bridge during the rush to cross it.[22]

Despite their sufferings the French soldiers were generally better off than the Russian and Turkish, who knew that a serious wound or disease meant death unless they could find some sympathetic civilian to care for them. Virtually the only doctors were on the staff of generals. After a fight, wounded would be collected and dumped somewhere to die; those who fell ill during a march were simply left behind in the nearest house or barn, where, generally, they too died. Surgery and medicine were static in principle, non-existent in practice.

Military doctors of the more progressive nations – England, Switzerland, Sweden, the United States after 1814 – were increasingly concerned with all aspects of military life, not merely administration, operative techniques and treatment of disease. Dr Henry Marshall's contribution was in the field of enlisting, discharging and pensioning soldiers. His advice to enlisting officers, especially, was standard practice for years, though it reads humorously today.

> Upon entering the inspection-room the recruit is to walk a few times pretty smartly across the apartment for the purpose of showing that he has the perfect use of his lower extremities. He is then to be halted and set up in the position of a soldier under arms with the knees about one inch apart, and examined in front and rear from head to foot. Should no material defect be discovered the examination may go on. The recruit is then to perform, in imitation of the hospital sergeant, the following evolutions: To extend the arms to right angles with the trunk of the body; then to touch the shoulders with the fingers; next to place the backs of the hands together over the head. In this position let him cough, while the examiner's hand is applied to the rings of the external oblique muscles. Let the inspecting officers examine the spermatic cord and testes; then pass his hands over the bones of his legs. The recruit next stands upon one foot, and moves the ankle-joint of each extremity alternately; when any doubt is entertained respecting the efficiency of this joint, or any part of the inferior extremity, he should be made to test his strength by hopping upon the suspected limb for a short period, and the size and aspect of the corresponding part of the opposite limb should also be accurately compared. He is next to kneel on one knee, then on the other, and subsequently on both knees; let him then stoop forwards and place his hands on the ground, and while in this position it ought to be ascertained whether he be affected with haemorrhoids. He is then to extend the superior extremities forwards for the purpose of having his arms and hands examined, and with this instruction he is to perform flexion and extension of the fingers, and to rotate the forearm. The head is next to be examined, including the scalp, ears, eyes, nose, and mouth. The surgeon is then to ascertain that he possesses the function of hearing and the faculty of distinct enunciation. In regard to the mental faculties, the inspecting medical officer should invariably ask a recruit a few short questions, as to what occupation he had previously followed, etc. etc., or adopt any other means which he may deem necessary to ascertain the condition of the intellect. . . .

There was, perhaps, something hypocritical in ascertaining the condition of the soldier's intellect when the intellect, intelligence and dedication of army commanders were so questionable during the period 1815–54. The army was allowed to deteriorate and officers devoted themselves to social activities rather than to training. Britain had garrisons in many parts of the world, but military action was desultory and inconsequential, though occasionally disastrous,*

---

* During the retreat from Kabul in January 1842 a force of 4,500 English and Indian soldiers and 12,000 Indian followers was continually attacked by Afghans. Only 800 survived to Khurd Kabul Pass; 200 reached Jagdalek. The last survivors were overwhelmed at Gundamak. One man, the regimental doctor, Brydon, reached Jellalabad with the news. Except for Brydon and a few prisoners the entire Kabul force perished.

and few people thought seriously about preparing for the medical problems which would occur in a major war. Here and there a medical inspector-general or a staff surgeon would write a caustic report about the need for more professionalism or improvements in the lot of the common soldier, but such people were regarded as eccentric. A few were genuinely eccentric, as was Dr James Barry. Dr Barry was a woman, but she more or less successfully concealed her sex for the forty-six years she spent in the army. A peppery little person, Dr Barry was devoted to her profession, which she practised for the benefit of soldiers in South Africa, the West Indies, St Helena, Malta, Corfu, the Crimea and Canada, surviving enmities, a court-martial, intrigues, diseases and discovery of her sex. During the course of her service in Malta in the late 1840s the troops suffered from a serious epidemic of cholera, and for her treatment of the sick she could boast that she received the thanks of the Duke of Wellington. Later, on Corfu, her methods of nursing sick and wounded soldiers evacuated from the Crimea were so successful that the recovery rate was the highest for the whole of the Crimea campaign; unfortunately they were never repeated on a large scale. Several commanding officers thanked her for her work on this occasion, as did the Royal Navy for the diagnosis of a malignant fever which had broken out on HMS *Modeste* and for 'successful treatment of the sick and the purification of the ship'.

Still later, in Canada, she made herself unpopular by urging a better balanced diet for soldiers, such as 'the cheering change of a roast instead of eternal boiled beef and soup'. She thought that drainage and sewerage should be improved, and she had 'the honour to submit' to the deputy quartermaster-general that hair mattresses and hair or feather pillows should be substituted for the palliasses and straw pillows. 'It must be evident what great comfort it would be to a poor sufferer to rest his emaciated and feverish limbs on something more genial than hard straw.' The significance of such an observation is that military doctors were now taking a wider interest in health, and while their suggestions were not always followed they were not now so actively resented. In short, there was tacit admission of their right to make such suggestions.

Dr Barry was appalled to find that Canadian barracks had no provision for married quarters; a soldier and his young bride were expected to share the common dormitory with a score or more of men. She saw this as deleterious to health as well as to morals.

Probably one of the causes [of drunkenness] and a great one, is the absence of separate accommodation for married persons . . . a room for each family would indeed be not only a great boon to the soldier but would diminish intemperance which is the chief cause of crime, punishment, sickness and death. This I have annually iterated and re-iterated. For example, a woman humbly born, but modestly and religiously educated, becomes the wife of a soldier, is suddenly placed in a barrack room with 10 or 20 men, perhaps some married, she becomes frightened and disgusted, next becomes habituated, or in despair has recourse to drunkenness and not infrequently the husband, a good man, joins with his wife and he becomes the occupant of a cell in a military prison, which, had a similar room been told off for each married person, they might live with decency and bring up their children in the fear of God, without being tainted by the awful and disgusting language of a barrack room.

Dr Barry* was not exaggerating about the evils of drink. Liquor was the direct or indirect cause of many diseases, ailments and injuries. It caused organic damage and it predisposed the system to chills and fevers. Many a drunken soldier died from exposure through sleeping off his stupor in bitter weather, or injured himself in falling or fighting. But neither Dr Barry nor any other surgeon on his own succeeded in notably mitigating the evil. Remedy followed decades of army education, the introduction of recreation rooms, libraries, games and – gradually – private accommodation for married soldiers.

---

* Following a severe bout of influenza in Canada she was pronounced unfit for service in July 1859, at the probable age of sixty-five. In the Army List she was the senior of the inspector-generals, with rank equivalent to major-general. Her sex was officially discovered after her death in July 1865; it had been unofficially discovered at least once during her army career.

CHAPTER TEN

Illness at Sea

For centuries naval physicians and surgeons had a greater range of problems than those encountered by army doctors; seamen were liable to many more injuries than soldiers, and a ship's surgeon was very much alone with his difficulties. It is a common misconception that the seaman lived a life much freer of disease than did the soldier; after all, he was isolated from shore-based diseases and he breathed fresh, clean air. The truth is that the seaman has been subject to diseases, disabilities and disasters not prevalent on land. His position when ill was critical, because some captains would not admit that illness existed – at least among common seamen. Under these commanders no man was allowed to be sick. Casualty statistics prove the seaman's vulnerability. Any warship of any nation in Tudor times could expect to lose half its crew in a six-month cruise. Many ships put to sea without a surgeon, for doctors were understandably reluctant to undertake sea service. Two centuries later, during the Seven Years War (1756–63), more doctors were serving, but disease was just as deadly; during those years, of the 185,000 raised for sea service in the Royal Navy no fewer than 130,000 died of disease, with scurvy the main cause. Crews went to action stations weak and listless, collapsing over the gun tackles and unable to drag themselves to the rigging. Only 1,512 were killed in action. During the Napoleonic Wars sea service remained dangerous and unhealthy. The total casualty figures, not allowing for peace-time losses, were 84,440 from disease and individual accident; 12,680 from foundering, wreck, fire and explosion; 6,540 from enemy action: a total of 103,660.

Heavy losses of men had long been accepted as inevitable, except by the more humane and purposeful doctors. But these men achieved reforms only with great difficulty. The navy was accustomed to frequent burials at sea. In 1679 Chaplain Teonge aboard the *Royal Oak* reported the burial of one man 'little better than starved to death with cold weather', and another 'eaten to death with lyce'. He saw 'pitifull creatures' sent ashore, so emaciated as to be useless for the rest of their foreshortened lives.

In most respects nobody in particular was to blame for the seaman's often poor state of health; medical science and knowledge of hygiene had simply not developed, although Captain James Cook, on his second voyage to the Pacific in 1772–5, despite a record period at sea, lost only one man through sickness.

The continuous scourge was scurvy, the seaman's most inveterate and merciless enemy. It 'beat-up' for him on every voyage and inflicted on his brine-sodden body a lingering death. The great figure in the fight against scurvy was Dr James Lind, 'the father of naval medicine', as his disciple Dr Thomas Trotter called him. In 1739, like so many Scots, such as Tobias Smollett, he joined the navy as a surgeon's mate, became surgeon of the *Salisbury* in 1747 and made the first controlled dietetic experiment on record to prove that lemons or oranges were the best available cure for scurvy. Lind's book on scurvy, 1753, ran through three editions and was translated abroad, but his treatment was not adopted by the navy until 1795, following persistent pressure by Lind's followers, Trotter and Gilbert Blane. This pathetic delay had appalling consequences; for instance, after a six-weeks' cruise in 1780 the Channel fleet landed 2,400 sufferers at Haslar Hospital, Southampton. At the time Lind was undistinguished and the naval medical service was considered the lowest form of medical life.

Captain Cook has been credited with the defeat of scurvy; in fact he postponed the introduction of lemon juice on the grounds of expense and Lind deserves more credit. His book was inspired by the fate of the seamen who accompanied Lord Anson in his circumnavigation of the globe, 1740–4; of the 1,955 who embarked, 1,051 died.

The Revd Walter, who sailed with Anson, described scurvy as 'surely the most singular and unaccountable [disease] that affects the human body'. The symptoms varied, but common ones included large discoloured spots, swollen legs, putrid gums and profound lassitude. 'This disease is likewise attended with a strange dejection of spirits; and with shiverings, tremblings, and a disposition to be seized with the most dreadful terrors on the slightest accident.' The Revd Walter observed:

Indeed it was most remarkable . . . that whatever discouraged our people, or at any time damped their hopes never failed to add new vigour to the distemper; for it usually killed those who were in the last stages of it and confined those to their hammocks who were before capable of some kind of duty. So that it seemed as if some alacrity of mind and sanguine thoughts were no contemptible preservatives from its fatal malignity. . . . It often produced putrid fevers, pleurisies, jaundice and violent rheumatic pains . . . sometimes an obstinate costiveness [constipation] generally attended with difficulty of breathing; and this was the most deadly of all scorbutic symptoms. At other times the whole body, but more especially the legs, were subject to ulcers of the worst kind, attended with rotten bones and such a luxuriancy of fungous flesh as yielded no remedy. The scars of wounds which had for many years been healed were forced open again by this virulent distemper. Of this there was a remarkable instance on one of the invalids on board the *Centurion*, who had been wounded above fifty years before at the battle of the Boyne; for though he was cured soon after, yet on his being attacked by scurvy his wounds broke out afresh and appeared as if they had never been healed. What is still more astonishing, the callous of a broken bone, which had completely formed for a long time, was found to be hereby dissolved; and the fracture seemed as if it had never been consolidated. Indeed, the effects of this disease were in almost every instance wonderful. . . . The havock which this dreadful calamity made in those ships was truly surprising. The *Centurion* from her leaving England, when at this island [Juan Fernandez] had buried 292 men and had but 214 remaining of her complement. The *Gloucester*, out of a smaller company, buried the same number and had only 82 alive. This dreadful mortality had fallen severer on the invalids [the Chelsea Pensioners who had been embarked in a desperate attempt to fill the complement of Anson's squadron] and marines than on the sailors; for on board the *Centurion*, out of 50 invalids and 70 marines there remained only 4 invalids, including officers, and 11 marines; and on board the *Gloucester* every invalid died and only two marines escaped out of forty-eight.[23]

Several progressive doctors, notably Sir Gilbert Blane,[24] Fought for the addition of citrus fruits to naval diet and because of their persistence scurvy began to lose it threat during the French Revolutionary and Napoleonic wars.* Lime juice was issued in 1792, but it did not become standard issue until 1795. However, seamen liked sourcrout (sauerkraut) much better, and in 1777 the Admiralty sent large quantities to the Newfoundland station. Much depended on the captain, the surgeon and the purser of individual ships. Pursers interested enough in their job and their men served green vegetables as well as fruit whenever they had the opportunity.

As scurvy was mastered† fevers took hold, since British ships and seamen were venturing farther and stayed longer in tropical climates, in the West Indies, South-East Asia and the East Indies and along parts of the African coast. The men's greatest fear was Yellow Jack; its onset was rapid and it quickly killed thousands of men. Sometimes only a few men of a crew would survive; on occasions the disease spread through a fleet. Men would be fit one day, dead the next night; at times nobody was left to bury the dead. One writer of 1800 notes that he, his wife and two other men were the only ones to return to England of an entire ship's complement.

Malaria was another prevalent disease, though it seems to have killed relatively few men, unlike typhus, often called ship fever. This dreaded disease resulted from unhygienic overcrowding.

For hundreds of years seamen of all races endured the stink of the bilge in the ship's bowels. When a ship was built, sand, shingle or stone was packed in the hold as ballast against the height and weight of the superstructure and masts. Gradually all sorts of filth drained into the hold, making it indescribably foul. After the blockade of Puerto Bello in 1727, when disease killed more than 5,000 men, the admiral, one of the victims, was buried in his own ballast.

---

* Blane noted that when the fleet was daily expecting action a general *stop was put to the progress of disease*, particularly of scurvy, 'from the influence of that generous flow of spirits, with which the prospect of battle inspires British Seamen'.

† But not permanently. A century after the publication of Lind's book the Admiralty decided to issue the cheaper West Indian lime juice, instead of Mediterranean lemon juice. Lime juice contains only half the number of milligrammes of ascorbic acid (Vitamin C), 20, compared with lemon juice, 40; rosehip syrup contains 200. By 1900 therefore, the cure for scurvy was less known than before Lind wrote. Scott and Shackleton suffered from it in the Antarctic. In 1916 there was an epidemic among British troops at Kut-el-Amara.

The men ate, slept and lived over the fumes that floated up from the stinking depths. Midshipmen, living on the orlop deck, were even worse off. Some captains had the bilge cleared and the ballast restacked, others stowed the ship's water casks there. But seamen had to wait until 1820 before the Admiralty ordered that all new ships would have iron or water casks for ballast, so that it could be removed, though with difficulty, for cleaning. However, it was many years before the older foul-bilge ships were paid off.

French ships were even more dangerous, and British officers and men detailed as prize crew were vulnerable to fever. The discipline and internal economy of French warships were much inferior to British standards. According to Blane their decks were never washed and there was 'a great defect in every point of cleanliness and order'. Air flow was obstructed by lumber and by bulkheads, which were not taken down even in battle. The gratings were covered night and day with tarpaulins, even in a hot climate. Even the scuppers on the lower decks were not opened as outlets for the water and filth which accumulated there; the only vent was a pipe passing from the decks along the ship's side into the hold, which became a common sink, 'inconceivably putrid and offensive'. The blood, the mangled limbs, and even entire corpses were thrown into the hold and lay there putrefying. The French sailors had a superstitious aversion to throwing bodies overboard immediately after death; the friends of the dead man wanted to perform a religious ceremony when an action was over. Increased sickness was inevitable.

Two admirals careful of health in the mid-eighteenth century were Boscawen and Hawke. Boscawen introduced a type of ventilator in his flagship, *Namur*, as early as 1747, and his enthusiasm for it carried ventilators into other ships. Hawke, in 1755, protested about lack of interest in naval health, especially care of the sick; his campaign was forceful enough to induce the Admiralty to put better medical equipment aboard ship. By insisting on adequate and regular re-provisioning for his squadron Hawke was able to maintain a long blockade of Brest during the Seven Years War, for his men stayed fitter.

Rheumatism and bronchitis, other perennial evils, were caused by the persistent dampness. All but a few doctors accepted this as inevitable. Here again Blane laboured for reform, urging the introduction of holy-stoning and hot sand to replace the continual washing. Many ships' doctors had urged captains not to have the decks washed so frequently, pointing out that 'tween-deck moisture was hard to eradicate. Blane even arranged for brazier fires to burn between decks in damp weather, though this measure was, naturally enough, resisted as a major fire hazard.

Lord St Vincent, when Commander-in-Chief in 1800, notified his captains that 'many consumptive cases might be prevented, and other mitigated, by timely application of flannel next to the skin, in catarrhs, coughs, and common colds'. He urged them to inculcate this doctrine in the minds of their surgeons who, 'from caprice and perverse opposition to every wholesome regulation, grossly neglect this important duty'. St Vincent's 'proudest boast' was the high standard of health in his fleets. He introduced soap into his ships in 1796 and he improved beds. Until 1801 the seaman had slept, within his hammock, on enveloped flock which was, apparently, nothing more than decayed wool. St Vincent insisted on a hair bed which was said to be 'wholesome and comfortable'. Many of his reforms lapsed when he was no longer a power in the navy.

Dr Trotter,[25] inspired by Lind, campaigned forthrightly for health-by-hygiene, urging that 'disordered and infectious or foul ulcerous persons' be not admitted aboard. Such men, he said, should be scrubbed and their heads shaved. Trotter especially disliked Irish landmen who, dirty and ragged, possessed 'neither the courage of an Englishman or Scotsman under disease . . . they sink from despondency when really ill while at other times with a servile, low cunning they are constantly pestering us with trifling or pretended complaints'. Whatever Trotter's bias, it was true that one dirty or infected man could quickly reduce a fighting ship to impotency; the records of naval surgeons are full of examples.

Trotter wanted the ships' officers, apart from the surgeon, to be conscious that sickness resulted from uncleanliness, from wet clothes and exposure, pointless exhaustion and many other factors within the officers' power to remedy. Among the many practices Trotter objected to was that of hanging fresh beef under the half-deck or under the booms in the waist, where it was exposed to the breath of the whole ship's company and often brushed by them as they passed.*

As in the Army, a doctor needed courage and decisiveness if he were to be much use to his patients – courage to gainsay the captain when necessary or to insist on hygiene, decisiveness in amputating, probing, bleeding. His treatment might be neither advanced nor effective, but it had to be positive, especially in action or in attempting to prevent a disease from spreading throughout a ship. That some doctors failed in their jobs is hardly surprising; everything was against them. The patient was the only man who had time for the doctor, and the moment he was cured or patched up he joined the others in criticizing him as a busybody. Some surgeons gave up being busybodies and took to the bottle as the only way of enduring a cruise that might keep them away from home for years.

No matter how much endurance the ordinary sailor had, his life, according to Nelson, was on an average 'finished at forty-five years'. Bad food and strenuous labour under extreme conditions sapped his vitals, aged him prematurely and exposed him to vocational ills. He 'fell down daily', to

---

* Trotter claimed to be the first to inoculate volunteers against smallpox in 1795, three years before Jenner evolved his method of vaccination in 1798. The first mass vaccination was carried out at Gibraltar in 1800, but it was not made compulsory in the navy until 1864.

use the old saying, in spotted or putrid fevers. At every meal he suffered acute indigestion. He was liable to a 'prodigious inflammation of the head, nose and eyes', occasioned by exposure.

He was racked by agues, distorted by rheumatic pains and often ruptured or double-ruptured. Rupture was such a common hazard that during the Revolutionary and Napoleonic wars possibly one British seaman in seven was suffering from it. The disability was so serious that the Admiralty issued trusses – an average of 3,714 of them annually between 1808 and 1815. The ruptures were caused by the great effort needed to heave and lift and push things – especially water-butts. Getting the casks from the hold, manhandling them ashore and then struggling with them back to the boats, hoisting them onto the ship's deck and manoeuvring them into the hold was probably the seaman's hardest job. Thousands of other seamen suffered from torn muscles caused by the strain of lifting the casks. Eventually somebody discovered how to fill them with a length of hosepipe leading from a watering barge alongside the ship. In its humble way it was a discovery comparable in importance to that of the breech-loading gun.

Dental decay afflicted many a sailor, partly because there was no such thing as an issue toothbrush, also because of unbalanced diet. The almost invariable treatment was crude extraction. Toothbrushes were not issued until the twentieth century, and in earlier times men's teeth were worn and blackened from nicotine and other agents. Other more or less minor health hazards were boils, carbuncles and blisters – chronic in all navies.

Insanity was relatively common from early times, but not until 1815 was any sort of research work done on the subject. In that year the industrious Blane showed that in the navy the incidence of insanity was seven times as great as in civilian life – 1 in 1,000 compared with 1 in 7,000. He suggested that intoxication, leading to men banging their heads violently while clumsily negotiating cramped spaces between decks, was one cause of the high insanity rate. Drunkenness, itself a naval occupational disorder, no doubt produced many cases of temporary insanity, but sheer worry, anxiety and frustration must have driven many a good family man around the bend. Dr Lind had referred to 'this vice of drunkenness' as 'one of the most destructive to our brave seamen, ought to be discouraged by all possible means, and severely punished by the officers'.[26]

There has been a tendency among naval historians to ignore venereal disease, but it is almost occupational and many seamen have contracted it. The girl the sailor had in every port was often a prostitute, her saving grace being that as a professional she was perhaps healthier than the enthusiastic amateur. In March 1795 Lind objected to the surgeon's standard fee of 15*s* for curing venereal disease. At Spithead, he reported, boats' crews brought medicine from shore, 'a medicine often fatal even in the best hands was a popular remedy with them – no other than *Hydrar. Muriat* [chloride of mercury]'. Some consulted itinerant quacks, who flocked to the seaports, and the men paid heavily for their advice while simple local complaints were converted into confirmed generalized ones. Others withheld the knowledge of the disease from the surgeon till the most excruciating and dangerous symptoms had supervened.

Dr Trotter attacked the avaricious brewers who bought up scores of pubs around the naval ports, notably Plymouth. 'A new mode of getting custom was observed by the publicans, who received into their houses all the unfortunate women, to the number of some thousands. These wretches flock to the naval seaports for the wages of prostitution, after being debauched in the interior of the country by the idle and dissolute soldiery. Thus, the populous town of Dock was apparently converted into a huge brothel.' The authorities closed 200 of the 300 pub-brothels, which Lind saw as a great triumph to the navy, since its men, when not under direct discipline, were no better than 'inconsiderate children'.

CHAPTER ELEVEN

Wounds at Sea

If the previous chapter appears to have dealt largely with disease rather than with wounds the balance is fair, for action was relatively rare. The surgeon's place in battle was in the after-cockpit, a dark hole of a place normally used as the midshipmen's mess. Here the surgeon, using the midshipmen's sea-chests as tables, wielded knife and saw. The chaplain and purser also worked in the cockpit during a fight. No anaesthetic existed, but most men bore their sufferings with extraordinary fortitude, though some, not surprisingly, screamed in agony. No man could remain conscious and bear the pain of a musket-ball or piece of iron embedded in the stomach. When the ship was tossing in a rough sea a surgeon would have to tie himself and his patient to the sick bay stanchions to perform an amputation or operation.

Shipboard battle wounds were frightful, since so many of them were caused by lancing splinters of wood, some of them very large. Such injuries were difficult to treat because they caused jagged, irregular wounds. Many men who survived these injuries were terribly disfigured. Others were crushed and maimed by falling masts and yards. Musket wounds were infrequent, but chain and grape shot and even heavy round shot caused many wounds. It was not infrequent for men to be decapitated by a cannon ball or for limbs to be wrenched from their sockets by one. It sometimes happened that no haemorrhage followed this violent loss of a limb. The surgeon of the *Fame* told Lind of an instance in which the thigh was cut through, except for a little flesh and skin, without the least haemorrhage. The surgeons thought this may have been owing to the near-severance of the limb, so that the blood-vessels contracted more easily than if they had been partly divided. The *Fame*'s surgeon sawed off the jagged end of bone and the man survived six days, still without bleeding, but died of lockjaw.

Boarding an enemy ship resulted in a crop of cutlass slashes and gaping wounds from pikes. Despite risk of infection a surprising number of men survived. A greater menace than 'natural' infection was that introduced by the surgeon's unclean instruments. If a musket-ball could not easily be extracted it was left, and many a British sailor survived for years with one inside him, suffering less than he would have done had the surgeon tried to dig it out.

Blane noted a 'singular species' of accident occurring in actions at sea due to what was known as the wind of a ball which could seriously hurt or even kill a man without any visible injury. He knew of two instances in naval battles in the West Indies, 1782, of a cannon-ball passing close to the stomach and causing instant death. In another ship a man had a ball pass close to his belly, so that he was 'without sense or motion' for some time and had a large, livid tumour rise on his stomach. Blane attended a seaman at Barbados who had the buttons of his trousers carried off by a cannon ball without any damage to the skin, yet his genitals were livid and swollen and he was unable to urinate without a catheter for three months. Blane reported the case of an officer stunned by a cannon-ball passing close to his temple. Even more strangely, Blane knew of a seaman who had two ribs fractured and died, though there was no mark on the skin. He thought that the phenomenon might be more accurately called the *brush* of a ball.

Until the advent of breech-loading mechanisms, the greatest number of wounds came from accidental explosion of gunpowder. In the sea battles of 1780 and 1781 a quarter of all casualties were due to powder explosions, which caused severe scorching at one end of the injury scale to incineration at the other. Dr Lind found the best remedy was linseed oil, which some surgeons mixed with lime water, others with ceruse, ointment of carbonate and hydrate of lead. Opium was used freely to alleviate pain.

Seamen were much more liable to accident than were soldiers. The sailor had to go aloft at any hour of the day or night, hundreds of feet up on masts and yards heeling 45 degrees and more, the ship pitching wildly. Frozen and soaked, he clawed at the heavy sails and ropes in obedience to yells from the deck. A slight injury was rare in a fall from aloft; it was instant crushing death or a broken back or a dive into the deep with, usually, no chance of rescue. A man might fall on somebody else and then both would be seriously hurt. Being washed overboard was a danger in a rough and breaking sea. Every time a man used the heads (toilets) in heavy seas he ran such a risk. Men went overboard with such frequency that by his thirtieth birthday Captain Marryat had won twenty-seven certificates for saving life.

Another hazard was that of guns and other heavy objects breaking loose in a storm. This was a serious emergency, almost as bad as fire. The great lump of wood and iron thundering from one side of the deck to the other would not only crush men to pulp but could smash clean through the ship's side. It had to be tackled as a mad animal and this took courage. A cool-headed seaman with the gun's swab or ramrod or shaft of some kind would try to lever the gun onto its side so that it could be grabbed and tamed.

Other accidents occurred when ships' boats were being lowered. A boat might overturn or one would jam as the other ran free, spilling the crew into the sea. Mishaps with oars were common too. There were also the dangers of falling downstairs, of slipping on vomit or excreta or blood, of being hurt by falling barrels, water-casks, boxes or shot.

In nearly all naval ships from the earliest times the sick bay – distinct from the cockpit where the battle casualties were treated – was at the forward end of the main deck, under the forecastle. It was fairly well situated, for it was over the galley and was warmed by the galley's oven-flue. Being well above the water-line the air was reasonably fresh except in the tropics, but for many years the pigsty was near the sick berths. Repeated agitations by Dr Andrew Baird resulted in the latter being moved elsewhere – by St Vincent again – in the 1790s. Under the general conditions of life aboard a warship the sick and wounded men had reasonably comfortable accommodation with much more space than in their normal living quarters.

The comfort of patients depends on the nurses, and naval nurses – until near the beginning of the twentieth century – were untrained and rough. Men who were not much use anywhere else in a ship were employed in the sick bay. Some were Loblolly Boys, young seamen serving in the sick bay. A few nurses were women, legal or *de facto* wives of seamen, but they were not trained and many had little gentleness or femininity.

A naval shore hospital was a more forbidding place than a ship's sick bay. The shore establishment, until the last quarter of the nineteenth century, was dirty, miserable and ill-staffed. Florence Nightingale improved conditions in army hospitals, but the navy had no such champion. Indeed, far from employing more women, the navy dismissed all hospital women in the 1850s feeling that men made better nurses. Some of the women were certainly rough, tough and immoral, but their presence among sick and wounded men had a beneficial psychological effect that outweighed their failings.

The risk of a sailor dying from disease varied from station to station; some places were deadly. The following tables contrast service in temperate regions and in tropical regions:[27]

stations	period of observation years	from	to	mean annual strength	annual ratio of mortality per 1,000	increase of mortality per 1,000 beyond that of Great Britain
Temperate						
Great Britain	10	1819	1828	46,460	15	
Canada	7	1816	1822	2,975	11	
Malta	8	1824	1831	2,226	15	
Gibraltar	7	1816	1822	3,267	20	5
Tropical						
Madras	4	1827	1830	11,820	48	33
Bengal	7	1826	1832	8,700	57	42
Windward and Leeward Islands	19	1810	1828	5,768	113	98
Jamaica	19	1810	1828	2,528	155	140

By 1856 the mortality was less but still high, with Australia the healthiest station and the East Indies and China the unhealthiest.

DISEASE ONLY

stations	mean death rate for the three years 1856–8 per 1,000
Home	7.8
Mediterranean	8.4
North America and West Indies	19.8
Brazilian	21.0
Pacific	6.9
West African	14.3
Cape of Good Hope	10.2
East India and China	37.7
Australia	3.6
Irregular	8.3

Sometimes, after medical discharge, the seaman had the added humiliation of being greatly feared by the general public, who believed that seafaring men, who were known to visit strange places, suffered from equally strange diseases.

By all accounts, the seaman met his end with astonishing stoicism and sometimes with wry humour. Towards the end of the nineteenth century a seaman dying in the sick bay is said to have expressed a last wish that the paymaster and ship's steward be sent for. He asked them to sit on either side of his bed and with apparent satisfaction composed himself for death. In fact he recovered, and when asked about his odd request explained that he could do no better than to follow the example of Christ – who died between two thieves.

Another example of fortitude was that of a stoker wounded in the action, in April 1917, between the British destroyers *Broke* and *Swift* and the six German destroyers they sank. This man had a shell splinter in his head, but did not report to sick bay until the following day. In explanation he said: 'I was too busy, sir, along of clearing up that rubbish on the stokers' mess-deck.'

Fewer men died as medical practice and hygiene improved, but progress was still slow, and as late as the 1840s an official report condemned the practice of having 500 men sleeping on one deck, with their bodies touching. In the 1850s various methods of ventilation were tried, but condensation defeated all remedies. More enterprising captains fitted a type of canvas funnel with a wide, open end which could be turned into the wind to steer air into the lower parts of the ship. Without wind – and there was often no wind in the tropics – the contraption did not work.

The march of mechanization led to improvements in naval health and to a lessening of the chance of fire and shipwreck. With fewer men needed to man an ironclad than a sailing-ship, overcrowding was not so serious.

Engines were developed to ventilate ships. A metal ship was less likely to catch fire, and more sophisticated equipment of all kinds made the seaman's life safer. Trained men were available for work in ships' sick bays, and hospital shore services were expanded. Between 1860 and 1900 the incidence of every disease decreased dramatically, and seamen had a life expectancy equal to that of men in any other job and a much greater one than the soldier on active service abroad. With the introduction of inoculation, vaccination and anaesthetics many more lives were being saved. Finally, in the war of 1939–45, the navy had more deaths from enemy action than from disease, a complete turnabout from the melancholy situation in the Seven Years War.

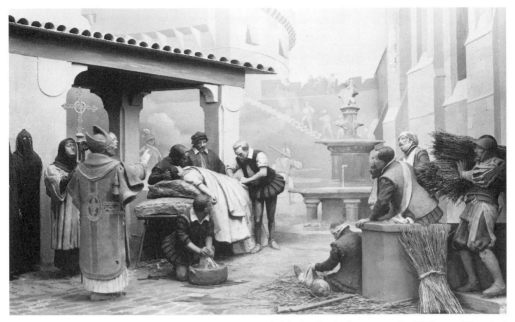

Ambroise Paré (1517–90) operating on a soldier wounded in battle. A diorama at the Wellcome Historical Medical Museum.

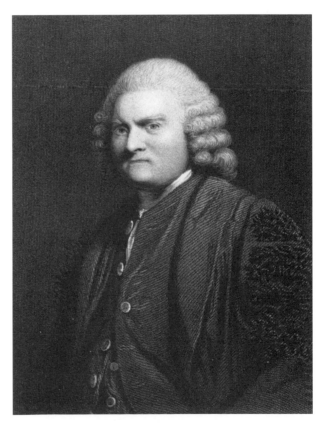

Sir John Pringle, 1707–82. (RAMC)

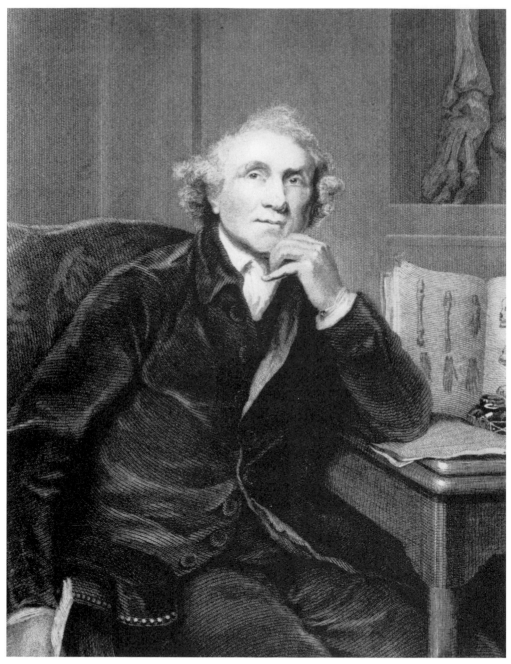

John Hunter, 1728–93. (RAMC)

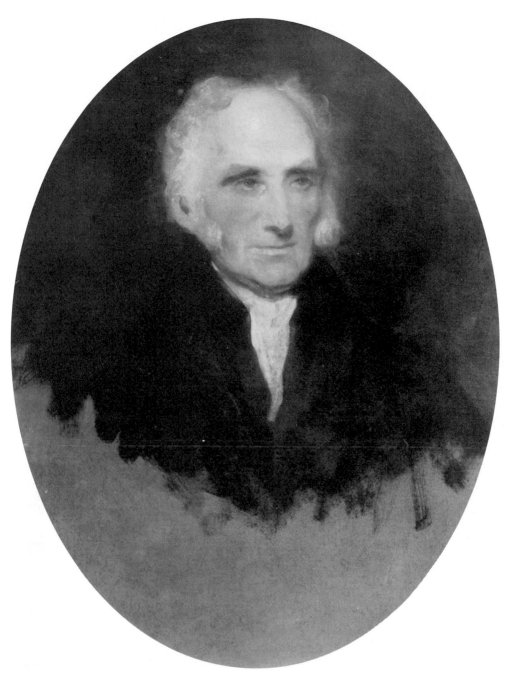

Sir Gilbert Blane, 1749–1834. (RAMC)

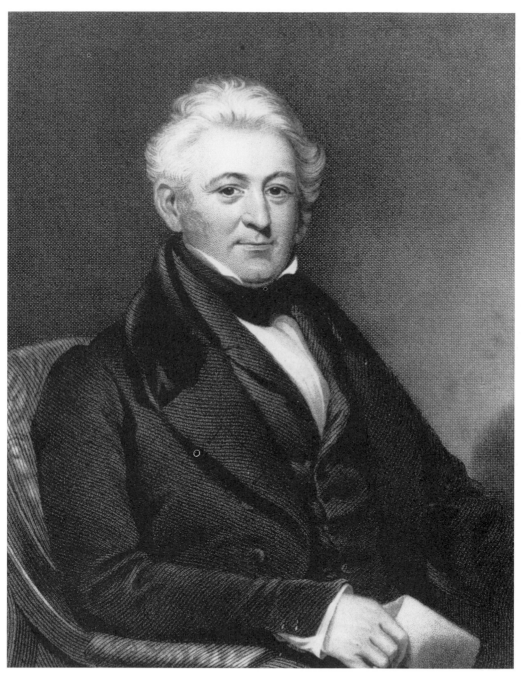

Dr George James Guthrie, 1785–1856. (RAMC)

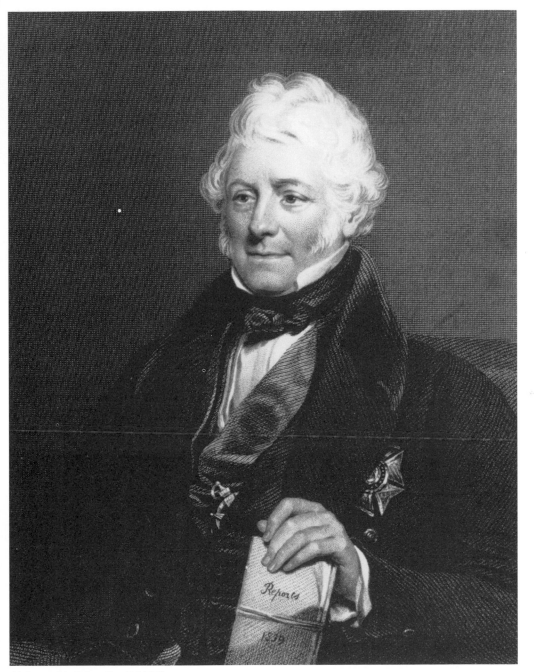

Sir James McGrigor Bt. (RAMC)

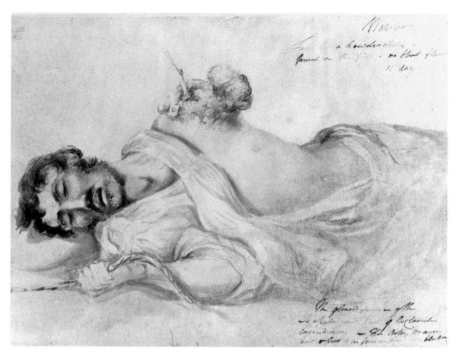

Five water-colour drawings made by Sir Charles Bell of men wounded at Waterloo and in hospital at Brussels. The left arm of this man was carried off by a howitzer shell, with the head of the scapula, the glenoid cavity and part of the clavicle. The artery was tied on the field and after eleven days the patient had suffered no haemorrhage. The wound was healthy and the man recovered completely. (RAMC)

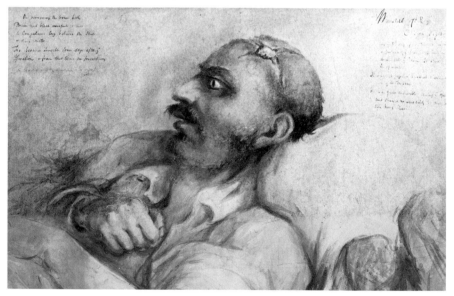

Gunshot fracture of the skull suffered by a man named Wanstell of the 17th Regiment. A portion of the bone was found driven into the brain and to remove it trepanning had to be performed. Insensible for five days after the battle and during the operation, he did not move until bled. Three days after the operation he became more sensible but died six days later.

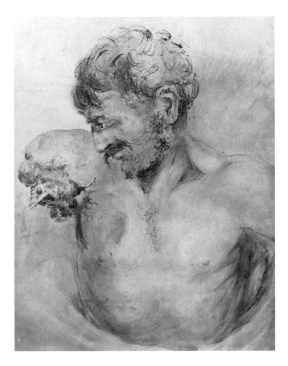

A soldier of the 16th Brunswick Hussars whose arm was carried off by a cannon ball. He lost much blood on the field but the bleeding stopped spontaneously. The arm was amputated by taking the head out of the socket, which Bell considered unnecessary.

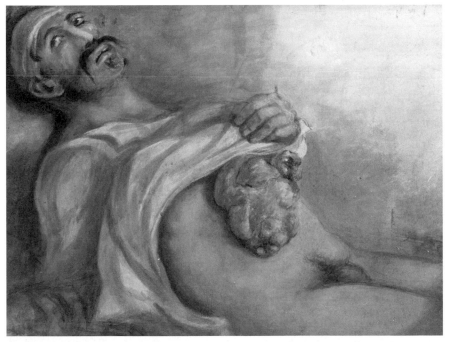

A soldier named Peltier of the 3rd French Lancers. His belly was opened by a sabre and the bowel immediately protruded. When he was brought into the hospital on the third day after the battle the mass was gangrenous. Dr Alexander Shaw of the Middlesex Hospital (Charles Bell's brother-in-law) noted that during lectures Bell spoke of the case as if recovery had taken place or might take place.

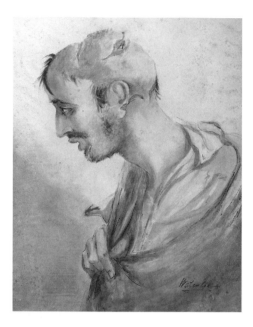

This trooper of the 1st Dragoons was wounded by a sabre and a portion of his skull was detached. He was brought into the hospital insensible and unidentifiable, since when he did recover consciousness he had no memory. Dr Bell advised that the isolated piece of bone be removed and it later reached the College of Surgeons, Edinburgh. It seems likely that the man recovered.

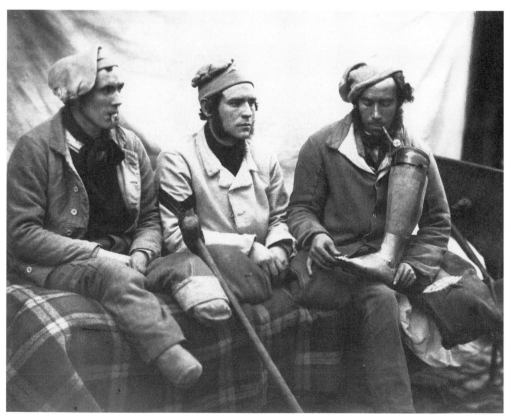

Crimea War casualties who were seen by Queen Victoria when she visited an army rehabilitation centre at Chatham Kent. From left: William Young, Henry Burland and John Connery. (RAMC)

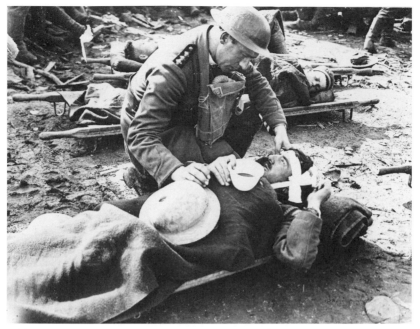

Chaplains worked closely with army doctors. This one comforts a soldier wounded in the head during fighting in France, 1917; a shrapnel ball had penetrated his steel helmet. The wounded man and others are awaiting removal to a field ambulance. (Australian War Memorial)

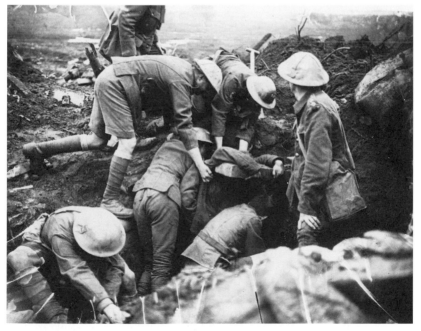

Battle of the Menin Road, near Zillebeke, 20 September 1917. Wounded are being dug out of the 13th Durham Light Infantry Regimental Aid Post that had been blown in by a shell. Some of the wounded suffocated. (Australian War Memorial)

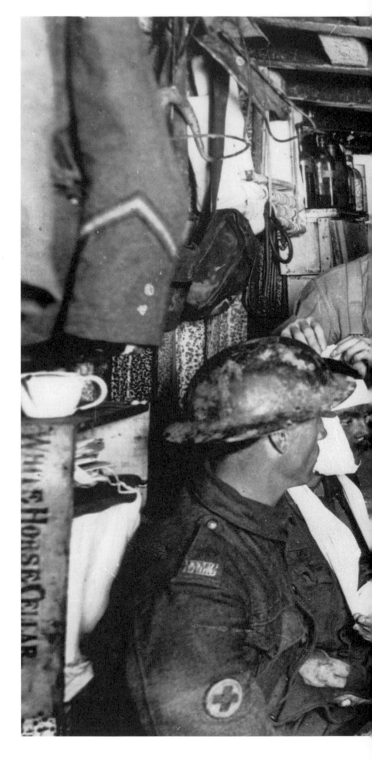

A doctor and his team tending wounded men at an advanced dressing station during the Third Battle of Ypres (Passchendaele) on 26 August 1917. They are in 'White Horse Cellar' and the man on the left is one of the post's bearers. (Australian War Memorial)

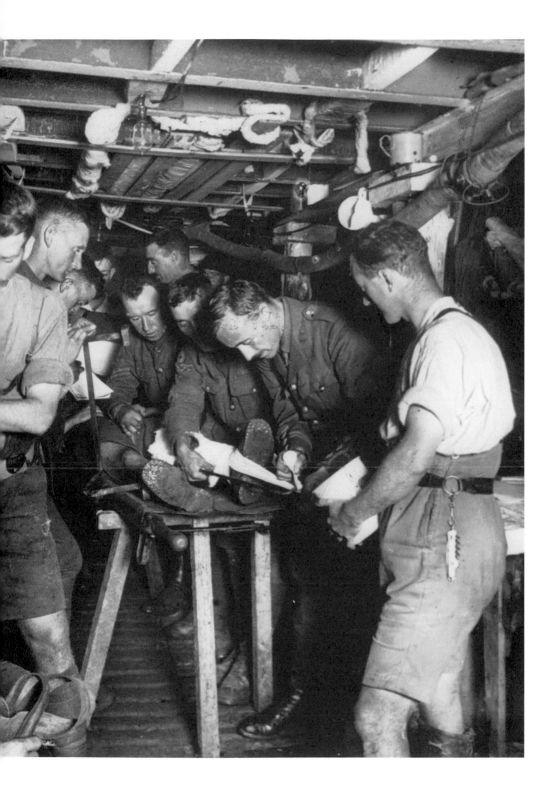

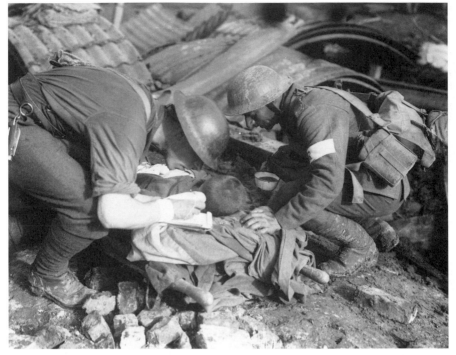

Stretcher-bearers attend to a wounded man during the Battle of the Menin Road, 20 September 1917. The bearer could be writing a note of the treatment given. (Australian War Memorial)

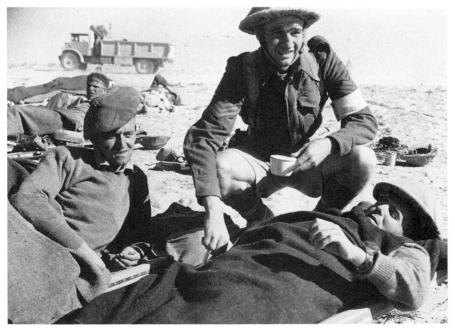

A medic sergeant attends two Black Watch soldiers wounded in the Western Desert, Libya, October 1942. (Black Watch records)

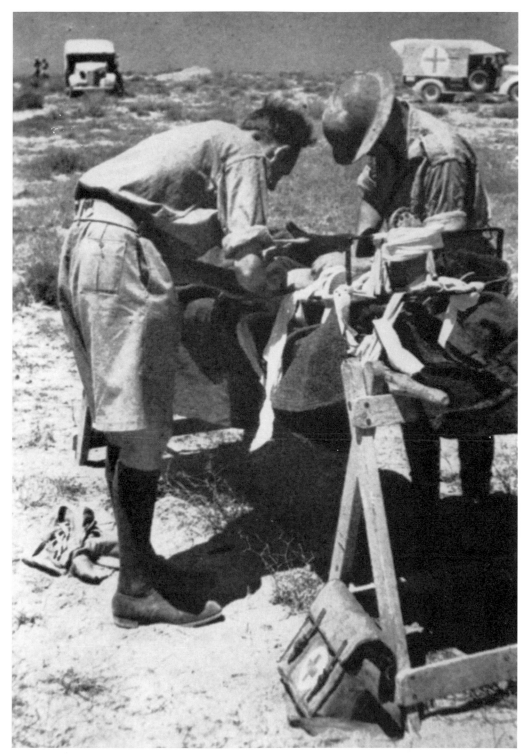

A surgeon and his orderly at work on a wounded patient during an action in the Western Desert, Libya, summer 1942. (Author's Collection)

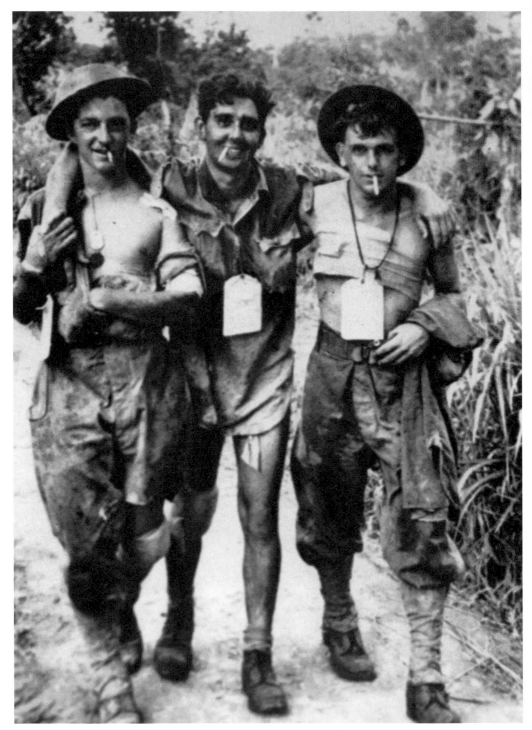

Many soldiers, having been given treatment, walked back to wheeled transport or to the next stage of their evacuation. These young Australian soldiers, wounded in Papua New Guinea in 1942, are believed to have died from their wounds, possibly because of infection. (Australian War Memorial)

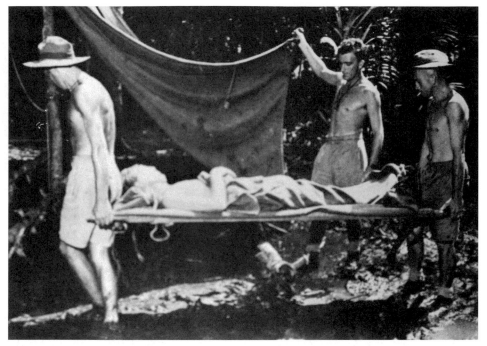

Doctors, bearers and patients had an additional enemy in jungle campaigns – mud. This man is being taken into a field station in Papua New Guinea, 1942. (Australian War Memorial)

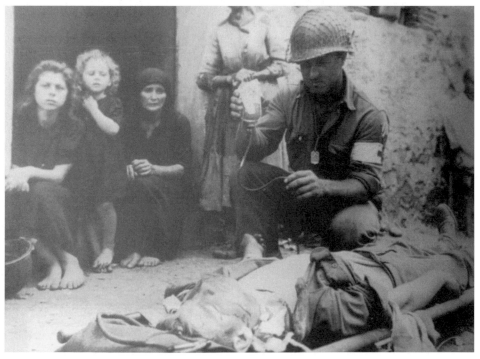

A casualty receives blood plasma in a Sicilian village, 1943. Plasma, the fluid part of blood with red and white corpuscles removed, saved many men's lives. (USMC)

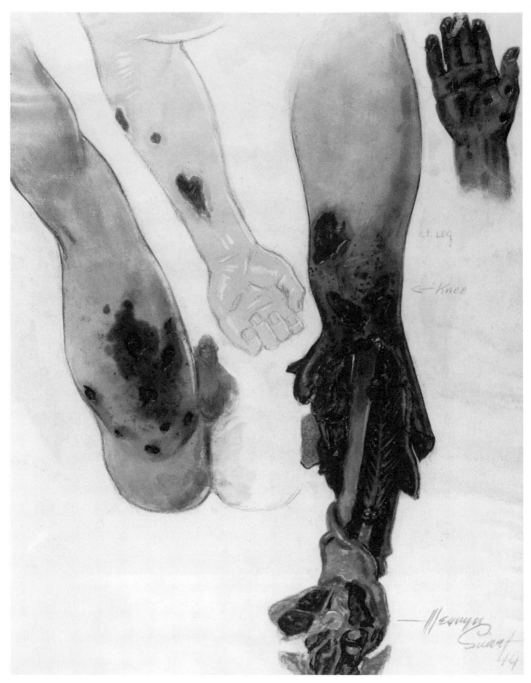

Wounds inflicted on a soldiers when he stepped on a mine in Italy, 1943. (RAMC field medical sketch)

CHAPTER TWELVE

The Surgeon and Service Punishment

For many years in most armies and navies it was the surgeon's duty to attend the punishment meted out to soldiers and sailors. From the mid-seventeenth until the mid-nineteenth century flogging was the most common form of punishment, inflicted for a long time with a rod but early in the eighteenth century the cat-o'-nine-tails reigned. The cat did not always have nine tails, though it rarely had less than six. Dr Henry Marshall, Deputy Inspector-General of Hospitals in the 1840s, noted that in his time the standard number was six. There was no uniform cat; some were of whipcord and some of leather. The tails were usually two feet long, but could be as short as sixteen inches, and often tied into three large knots, to cause more pain. The martial laws of England, Robert Southey observed in 1807,[28] were the most barbarous in Europe. It was true enough. Other nations punished their soldiers and sailors severely, perhaps by the universal method of tying a man to a cavalryman's stirrup and making him run or by spread-eagling him on the wheel of a gun limber and slowly turning it, or by imprisoning him in the black hole. But few were so intent on drawing blood or mutilating the serviceman's body as were the British. In no other army or navy was the lash so much in use.

John Shipp, in Jersey in 1808, found the sentence of 1,000 lashes rigidly enforced 'with the additional torture which must have resulted from the number five (or ten drum taps) being slowly counted between lashes . . . many of the poor creatures fainted several times. . . . Numbers of them were taken down and carried from the square in a state of utter insensibility.'[29]

The mechanics of flogging were simple. In the centre of the parade ground were the triangles – sergeant's halberds lashed tripod-style or, on a ship, a grating. The defaulter when lashed had his arms and legs spread apart, and the ropes were often so tight that a man's hands turned black and were numb for days. The hands-high position was also damaging to circulation and greatly strained the heart. Occasionally, if a man were so tied that he could twist about in pain and if the cat-wielding drummer or boatswain's mate was inaccurate, the thongs would twist around the victim's neck and damage his face. Every available man was paraded to watch the performance. The drummers relieved one another after twenty-five lashes, so that their arms would not become too tired. Usually only a few lashes would draw blood and by fifty a man's back could be a jelly, though some tough characters withstood a lot more without showing more than bruises. If the officer supervising the flogging believed that the drummers were not putting their weight into it he would speak sharply to the drum major or even lash him with his rattan cane. The drum major would then cane the drummers and incite them to renewed efforts.

The surgeon was supposed to stop the punishment if he considered it excessive, but this rarely happened. Even when a soldier showed signs of collapse the surgeon would merely bring him round so that the flogging could continue. Should the flogging be interrupted – and there *were* surgeons who insisted that it stop – the respite was only temporary. When his wounds had been healed the man was brought out for completion of the punishment.

No soldier was ever sentenced to less than twenty-five lashes; even one hundred was considered light punishment by many a victim. Sentences of 300 to 500 lashes were fairly common and others of 800 to 1,500 lashes not infrequent. Four hours were needed to inflict 1,000 lashes, and it is on record that in 1788 a soldier was sentenced to 2,000 lashes. In 1814 three men of the Bengal European Infantry were sentenced to 1,500 lashes each, and one victim in desperation grabbed the drum major's sword and shouted to his comrades in the ranks to rescue him. The man was overpowered by the sergeants, received every stroke of his 1,500 lashes, was court-martialled for mutinous conduct – and shot.

There is no need here to elaborate the sanguinary details further; we are concerned with the surgeon's part in punishment and his attitude towards it. This can be seen clearly through regimental-surgeon Hamilton, who had studied punishment.[30] Hamilton conceded that British discipline might be called severe, but pointed out that it was more lenient than what the soldiery of some other nations experienced. In Prussia, certainly, a soldier was flogged if the wind blew his hat off. So was a dragoon who fell from his horse – if he managed to avoid being trampled to death. But in Britain, 1759, Anthony Gregory of the 10th Regiment was given 100 lashes for allowing the queue (the artificial tailpiece) of his hair to drop off. This was not particularly lenient.

Hamilton confessed that the duty of supervising punishment was 'most disagreeable'. The surgeon had to be alert, for a soldier or sailor, naturally enough, would try to feign a fainting fit or convulsions or some other form of collapse. 'The surgeon will sometimes find the sufferer fall . . . before receiving his first twenty-five lashes. . . . He should not be taken down at this period; there are few that cannot bear double or treble this number. . . . The first few strokes in lacerating the skin give more pain than a great number afterwards. . . .'

Anatomically, Hamilton observed that the shoulder muscles, which lay most in the way of the cat, had few nerves and did not feel so acutely as many other parts of the body. He thought that drummers should be taught to avoid the ribs and other parts more vulnerable to damage. Injury was not merely superficial. Soldiers contracted pneumonia, lockjaw, asthma and other diseases after flogging.

Surgeons who did not insist that a man be taken down when he had fainted or had fallen into a stupor were not necessarily showing fear of the commanding officer or lack of humanity. They realized that in this state he was probably suffering less than if fully sensible. Besides, as Hamilton said, 'the continuation of the stimulus of flagellation is one of the best means of recalling the patient to sensibility'.

Nevertheless, if a man was not aroused in a few seconds, or if he turned cold or sweated profusely, the surgeon would be more likely to ask for the punishment to be suspended while the man was given a drink – soldiers and sailors enduring flogging almost invariably called for drink – or had cold water thrown over his face. The surgeon might hold volatile salts under his nose or rub volatile alkaline spirits on his temples. The average surgeon believed it better for a man to have all his punishment in one session – short of risking his life – than for him to be forced to anticipate a second dose, which taken on barely healed skin would be much worse than the original instalment.

Hamilton's observations on the surgeon's decision to take a man down give an insight into the attitude of a subordinate towards the godhead and towards the common soldier or sailor.

> When the Surgeon finds it incumbent on himself to take a man down he ought carefully to represent the severity of a second or third punishment, and endeavour, if possible, to procure the man's release. This he may do privately, without its being known to the delinquent from what source his pardon comes, for it is better that mercy should seem to proceed always from the commanding officer, whose duty it is to keep the privates in due subjection, and from villainous actions, than from any other. This clemency may have a proper effect on some, and from a sense of gratitude make them behave well, while it will, at the same time, gain him a good name in the regiment. Yet, we confess, the evil-disposed may take advantage of such mild treatment, and commit bad actions through hopes of experiencing similar mercy.

Surgeons knew, with experience, what various builds of man could stand. Those of red or fair hair, with ruddy complexions and of a small or tall or 'genteel shape', or those who had a tendency to diseases of the chest, would be more readily affected. It was useful too to know a man's background; a tailor, being tender from indoor living, took his punishment badly. Men of dark complexion, with black, hard hair or reddish-brown and curly hair were noticed to be more robust. Similarly, men who had a lot of body hair were stronger than those with little or none. Those who had a melancholic temperament were better able to stand punishment than 'the sanguine or choleric'.

It did not always pay to take the lashes without complaint. In France in 1780, after a soldier received 200 lashes without flinching, the officer in charge ordered the flogging to stop and stabbed the soldier with his sword to make him cry out, which he did – and died.

Hamilton, in October 1782, saw a grenadier named Sergeant given 200 lashes for theft without his skin showing a cut, though the drummers, strong men, used all their strength. The adjutant told Hamilton, with satisfaction, that he had never seen lashes 'better laid on'. A hard man, aged twenty-seven, and seven years in the Army, with black hair and brown skin, Sergeant was apparently made in the right proportions to withstand punishment. Hamilton also saw two men, Shepherd and Hall, punished for house-breaking. Shepherd took 500 lashes and was well in three weeks; Hall had 400 and was in such distress that he was taken down and spent six weeks mending before the surgeon could send him back for the balance of his sentence. The difference in reaction was due to differing physique, in Hamilton's judgment.

Hamilton urged surgeons to inspect the method of tying the man to the halberds, so that a man's circulation was not permanently damaged. For the victim's own sake his thighs should be much more tightly bound than the hands, for if he swayed too much he only aggravated the punishment. Men should be admonished to stand as firm as possible, for the more they tossed the greater the punishment. Hamilton cautioned surgeons, since they could not evade the duty of being present on these occasions, to check the size and weight of the cats.

> The cords should be small, by which means they will cut cleaner and bruise less; nor should the same cat be long used at one punishment; for by the additional weight of blood, with which they are loaded, the severity of each stroke is greatly augmented. They fall now on the sufferer's back like so many flails, to use the poor men's own expression. They have often afterwards, on my dressing them, declared, that one stroke from a cat loaded with blood, gave them more pain than four from a dry one; it is evident it must be so.

In an age when a surgeon's career could be ruined should he anger his commanding officer Hamilton was a courageous man. He criticized his fellow surgeons for using 'too much delicacy' in not pressing their opinion and authority. The surgeon's business, as he saw it, was to save the patient's life and to absolve the regimental officers from blame. Though contrary to the opinion of the whole corps, the surgeon should exercise his authority and take down the defaulter. 'An apology is often offered, by surgeons, that officers may be offended when it may appear to them that scarcely half enough has been inflicted . . .' Indeed, officers were very easily offended, partly because the surgeon was considered to be not quite socially acceptable, an attitude sometimes fostered by royalty. In 1778, when George III reviewed the army camps, no surgeon was permitted to kiss his hand, a privilege granted that day to every officer, including youthful ensigns, down to chaplain; the surgeon ranked after the chaplain.

From the vast quantities of lashes inflicted and the number of men who died from them it is clear that many surgeons lacked Hamilton's strength of character and, no matter how much they detested flogging, were prepared to condone it.

Surgeon Parkin, giving evidence before a royal commission on punishments in 1835–6, claimed that statements that flogging was degrading were specious because it would be almost impossible morally to degrade most of the men sentenced to the cat. 'The man who is picked up drunk from the kennel, kicked out of a bagnio, bleeding from wounds in the head and face and brought almost insensible into the barracks and hospital; or has been one of five – two of his comrades and two prostitutes – wallowing in the same bed together for a night, cannot suffer a moral degradation from the lash.'

The French Army at that time had no corporal punishment, but the commission noted that 'after all . . . the French code does not produce, even in times of peace, a discipline in any degree equal to that which is enforced in the British Army. . . .'

Flogging round the fleet, an awesome spectacle, continued until well into the nineteenth century. When the weather permitted the commander-in-chief would order the sentence – 300 to 500 lashes – to be carried out, with each ship of the fleet sending a boat with a guard of marines. The convicted man was taken aboard a large boat and there lashed by his wrists to a capstan bar. The officer in charge read the sentence and ordered the boatswain's mates to 'do their duty'. Each mate would use the cat vigorously – having had much practice on a ship's barrel – but after six strokes, so as not to weaken his blows unduly, he would pass the cat to another boatswain's mate. About twenty-five to thirty lashes completed, the prisoner would be taken down from the capstan and rowed to one ship after another until he had received his total, small boats accompanying him while musicians played 'The Rogue's March'. The whole business could last half a day, and the victim would often be in a state of collapse.

Flogging around the fleet frequently took place in front of astounded foreigners. One such punishment in Port Mahon, Minorca, was seen by thousands. An old monk said to one officer:[31]

> You boast of humanity. What is there in all the tortures that your nation truly or falsely impute to the tribunal of the Inquisition more protracted or inhuman than this proceeding? Why do you suspend the lashes but to increase the agony? The culprit has already fainted twice, yet your surgeon authorized a continuance of the whipping. Is not the poor wretch's back entirely flayed from his neck to his loins? Yet the scourging still goes on.

It went on until 1868, but only in 1881 did an Act of Parliament officially forbid it. It is probably true that more soldiers and sailors suffered at the hands of their own officers than they did from enemy action, which means that doctors found their most constant employment in patching up the bodies of defaulters. I have dwelt on flogging, but there were many other corporal punishments. Picketing for instance; that is, a man was suspended by one wrist from a tree-branch or something similar while he stood with bare heel resting on a pointed stake. A man might be tied neck and heels with a musket under his hams and another over his neck, the muskets being tied together so that the man had his head between his knees. In this position many a man sat until blood gushed out of his mouth, nose and ears or until he had a rupture. There was the wooden horse, a thick plank of wood standing on four legs; the defaulter, wrists tied behind, was made to mount this contraption and sit astride it for a set period. To make the position even more painful weights were tied to his ankles. The strappado was another severe punishment. The victim had his arms fastened behind his back and then was hoisted high by a system of pulleys before being dropped with a jerk. Since this happened three or four times dislocation of the shoulder joints was frequent. In the navy there was for a time branding or keelhauling, being strung up by the heels or being gagged by a bit-like gadget with spikes to damage the tongue. All these punishments kept the surgeon busy trying to restore the victim to a fit enough state to fight for his monarch and country. Surgeons must have felt they had enough to do in treating disease, battle wounds and normal injuries without being saddled with deliberate mutilations.

CHAPTER THIRTEEN

Crimea – Administrative Chaos

Despite the advances in military medical practice up to 1815, when the Crimean War commenced in 1854 it seemed that no permanent improvements had been made and that medicine, surgery and administration were stagnant. Physicians and surgeons of all the European nations and in the United States had not been without opportunity for improving their professional skills, for, while Europe was relatively quiet, military campaigns were in progress in many parts of the world, as can be inferred from Dr Barry's service. Unfortunately doctors' professional experiences in India, Africa, the Far East and the American West were rarely reported in the medical centres of the world, so that their findings and conclusions were wasted. Oddities rather than the results of research drifted back. For instance, it was learnt, or relearnt, that arrow-heads were difficult to withdraw. On 10 January 1832 a hill tribesman fired an arrow which struck a sepoy of the 50th Regiment Native Infantry in the right antrum (the cavity in the upper jaw bone). Dr Tytler and Assistant Surgeon Griffith enlarged the wound and together tried to withdraw the arrow, after which a captain known to be very powerful finished the extraction. It was not reported how the patient stood up to this agony. Similarly, Edinburgh University Medical School acquired the breech of a gun and a screw-nail, which had lodged for nearly eight years in the head of a Lieutenant Fretz of the Ceylon Regiment. The barrel had burst and the breech entered the officer's forehead between the eyebrows, then lodged in the region of the nasal cavity and projected partly through the palate, apparently without greatly inconveniencing him.

During these pre-Crimean years it was commonplace in British practice for a regimental medical officer to undertake the removal of a cancerous breast, yet leave the removal of an abscessed tooth to the regimental farrier. The service seemed to attract some medical eccentrics, though usually they found their way into regiments of high social standing. One of the most idiosyncratic of all was Frank Buckland, a well-known naturalist and medical officer of the 2nd Life Guards pre-Crimea. Buckland would hang dead rats and other specimens among his clothes and in hot weather his quarters had an evil smell.

For the first half of the century British, French, Prussian and American practice was decidedly superior to that of all other nationalities. The greatest output of doctors came from these countries and the others, generally speaking, learnt from them. Not until after Solferino (1859) were great improvements made in many other countries. The whole picture of military medicine up to this time was one of improvisation and compromise, of failing to prepare for an emergency. There was, as yet, no public outcry about war casualties; men were still expendable, war was still glorious. War correspondents were not yet on the scene to depict war in all its horror, and the general public, unless it had itself been overrun during conflict, had no conception of the misery and pain of war diseases and wounds. The whole fight for a more humane and efficient approach to the problem of casualties still rested with the doctors. But the doctors needed encouragement and massive help from ministers for war and from commanders-in-chief. Because of the mentality which saw an ill-conceived cavalry charge as gallant when it was nothing more than the deliberate throwing of hundreds of men onto a butcher's block, they did not get this help. Doctors seemed to be only people who saw casualties in perspective.

Hamilton had said:

When we consider the value of a man to Government, a political and patriotic principle, as well as humanity, should influence us to procure everything the army can afford for his welfare. The death of a private is a loss to the nation, since he costs considerably before he is fit to act as a soldier in the defence of his King and country. . . . Every death must affect the service . . . and, we hope, humanity will be sufficient to enforce what politics demonstrates as necessary. Hence every degree of encouragement should be given to the medical department, where so large a share of the soldier's welfare is placed.

In Britain a soldier was still required to pay for his own means of treatment. Milk, vinegar, bread and oatmeal for poultices, and oil were often used in regimental practice. A soldier with a bruise or sprain would be sent away with advice to bathe it in vinegar, but if no vinegar were given to him he could not afford to buy it. In some regiments soldiers were expected to buy their own bread and milk for poultices – costing as much as 1½d a day perhaps for weeks, leaving him at most 2½d. When a patient was sent to the regimental hospital half a crown a week was allowed, this money being given to the hospital sergeant and spent as the surgeon directed. Similarly, flannel was often prescribed for wrapping around rheumatic limbs and shoulders. A soldier could not possibly afford to buy flannel, and Hamilton and others campaigned for years for a stock of issue flannels to be kept in the regimental dispensary and lent to soldiers. Such doctors also urged that the surgeon, representing the army, should pay for poultice-beer and poultice-oatmeal and for the oatmeal or stale beer which some doctors applied to difficult sores, apparently with good effect. Hamilton thought that the soldier should be charged only for special food ordered by the regimental doctor.

Perhaps the most neglected problem was that of getting wounded soldiers from the field to a hospital. Throughout history no satisfactory method had been found; after all, only three basic forms of land transport existed – the soldier's own legs, an animal such as a mule and a cart pulled by an animal. All doctors knew that many a soldier might as well be left to die where he fell rather than be jolted to death by rough portage. F.C. Cherry, an army veterinary surgeon, invented a spring-fitted cart, and twelve of these carts were used by the British Legion which served in Spain in 1835.[32] Raised by Sir De Lacy Evans and others to help Queen Isabella against the Carlists, the Legion used these carts extensively, and the principal medical officer, Sir Rutherford Alcock, reported them satisfactory.[33] But they did not become standard equipment in the British Army, which still remained remarkably proof against the obvious advantages of French medical transport. In 1843 Inspector-General William Ferguson was writing plaintively that the British means of transporting sick and wounded 'has ever been deficient and cruel, as all can testify who attended the bullock-carts of the Peninsula'. Another great military surgeon, Sir George Ballingall, was urging that plans to deal with sick and wounded should not be left to some spur of the moment, but should be established and organized on a 'liberal scale' before some crisis occurred.[34]

The crisis was to be the Crimean War of 1854–5. It found the British service as deficient as ever in transport for casualties; for that matter, almost every aspect of the army medical service was inadequate except for the continuing skills of the doctors themselves. Few of the deficiencies and anomalies which confronted them were of their own making.

We need to see the medical service at two levels – that of the director-general and of the principal medical officer in the Crimea, and that of the regimental surgeon.

Sir Andrew Smith, a far-sighted, energetic man, had succeeded Sir James McGrigor as Director-General in 1851. In this post of tremendous responsibility – the British Army was a vast organization in 1854 – Smith was paid £1,200 a year and had only twelve clerks to administer all the affairs of the department. The purveyor's department, also largely responsible for the health of the army, had been reduced to a staff of four. The Commissary-General, Filder, a veteran of the Peninsular War nearly half a century earlier, had to conduct and record the whole business of supplying the British Army in the Crimea, with the help of three clerks whom he regarded as incompetent.

The whole system was complicated to the point of absurdity. The commissariat were the army's caterers, carriers and storekeepers, buying and delivering the standard daily rations of the men whether in barracks or in hospital. All 'medical comforts' – that is, invalid foods – were the responsibility of the purveyor, yet all the purveyor's contracts were made through the commissariat. At the same time, though the commissariat bought and delivered the daily standard rations, the purveyor cooked and distributed

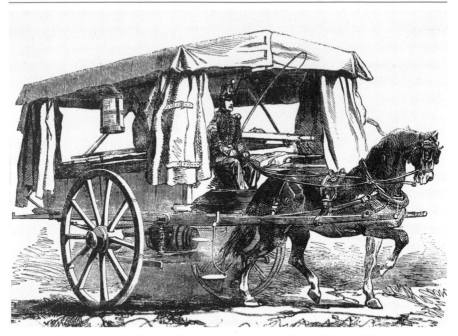

The ambulance cart which George Guthrie designed for use in the Crimean War 1854–5.

them. Nobody knew the dividing line between the two departments, nobody knew the precise relationship between purveyor and doctor.

On 10 February 1854 Smith received instructions to prepare medical services and stores for an army of 10,000; in fact it numbered 26,000. His complete list of medicines was ready the following day, and the ordnance department received his total list of stores within a week, but they stayed in pigeon-holes, and long delays occurred. Smith urged the need for a trained ambulance corps and evolved a plan for a hospital conveyance corps. This brigade of hospital vehicles was formed under the direction of an artillery colonel and the ever vigorous George Guthrie, and consisted of twenty carts, each drawn by two horses; five store wagons, each drawn by four horses; one forge cart and one portable forge each drawn by two horses. Ten of the carts were built to carry sixteen wounded sitting, the other ten to carry two men lying on stretchers, nine men sitting before and behind, while a twelfth could lie on a stretcher slung from the roof. The brigade was calculated to be sufficient for two army divisions.

No doubt many defects will be discovered [Smith wrote[35]] therefore the medical officers will have an opportunity of improving upon appliances that are known theoretically only to the British Army, though practically to the French since 1792. . . . Notwithstanding the French have used so long what we are now only beginning to employ still there is reason to believe that much must yet be effected before we shall be able to consider the object in view to have been satisfactorily obtained.

It was not obtained at all, mostly owing to the complete lack of training of the men the army employed for the hurriedly enlisted Hospital Conveyance Corps. They were not accustomed to working together, they were drunken, disorderly, too old, too feeble and too ignorant.

The two four-wheeled wagons which did reach the war theatre were dumped on the beach at Calamita Bay with no harness or drivers; a staff officer sent them back to Bulgaria because he considered officers' horses had priority in deck space for onward movement to the war.

There were no trained stretcher-bearers to carry the wounded off the battlefield and provide attendants for general base hospitals. Smith had asked for intelligent, able-bodied men for such strenuous, responsible duties, but the army enlisted aged and feeble pensioners and other ineffectives. Few reached the battlefront, so the regimental surgeons, their orderlies and the bandsmen were left to bring in the wounded under fire; the three Victoria Crosses these doctors won attest to their bravery.

In hospitals the surgeons too often found their hospital attendants – ordinary soldiers detailed from regiments – lacking intelligence, sympathy, activity. Obviously a commanding officer of an infantry or cavalry regiment was disinclined to part with men who had these qualities – they would be his best men.

The man chosen for the unenviable job of principal medical officer was John Hall, with a distinguished record of service in peace and war in India, the West Indies and South Africa. This man was to suffer blatant obstruction and unjust vilification which has continued to the present day. Landing at Varna on 27 June 1854, with no inkling as to the plan of campaign or the resources at his disposal, Hall was confronted by the leaders of the expedition, the Duke of Cambridge, Lords Raglan, Cardigan, Lucan, Sir George Brown, and others. It was an unhappy introduction. The hospital accommodation allotted at Scutari was a square of an old Turkish barracks, 'alive with fleas and quite uninhabitable. The whole place was in great confusion', largely because a flood of cholera cases was pouring in from Devna, ten miles to the north. Hall had visited this place, a notorious plague spot, and had reported adversely, but Sir George Brown insisted on remaining there with the Light Division because of the beauty of scenery; commenting acidly that the duty of medical officers was limited to the treatment of the sick and wounded.

Much of the Crimean tragedy might have been avoided had Hall's advice been taken. On 4 July, a week after his arrival, he wrote: 'It is very unwise of the Allied Commanders to put off their operations until the sickly season arrives, when half their force would soon be crippled by disease . . . what would be the use of going to the Danube to get fever . . . far better to transport the army by sea to Odessa if they really want to get near the enemy.' His advice was ignored. On 31 August Hall noted in his diary: 'Lord Raglan talks of embarking the army soon but whether he will be able to do so with this terrible scourge raging I very much doubt.'

In spite of all, Raglan decided to make a landing, and a convoy of 450 craft carried three armies to the coast of the Crimea on 9 September. Even then the PMO was not informed of the destination. There were no hospital ships to receive casualties, and on 15 September Hall estimated that there were probably 600 British sick still on the transports.

The hopeless confusion of the landings was only a beginning. Hall, with little or no executive authority, went from ship to ship trying to induce the staff to take the casualties to Scutari. It was at this point he found the two ambulance wagons horseless, harnessless and driverless on the beach. He had asked for 42 wagons for stores and wounded men, 336 stretcher-bearers and 672 other men.*

Hall made repeated appeals to Raglan and his staff and was rebuffed. Conditions in the forward areas were appalling. Hall found misery and discomfort everywhere, the men fearfully overworked, ill-fed and reduced to eating their rations of pork raw in the trenches.

Hall was no more horrified than the regimental medical officers. When the army disembarked at Calamita Bay on 14 September, Dr Alexander, staff surgeon to the Light Division, exclaimed: 'My God! They have landed this army without any kind of hospital transport, litters or carts or anything.'

The doctors faced almost insuperable difficulties from the start. Surgeon Thomas Longmore of the Green Howards Regiment landed at Calamita Bay to find that his medical panniers had been returned to Malta, and went into the battle of Alma carrying one small haversack and his pocket case of instruments. When the 5th Dragoon Guards were disembarked at Varna the CO saw medical panniers being unloaded, described them as 'useless encumbrances of war' and left them at base; a few weeks later men were dying in hundreds from cholera, and the only treatment the surgeon, William Cattell, could muster consisted of brandy from the officers' mess – mixed with cayenne pepper – and whatever he could beg from the private supplies of his brother officers.

When the British and French won the battle of the Alma, 25 September 1854, the wounded paid a heavy price for their superiors' neglect.

---

* In his post-mortem surgical history of the campaign, the director-general wrote: 'of those [peculiarities of the Crimean War] the first felt was the deficiency of conveyance for wounded, and for transport of hospital stores. . . . It is now pretty generally known that the army landed with no other hospital transport or ambulance than one pack pony per regiment, for the conveyance of . . . the small basketwork cases containing the surgeon's instruments, a few dressings and appliances, and a few medicines most likely to be needed on an emergency, the whole being limited by the weight-carrying powers of the sorry animal generally furnished for this duty. To this were added ten canvas stretchers per regiment for the conveyance of sick or wounded men on the shoulders of their comrades. For all other means of transport, whether of wounded, of instruments, of medical comforts, or surgical appliances, the army was left entirely dependent upon the resources of the country. These, it is now a matter of history, failed to supply what was needed.'

Bandages, splints, chloroform, morphia – nothing. The wounded could only be laid on the ground or on straw soiled by manure. A man about to have a limb amputated would sit on a tub or lie on an old door while the surgeon operated, often by moonlight since no candles or lamps were available. Of course no anaesthetic had arrived. Chloroform had been discovered in 1831* – but it had found its way only slowly into army medical practice. Conditions on 'hospital' ships – they were nothing more than ordinary transports – were horrible. One, the *Kangaroo*, fitted to receive 250 sick, had almost 1,500. Too weak to withstand the ships' movement, the men rolled about in the excreta and vomit. Amputees screamed with pain as they were flung about the decks.

In the grim, forbidding Crimea the men faced the start of winter without warm clothing, fuel or sufficient food; there were only just enough huts and tents for headquarters staff. Sanitation was rudimentary. Apart from cholera, dysentery and typhus swept through the Army and within a few weeks there were more soldiers on the sick list than fit for duty. Doctors were unanimous in condemning the commanders' lack of interest in their men. From Sebastopol, Dr Marlow of the 28th Regiment noted that 'very tolerable structures have been raised for the occupation of individuals while men labouring under disease are left on the damp ground under a leaky tent'.

In mid-October Sidney Herbert, Secretary at War,† writing to Florence Nightingale, claimed that the number of medical officers with the force amounted to one to every ninety-five men, 'being nearly double what we have ever had before, and 30 more surgeons went out 3 weeks ago. . . .' He advised her that medical stores had been sent out 'in profusion' – lint by the ton, 15,000 pairs of sheets, medicine, wine, arrowroot and much else. Because of inept staff work months elapsed before the troops saw any of these stores.

---

* See page 107.
† Not Secretary *for* War. Administration of the British Army was divided between the two ministers. Herbert was responsible for financial administration, his colleague for the purely military side of war. Herbert's figure is suspect.

CHAPTER FOURTEEN

Crimea – Regimental Pathos

The battle of Balaclava took place on 25 October 1855, followed by the great slaughter of Inkerman on 5 November. By this time Florence Nightingale and her party of thirty-eight nurses were arriving and soon after they reached Scutari a flood of sick and wounded men rolled in. The hospitals of Scutari had been designed for 1,000 patients; many times that number reached them and the later arrivals lay in rows along the floors and overflowed into the passages. Amputations were carried out in the wards themselves as sick men watched. The Revd Sidney Osborne assisted at an amputation of a thigh, during which the patient's position became so uncomfortable that the clergyman had to put his arm beneath the man while a surgeon on the other side held Osborne's wrist.

Every medical necessity was scarce; the staff, who had been trained merely to minister to the sick, were out of their depth, and the treasury clerks responsible for supply were obstructive in the issue of stores. A soldier was supposed to carry a change of clothing and his eating utensils, but most of the men reaching Scutari had obeyed their officers' orders to abandon their packs so they now had no equipment. Yet the purveyor refused to consider any requisitions for these articles.

Deep beneath the enormous Scutari building, in smelly, damp cellars, lived 200 women, who through an oversight had been allowed to accompany the army. In their dens they ate too little food, soaked up too much liquor, plied as prostitutes, gave birth to infants and died of cholera.

The Nightingale party, which was to remedy all these evils, was the result of public opinion made vocal by vehement articles sent to London by W.H. Russell of *The Times*. Russell often exaggerated and was sometimes inaccurate, but almost any means would have justified this particular end of bringing sane, competent treatment to the unhappy troops.

We are lucky in our Medical heads [Miss Nightingale wrote on 14 November]. Two are brutes and four are angels – for this is a work which makes angels or devils of men. . . . As for the assistants, they are all cubs, and will, while a man is breathing his last under the knife, lament the annoyance of being called up from their dinners by such a fresh influx of wounded. But unlicked cubs grow up into good old Bears, tho' I don't know how, for certain it is the old Bears are good.

It is needless here to repeat the details of Miss Nightingale's work, but with 10,000 men under her care she managed to reduce the death rate from 42 per cent to 2 per cent in four months; even so, in the barracks hospital alone 9,000 men died in three months. Miss Nightingale was able, after initial difficulties, to get her own way in everything, while Hall had been crippled. When Hall transferred a member of the nursing staff from one hospital to another Miss Nightingale induced Lord Raglan to order that only she had the authority to transfer nursing staff. Through *The Times* fund she was able to amass vast stores.

Civilian sanitary inspectors were visiting army camps and reporting direct to London, Members of Parliament were ferreting out hospital scandals for political purposes, private hospitals were setting up without reference to Hall, who knew that he was to be made the scapegoat for the medical débâcle. It is beyond the scope of this book to trace Hall's troubles, but after much difficulty he was absolved from blame and awarded a knighthood.

Hall was made aware of his difficult position by Raglan's sudden interest in what was happening to some of the casualties. At midnight on 1 December the adjutant-general arrived at Hall's tent with an angry letter from the commander-in-chief saying that an officer had reported the case of a man found on the deck of the *Avon*, with both legs lost and covered only by a blanket. He directed the adjutant-general and PMO to investigate the

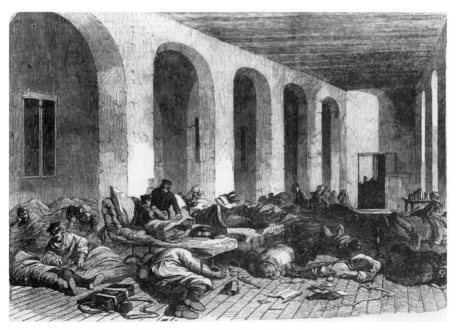

The dreadful condition of British wounded in the hospital at Scutari, Turkey, before Florence Nightingale's arrival, 1854.

matter. They found the man was receiving proper attention, but he was hopelessly ill with gangrene. The *Avon*, which contained twenty-two wounded and 275 sick, was in poor condition. Hall recorded: 'His Lordship is still angry . . . and says he must have the matter investigated by a court of inquiry. "Straining at gnats" when men are dying at the rate of 100 a day in camp from exposure, want of clothing, fuel and food.'

At the end of 1854 Hall was desperate, as a diary entry shows:

> Captain Chapman of the Engineers came over about the huts for the sick and I went with him to Lt. Col. Gordon, the Q.M.G., about them. Timber is required to cover the huts and I asked if two ship-loads had not arrived at Balaclava. He said 'Yes', but Lord Raglan desired that cavalry horses and those of the artillery are to be put under cover first. When I applied for the sheds at Karani it was the commissariat donkeys that were to have preference over sick soldiers and now it is the horses, asses then horses! No provision has been made for sheltering any portion of the army. They are overworked, badly fed and have no fuel to cook their food with. They have no camp kettles, only one blanket, many of them no shoes and they are dying by hundreds of exhaustion . . . he cannot expect me to keep silent when the men are 12 hours in and only 12 hours out of the trenches, are half fed and nearly naked and have only scant protection against the weather from their canvas tents.

Hall's problems with overall policy and organization and at the base hospitals were serious; those of the regimental surgeon were probably worse, for he was in the firing line. The life of a surgeon – and by reflection, that of the soldier – can be seen through the experiences of William Cattell of the 5th Dragoon Guards.[36]

At Devna Cattell found that no sanitary precautions had been taken at a camp site notoriously unsuitable for a camp, but observes that the accepted job of medical officers was to tend the sick, not to attempt to *prevent* sickness. The river water was good, but no care was taken to keep it so. Horses were watered at the springs, which were soon muddy puddles; men already suffering from diarrhoea would lap up water from these puddles, despite severe warnings. The latrine was a deep trench, partly sheltered by the thrown-up earth and surmounted by a screen of brushwood. Mosaic sanitation or the use of dry earth was unknown and the pit was a breeding ground for flies. They formed dense black clouds in the tents and attacked the men's eyelids particularly.

In summer diarrhoea was prevalent because of injudicious eating of fruit, especially Killjohn apricots, and because of vegetable deficiencies. The men still washed themselves and their clothes in the same river and the commissariat, established on the bank, threw offal into it. One of Cattell's dragoons fell ill immediately after bathing in the river and died in fifteen hours. It was the chief supply for cooking for the infantry – and this at a temperature of over 100 degrees. Yet troughs and tubs could easily have been used to provide water so that the river itself would not be contaminated.

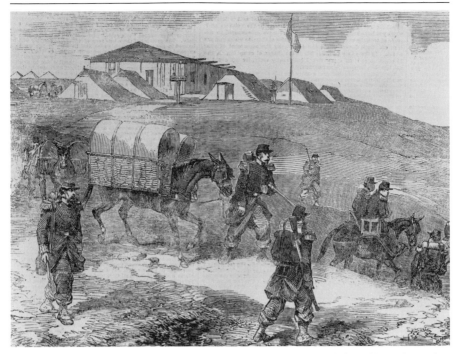

French wounded in the Crimea, 1854–5, being evacuated by panniers (left) and by mule cacolet.

Flogging was commonplace during the Crimean campaign. A defaulter would be lashed to a triangle to receive lash after lash from the farrier and trumpeter alternately, the weals crossing each other until the back was scored by purple, bleeding bands. A man would often be handcuffed and strapped to the stirrup alongside a mounted man and was expected to keep up at the trot.[37] The surgeon had enough troubles without the delicate treatment of maltreated soldiers.

Weather conditions were as harsh as the punishments. In winter even in the tents men's breath caused icicles to form in their beards, which froze to the blankets. Officers were more fortunate than the men, for they had servants who, last thing at night and first thing in the morning, handed in bowls of fire which the officers used to release their beards. New tents were fitted with hooks and eyes and, without dragging out a peg, it was impossible to open them from the inside because of contraction. For Cattell this 'occasioned great distress, the impracticability causing urgent desire to relieve the bladder'.

Supply was woefully incompetent. Coffee arrived in the form of green beans, puddings were hard as iron, the biscuits weevilly. The French allies had a much better grasp of the situation; they had excellent bread rolls and they made appetizing soups and salads from dandelions and other plants which the British trod underfoot, though the eating of such things would have lessened the scurvy which afflicted the army. French treatment was decidedly better in all ways – better organization and supplies, more doctors – and, most important, the French soldiers had the service of the devoted Sisters of Charity, all highly efficient nurses.

In summer, harassed and worried by constant work from 4 a.m. until 8 p.m. under a very hot sun, the men had no rest, no regular hours of duty. Cholera was prevalent and the Turkish soldiers suffered from a fever called sisina tittera, from its cold rigors. The cholera cases had few premonitory symptoms; the slight diarrhoea would pass unnoticed, then there would be sudden violent spasms with little pain, followed by collapse. At one camp site Cattell, having no medicine except a little red pepper, rode to Monastir to try to beg or borrow opium. On one day his regiment suffered nine deaths and he admitted twenty-five cases to the hospital. He found that in the tents the men were, unusually, reading their Bibles. 'If seized they at once gave themselves up for lost and terror increased religious receptivity. So great was the fear that on 8 August it developed into panic and, led by the CO, many men galloped madly for a conical mound, and the only high spot, about a mile and a half distant. Left with the sick and dying and without rations, Cattell went to General Scarlett, commander of the Heavy Brigade, for orders. The unflustered Scarlett said: 'I am staying with the hospital and so do you.' That evening the hospital, Cattell's tent and Scarlett's tent were the only ones standing.

Burial parties were the busiest groups in the Crimea, though a man who dug graves in the morning might well occupy one in the afternoon. On one occasion the funeral service was being read by the 5th Dragoon's adjutant, Godman. As he was about to begin the hospital sergeant, Fisher, ran up and said: 'Wait a minute – another is almost ready.' The adjutant asked if the man were dead. 'Not quite', Sergeant Fisher said, but a few minutes later brought out the victim and put him in the grave with the rest.

Cattell was bitter about lack of supplies. For weeks he had battled against the devastating outbreak of cholera; patients were treated in unserviceable bell-tents, for there was no evacuation to general hospitals; he had no medicines and he had been treating cases with spoonfuls of brandy, sometimes reinforced with cayenne pepper. Finally, following several urgent requests for supplies, he received some instructions on how to treat cholera:

The patient is first to be put flat in a bed and to take six pills No. 1. These consist of:

Camphorae ½ Drachm
Opii pulv gr xij
Pip Cayenne gr ix
Spt Vini Rect
Conserva Rosar q.s.
In pilul. xij divide

Next follows an ounce of Mixture No. 11:

Sp Aetheris Sulph
Spt Ammon Aromat
Tinct Camphorae
Tinct Opii aa 1 Dr.
Aq. Cinnamon Oz ij

The mixture may be washed down with a cordial, spirits flavoured with cloves or ginger, or, if the stomach can bear it, he may get a strong brandy punch, very hot. If necessary he can have an enema of 4 ounces of boiled starch with an aqueous solution of six grains of opium. When sweating has occurred for a few minutes he is to be given copious draughts of warm whey, ginger tea, toast water with ginger, mint or balm tea. . . .

   In the later stages he is to receive wine, light broths and beef tea and a healthy tone is restored to the stomach by aromatic bitters. Finally, when he has resumed a natural appearance, he is to have roast beef, steak and chops.

What Cattell, exhausted from lack of sleep and bereft of medical supplies, thought about this can be imagined. A true field doctor, he made do with alcohol. By giving his sergeant, Elliott, a quantity of champagne drop by drop he cured the man of all the symptoms of cholera. Again, he cured diarrhoea with port wine. Red Tenedos wine was believed to cause or aggravate cholera, but Cattell and others drank it regularly as a change from the charcoal coffee; in any case it was safer than the water.

   Cattell's description of the evacuation of men from the front to Scutari is the most vivid on record.

Towards the end of the month there were nearly 8,000 men in hospital. Wrapped in wet blankets they were taken from the muddy tents and placed on horseback, a dismal troop as of mounted corpses, with closed eyes and lurid cheeks, some fever-stricken, glaring with wide eyes void of observations. . . . Bound for the great hospital at Scutari the cavalcade would roll on, wading through and slipping past the dying horses, the half-buried bullocks and skeletons and carcasses in various stages of decay. On . . . to the place of embarkation. . . . Lying among crowds of other sick and wounded, on bare planks, in torture, lassitude and lethargy, without proper food, medicine or attention, they were launched on the wintry sea. Their covering was scanty and the roll and plunge of the ship was agony to the fevered and maimed. . . . In place of the hush, cleanliness and quiet and the silent step which should be around the sick were sounds such as the poets have feigned for the regions of the damned – groans, screams, entreaties, curses, the strain of the timbers, the trampling of the crews and the weltering of the waves. The sick flocked in faster than the dead were carried out till the hospitals overflowed, while still faster flowed the misery-laden ships from the Black Sea as they went on feeding the fishes with their dead.

Conditions were little better on the ships themselves; the navy had hoped to escape cholera, or at least to reduce its effect, by putting to sea and staying there. But HMS *Britannia*, the flagship, lost 139 out of 885 men; 55 of the first 60 cases died within twenty hours.

The story of the treatment of wounds in the Crimea is as melancholy as that of disease, though it is difficult to blame the surgeons, who were overwhelmed with work under the worst possible conditions. Treatment of chest wounds was particularly unsuccessful, oddly so in view of surgical advances. Patrick Fraser, physician to London Hospital and staff physician to the army in the Crimea, gives the mortality of chest wounds – that is, of those admitted to hospital – 28.5 per cent, but the mortality of those with an actual lung wound was 79.2 per cent. The director-general's report of the time, however, indicates that it was rare for any soldier to survive if the ball was lodged within the pleural chest lining. It was astonishing enough that soldiers survived to reach the hospital.

In January 1855 W.H. Russell saw wounded arriving at Balaclava, strapped to mules lent by the French.

> They formed one of the most ghastly processions . . . with closed eyes, open mouths and ghastly attenuated faces, they were borne along two by two, the thin stream of breath visible in the frosty air alone showing that they were still alive. One figure was a horror, a corpse, stone dead, strapped upright in the seat. . . . Another man I saw with raw flesh and skin hanging from his fingers, the raw bones of which protruded into the cold, undressed and uncovered.

The compassion and general competence shown by regimental surgeons throughout the Crimean agony was exceeded only by their courage. If wounded men could not be brought to them they went to the wounded, often under heavy fire. The first surgeon to win the Victoria Cross* was James Mouat of the 6th Dragoons, who went to the assistance of the CO of the 17th Lancers, lying dangerously wounded in an exposed place after the retirement of the Light Brigade at Balaclava. Under fire from the Russians, Mouat stopped serious haemorrhage and saved the officer's life. In September 1855 Assistant Surgeon Thomas Hale, Royal Fusiliers, remained with an officer who was dangerously wounded at Sebastopol and, going beyond his medical duties, helped to rally the troops demoralized by artillery and musket fire. Later, after the infantry had retired, he rescued several wounded men lying in the open and carried them into a trench, where he treated them. The same day, Assistant Surgeon Henry Sylvester went out under continuous fire to dress the wounds of an officer, mortally wounded as it happened.

Surgeons could achieve much by risking their own lives under fire or through high risk of disease infection, but they could only remain frustrated by lack of transport for wounded, frustration made all the more acute by observation of the efficient French system.

---

* The decoration was instituted 29 January 1856.

General Lord Strathnairn, as Commissioner at the French headquarters, had opportunity to observe the importance of their well-organized system of ambulance transport. 'Transport of the wounded from the field of battle . . . besides satisfying the right of humanity and sustaining that spirit of confidence in the soldier . . . has another admirable effect; it obviates the incalculable disadvantage of troops engaged in action leaving their ranks for the purpose of carrying off the wounded.[38]

Indeed, in any action, few things are more likely to cause a reverse than men leaving the ranks to help wounded to the rear; among British troops in the Crimea it was not unusual to see four or five men supporting one man towards the rear, while among the French one trained attendant was sufficient.

Some attempts were made to improve administration and organization, including evacuation of wounded from the battlefield. In 1855, after the railway between Balaclava and the camp before Sebastopol had been completed, it was occasionally used to transport sick from the camp hospitals, but only ordinary wagons were available and no seriously incapacitated cases were sent by it. This was the first time that any railway was used for transporting sick and wounded soldiers from an active battlefront to the rear.

On 21 July 1855 an efficient Hospital Conveyance Corps was incorporated into the Land Transport Corps. A month earlier the Medical Staff Corps had been formed. This unit, which was to grow into the Royal Army Medical Corps, was recruited from civilians, regimental NCOs unfit for further field service and some men of the Land Transport Corps who could read and write. Nine companies were raised initially, a tenth being added three months later. Their headquarters and depot were at Fort Pitt, Chatham, then an important medical centre with three hospitals and an invalid centre. With a quasi-military character only, discipline was poor for there was only one officer, who combined the functions of OC depot, adjutant and quartermaster.

During the second winter the army, now grown to 80,000, was much better cared for, but when peace was proclaimed to the troops on 29 April 1856 the British Army had 126 well-filled cemeteries; of the 23,000 British dead more than 19,000 had died of disease.

It was perhaps some consolation that the Russians had suffered even more – losing at least 100,000 dead and probably more.* The Russian medical administration was virtually non-existent, especially in its lack of systematic removal of casualties. On 13 September 1855, two days after the final taking of the great fortress and arsenal of Sebastopol, the allies found

---

* Records were poorly kept and figures for the Crimea are unreliable; those given here are conservative estimates.

2,000 Russians in a great vault; wounded and immovable, they had lain helpless for forty-eight hours with no food or water and when found fewer than 500 were alive.

The whole Crimean episode was so much a blunder, medically as well as militarily, that a thoughtful man might well have believed that another sort of crisis or climax was being approached, a climax which would transform military medical services.

CHAPTER FIFTEEN

Solferino and Henry Dunant

On the night of 23 June 1859 an Austrian army of 175,000 men and 500 guns and an allied French, Piedmontese and Sardinian army of 150,000 men and 400 guns were moving in the dark, towards each other, along every road of a twelve-and-a-half-mile front. The commanders expected battle in three or four days' time; in fact they were within hours of contact and what would be known as the battle of Solferino was to become the tragedy which forced all the military nations to revise their attitudes to casualties and to reform their military medical services.

Properly to appreciate the horror of Solferino it is necessary to understand, if only superficially, a little of the military situation.

Despite French superiority in organization the Austrians were the first to react to the battle contact and early on the morning of the 24th they occupied many vantage points from which their artillery swept the French with shells, case-shot and grape-shot.*

Rank decided priority of treatment – officers, non-commissioned officers, men. This was common practice in most armies, though in the British forces only senior officers could count on priority. Not until the war of 1914–18 did it become customary for surgeons to take wounded as they came.

The French surgeons that day at Solferino worked with feverish haste on battered bodies. Two, working in the field hospital directed by Dr Méry, Surgeon-in-Chief of the Imperial Guard, had so many amputations and dressings to attend to that they fainted. Another was so exhausted that two soldiers had to steady his arms as he worked.

Slowly and painfully the French won the lower slopes of Solferino's cone-like hill, but the Austrians clung to the spurs and commanded the valleys. They broke up one major French attack, then French artillery smashed holes through the convent and cemetery walls and French infantry poured through to take Austrian positions with the bayonet. Finally, dense columns of French were formed up and sent pounding up the hill. Shells, musket-fire, yells and shrieks made a frightful din and casualties were heavy, since the French had to take every house, garden and vineyard by force.

---

* Case-shot contained ordinary musket balls, grape consisted of small pieces of iron scrap. Case-shot was similar to shrapnel – invented by General Shrapnel and first used in 1806 during the Peninsular War – which, on bursting in the air, scattered balls.

The day was hot. The Austrians had been marching all night, the French had been on the move since before daybreak and had had nothing but coffee. All the men were tired before the fighting started.

The hill of Solferino, the key to the position, was a formidable stronghold and became a nest of miniature Austrian strongpoints which could only be breached by cannon or taken by escalade. At another point, the farm of Casa Nuova, surrounded by ditches, walls, hedges and trees, Austrian engineers had made a major strongpoint. The French used forty-two guns to batter it, then sent in infantry, and fierce hand-to-hand fighting occurred.

When the battle started field hospitals were set up in farms, houses, convents and churches – even under trees. A prominent black flag in those days marked the location of first-aid posts and field ambulances, and belligerents usually respected them.

All round Solferino, by two o'clock when the French had control of the place, the ground was littered with broken weapons, helmets, mess-tins, belts, remnants of blood-stained clothing. The hand-to-hand struggles were appalling in their ferocity, with Austrians and allies trampling one another underfoot, killing one another on piles of dead and dying with butt, bayonet and sabre. Many a man, wounded or without weapon, used rocks, his fists, even his teeth. Some picked up enemy soldiers and threw them into ravines. The Croats of the Austrian army clubbed to death every wounded man they encountered; the Algerian sharp-shooters gave no quarter to wounded Austrians.

By mid-morning the heat was torrid; soon after noon it was fierce – and water was scarce. Artillery constantly changed position with horses, guns and limbers pounding over dead and wounded. The French grape-shot, effective at distances hitherto unknown, inflicted casualties even on distant Austrian reserves. Some Sardinian columns came under practically point-blank grape-shot fire and were so badly broken that the survivors fled. Of the 25,000 Sardinians and Piedmontese engaged around San Martino and Pozzolengo 179 officers and 4,428 men were killed and wounded.

The wounded men who were being picked up were pale and exhausted. The most badly hurt had a stupefied look as though they could not grasp what was said to them and stared out of haggard eyes, but their prostration did not dull their pain. Others, anxious and excited by nervous strain, were shaken by spasmodic trembling. Some, with gaping wounds already beginning to show infection, were almost crazy with suffering and begged to be put out of their misery. There were men who had not only been hit by bullets or knocked down by shell splinters, but whose arms and legs had been broken by artillery wheels passing over them. The impact of a cylindrical bullet shattered bones into many pieces, and wounds of this kind were always very serious. Shell splinters and conical bullets also caused painful fractures, and often severe internal injuries. All kinds of splinters, pieces of bone, scraps of clothing, equipment or footwear, dirt or pieces of lead, aggravated the severity of a wound.

Fighting was still continuing when a violent storm, soupy with dust, broke up the battle and gave the Austrians cover while they withdrew east of the Mincio River. The battle had raged for fifteen hours. Not until sunrise on the 25th did anybody discover the full horror of the vast battlefield, littered by dead, dying and wounded men and animals and the ghastly debris of war.

Solferino was fought at the height of the tourist season, and though most visitors fled some remained. One of these at Castiglione was Henry Dunant,★ a Swiss, who exhausted himself in his efforts to help the wounded. The townspeople and the able-bodied troops could not cope with the situation. There was food and water, but men died of hunger and thirst; there was plenty of lint, but not enough hands to dress wounds, which were soon infected by flies and dust. On the floors of churches lay Frenchmen and Slavs, Germans and Arabs, Rumanians and Croats, Sardinians and Algerians.

The medical services were inadequate to deal with the casualties. The total number of French *infirmiers militaires* sent to Italy during the 1858 campaign was 2,186;[39] some of these became ineffective through injuries or sickness and the remainder were distributed among regiments and the numerous small hospitals – more than 200 according to one report. But the allotment of 2,000 attendants to 128,225 fighting men was too thin.

At Castiglione, the most important rescue centre, overcrowding became dreadful as mule-carts came jolting in with loads of wounded men, many of them crying out with pain. One man had a leg so badly broken that it seemed to be almost severed from his body. Dunant saw a corporal whose arm had been pierced by the stick of a Congreve rocket,† he had pulled out the stick and used it to walk to Castiglione.

Search parties of troops and Italian civilians probed the ravines and ditches, the woods and vineyards for days after the battle. Wounded, by now nearly dead, were being brought in as long as seventy-two hours after the battle. Three weeks elapsed before all the dead were found and buried and, in Dunant's opinion, many soldiers were buried alive. Perhaps, in most cases, they were only technically alive.

The townspeople of Castiglione gave all the blankets, linen and mattresses they could spare, but the hospital, the church, the San Luigi monastery and barracks, the Capuchin church, the police barracks, the churches of San Maggiore, San Giuseppe and Santa Rosalia, were all filled with wounded men, piled on one another and with nothing but straw to lie on. Straw was also spread in the streets, courtyards and squares, and here and there wooden shelters were hastily erected or pieces of cloth stretched, so that the

★ Generally referred to as 'Henri Dunant'; however, he himself signed and published the original of his manuscript, *Un Souvenir de Solferino*, as 'J. Henry Dunant'.
† This rocket, invented by Sir William Congreve, had a range of 3,500 yards and was first used during the battle of Leipzig, 1813.

wounded might have a little shelter from the sun. Private houses were taken over and the better-off citizens welcomed officers and soldiers, and did what little they could to relieve their pain. Some ran through the streets, looking for a doctor for their guests. Others begged to have corpses taken from their houses.

Faces black with flies that swarmed about their wounds, men gazed around them, wild-eyed and helpless. Dunant saw others who were 'no more than a worm-ridden, inextricable compound of coat and shirt and flesh and blood'. Many were shuddering at the thought of being devoured by the worms, which they thought they could see coming out of their bodies; they came, of course, from the flies. Dunant noticed one mutilated man with a broken jaw and his swollen tongue hanging out of his mouth, tossing and trying to get up. Dunant moistened his dry lips and hardened tongue, dipped a handful of lint in a bucket and squeezed the water into the deformed opening that had been the man's mouth. Another man had lost his nose, lips and chin to a sabre cut. Half-blind, unable to speak, he made signs with his hands and uttered guttural sounds to attract attention. Dunant gave him a drink and poured a little fresh water on his bleeding face. A third, with his skull gaping open, was dying, 'spitting out his brains on the stone floor'. His companions in suffering kicked him out of their way, as he blocked the passage. Dunant sheltered him as he died.

An old sergeant, with several service stripes on his sleeve, said to Dunant with the utmost suddenness, with conviction, and with cold bitterness: 'If I had been looked after sooner I might have lived, and now by evening I shall be dead!' And by evening he *was* dead.

Long waits were inevitable and not everybody could be attended to 'sooner'. Surgeons fell down with exhaustion. Two surgeons-in-chief, Leuret and Haspel, and two Italian assistant surgeons, Riolacci and Lobstein, worked as a team for forty-eight hours without sleep.

A few Austrians would not accept the help of French army surgeons and tore off their bandages, causing fresh bleeding. Dunant saw one Croat grab the bullet just extracted from his wound and throw it in the surgeon's face. According to Dunant another wounded prisoner, an Austrian aged twenty, turned white-haired during the battle.

Dunant wrote:

Up at the end of the church, in the altar recess on the left, a trooper of the African Light Infantry lay on straw, uttering no complaint, and hardly moving any longer. Three bullets had struck him, one on the right side, one in the left shoulder, and the third in the right leg. . . . It was Sunday night, and he said he had had nothing to eat since Friday morning. He was a revolting spectacle, covered with dry mud and clotted blood, his clothing torn, and his shirt in shreds. We washed his wounds and gave him a little soup, and I covered him with a blanket. He carried my hand to his lips with an expression of inexpressible gratitude. At the entrance to the church was a Hungarian who never ceased to call out, begging for a doctor in heart-breaking Italian. A burst of grape-shot had ploughed into his back, which looked as if it had been furrowed with steel claws, laying bare a great area of red, quivering flesh. The rest of his swollen body was all black and green, and he could find no comfortable position to sit or lie in. I moistened great masses of lint in cold water and tried to place this under him, but it was not long before gangrene carried him off . . . Over against the wall, about 100 French non-commissioned officers and soldiers were stretched in two lines, almost touching. . . . Calm and peaceful . . . they suffered without complaint. They died humbly and quietly.

But many died in desperate agony from untreatable wounds or while having a limb amputated without anaesthetic. Dunant has left a vivid account of an amputation – that of a mangled leg from a young Frenchman. Without anaesthetic such an operation could be emotionally exhausting to a surgeon. In this case the patient cried out in terror: 'Don't drop me!' as an orderly was trying to get him onto the low operating table and threw his arms around the young surgeon who was himself 'pale with emotion and almost as upset as the patient'.

The surgeon turned up his sleeves almost to the shoulder and donned a white apron. Dunant wrote:

With one knee on the ground and the terrible knife in his hand, he threw his arm round the soldier's thigh, and with a single movement cut the skin round the limb. A piercing cry rang through the hospital. The young doctor, looking into the suffering man's face, could see in his drawn features every detail of the frightful agony he was undergoing. 'Be brave!' he said to the soldier under his breath, as he felt the man's hands stiffen against his back 'Two more minutes, and you will be all right.' The surgeon rose, and began to separate the skin from the muscles under it, which he thus stripped. Then he cut away the flesh from the skin, and raised the skin about an inch, like a sort of cuff. After that he returned to the main task, and with a vigorous movement cut through the muscles with his knife, as far as the bone. A torrent of blood burst from the opened arteries, covering the surgeon and dripping on to the floor . . . Quiet and impassive the surgeon said nothing until . . . he said angrily to the orderly: 'You fool, can't you compress an artery?' the orderly had had little experience, and did not know how to stop the haemorrhage by applying his thumb to the blood vessels in the right way. The patient, in an ecstasy of pain, muttered weakly: 'Oh, that will do, let me die!' and cold sweat ran down his face. But there was still another minute to go through, a minute which seemed like eternity. The assistant, kind as ever, counted the seconds, and looking from the operator to the patient's face and back again, he tried to sustain his courage, and seeing him shaking with terror, 'Only one minute more', he said. It was indeed now time for the saw, and I could hear the grating of the steel as it entered the living bone, and separated the half-rotten limb from the body. . . .

The patient fainted at this point but although broken and exhausted he survived the ordeal. One can only wonder what this operation cost the surgeon.

Lack of adequate transport hampered attempts to evacuate sick and wounded to base hospitals. The Austrians, the losers, were worse off than the French. As the railroad to the Tyrol could not be used because of strategical reasons the sick were sent circuitously by Casarsa and Palmanuova to Nabresina; 1,200 sick and wounded daily used this road. The railway from Casarsa to Nabresina broke down and the men were conveyed on rough country carts, then the cattle sickened and transport became still more difficult. At Palmanuova Dr Felix Kraus saw 1,300 men, almost all wounded, who had no shelter and for whom nothing had been prepared; only two surgeons were available and they lacked medical material of all kinds.

The losses at Solferino were: allies, 14,415 killed and wounded and 2,776 missing; Austrians, 13,317 killed and wounded, 9,220 missing. Two months later the total figure was practically doubled by men dead of wounds or disease and those in hospitals from post-battle sickness, fever, sunstroke or exhaustion.

Figures could have been even higher had not Baron Larrey* gone to much trouble to scatter his sick and wounded in small groups as widely apart as his transport would allow; in this way he reduced the incidence of gangrene, pyaemia (blood-poisoning) and typhus.

Henry Dunant was so moved by the plight of wounded soldiers that he became the spirit that brought the Red Cross into being. The publicity which attended its formation, as well as the writings of Dunant and others who had seen the aftermath of Solferino, forced upon military commanders and their governments the realization that conditions must improve. From this point progress was steady but slow. Even more important, the military hierarchy no longer merely tolerated doctors at war, but recognized them as indispensable in the army system.

* The second baron, son of Napoleon's medical chief.

CHAPTER SIXTEEN

American Civil War, Franco-Prussian War – and Massive Casualties

Progress was necessarily slow at this time because the inventors were outstripping the surgeons, and armaments manufacturers were able to spend more money than the humanitarians of the infant Red Cross Society. The American Civil War 1861–5 introduced a remarkable range of martial innovations or improvements, all calculated to increase the killing and wounding capacity of an army. There were the repeating rifle – the Spencer initially – wire entanglements, land-mines and booby-traps, more sophisticated grenades, mortars, explosive bullets and flame-throwers, submarines, naval mines and torpedoes, railroad artillery, revolving gun turrets, telescopic sights, trench periscopes, Requa's machine-gun – one of the first of its kind. The rifle made the defensive the stronger form of warfare; the offensive became more difficult and more costly in terms of human life. This in turn led to armies of greater size, for more men were needed to tackle a job. In 1864 the Union forces were 683,000, a large army by any standards.

Normally years are needed to raise, train and equip the medical services to support such large forces. The American medical administrators and surgeons of both North and South had to improvise as the war progressed, facing one crisis after another in their efforts to deal with problems set by the large area over which the campaigns were fought – 1 million square miles – the great numbers of sick and wounded and the complexity of wounds.

Much suffering and loss of life resulted early in the war from lack of an efficient ambulance organization; this deficiency so aroused public opinion that great efforts were made to remedy it. In time the ambulance system of the Northern armies became thoroughly organized, but the Confederate forces throughout the war had only rudimentary ambulance services.

Medical administrators of the army were agitating publicly for better organization – and using straightforward language. On 4 October 1862 Surgeon-General Hammond of the Union Army reported,[40] 'In no battle yet have the wounded men been properly looked after; men under the pretence of carrying them off the field leave the ranks, and seldom return to their proper duties.' Just after the battle of Bull Run, 30 August 1862, he had written:

> The frightful state of disorder existing in the arrangements for removing the wounded from the field of battle, the scarcity of ambulances, the want of organization, the drunkenness and incompetency of the drivers, the total absence of ambulance attendants, are now working their legitimate results. . . . Wounded remain on the battle field, in consequence of an insufficiency of ambulances and the want of a proper system for regulating their removal. . . . Many have died of starvation, many more will die in consequence of exhaustion, and all have endured torments which might have been avoided.

Dr Agnew, a member of the United States Sanitary Commission, estimated that 500 lives were lost from want of proper transport at the battle of Antietam, 15 September 1862, alone.

By the time of Gettysburg, 1–3 July 1863, transport was better. More than 15,000 wounded were sent back from the advanced positions by railway to Baltimore, York, Harrisburg and Philadelphia. A large proportion of these men were transported in goods wagons containing straw. After the battle of Olustee, 20 February 1864, 1,100 were transported in goods

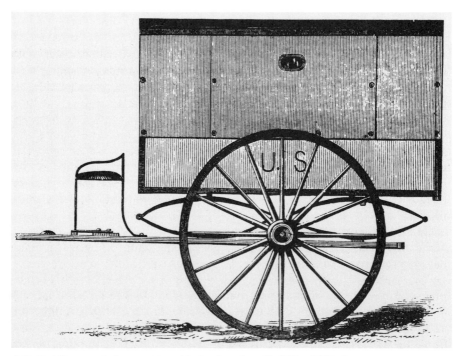

A United States ambulance cart used in the American Civil War, 1861–5.

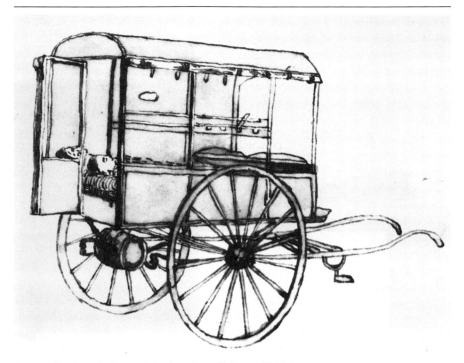

A type of early ambulance of the American Civil war, 1861–5.

wagons, lying on branches of pine and a little straw, and covered with blankets. The train was driven to Jacksonville, a distance of nearly fifty miles, and Assistant-Surgeon Janeway, who was in charge, reported that the patients who had undergone amputation and received severe wounds did not complain very much of this rough method of transport. In 1864 there were three ambulance trains, each of ten or twelve wagons, which joined the advanced force at the front of the railway line. Each train had a kitchen wagon, a second for a dispensary with medical comforts and apparatus.

The battle of Gettysburg resulted in 54,807 casualties – a harvest to dismay even a well-staffed, well-equipped medical service. There was no time for surgical refinements, though in fact refinements such as asepsis had still not reached the operating table.

For that matter, anaesthetic had not long reached it. Humphry Davy had described the properties of nitrous oxide as early as 1800 and suggested its use during operations, but his advice was ignored. Chloroform had been prepared almost simultaneously by Samuel Guthrie in the United States, J. von Liebig in Germany and E. Soubeiran in France in 1831, but its first use as an anaesthetic occurred in 1847 – at the hands of Sir James Young Simpson in Edinburgh. It had several dangers, including damage to the heart, and fell into disrepute. It became respectable largely because Queen

Victoria accepted it at the birth of Prince Leopold. Ether was first used in the United States in 1846, ethyl chloride in 1848, and during the 1850s many American doctors had become experienced in administering some form of anaesthetic. In view of the vast amount of surgery during the American Civil War the new skill had not come any too soon.

During General Grant's attack at Coldharbour, 1864, over 10,000 men were wounded (besides the killed), the greater part in ten minutes and all within an hour. Under such pressure a man with a bullet in the small intestine was passed over as hopeless. If a man's wound justified surgical attention he was taken in charge by surgeons whose bare arms and aprons were smeared with blood, their knives held between their teeth while they helped the sufferer onto the table. If the chief surgeon decided on a major operation, ether or chloroform was administered. The surgeon then wiped his knife across his apron and went to work. He worked under conditions that were poor even for those days; on operating tables made from barn doors or planks of wood, in poor light, for hour after exhausting hour. The severed arms and legs would reach level with the tables. A soldier might have a competent job done on him, but things could go very badly wrong within a few days. A man who had lost an arm or leg would come out of the operation with from five to thirty whip-thongs or, a little later, silk strings hanging out of the stump. These were the ends of ligatures, some with knots to identify ligatures of large blood vessels. A few days later the plain strings were pulled to see if the tissues had rotted away sufficiently to allow them to come loose. After a longer period the knotted strings were pulled; often a gush of blood followed, indicating that the vessel had not healed. The wound had then to be reopened or the vessel tied higher up; another amputation might be necessary. If the patient contracted pyaemia his chances of recovery were then only three out of a hundred. There was still the great danger of gangrene.

Apart from complete ignorance about prevention of wound infection there was the constant danger of bacteria being introduced through the lint used as dressings. Lint-plucking was for any homeland what the camp fire was for the soldier. As war commenced every cupboard was ransacked and all old and worn linen plucked to threads by the women of every house. Great piles were put into coarse sacks and sent to the military hospitals. In peace-time lint-plucking did not have quite the same appeal, and prosperous citizens would send their old linen to the hospitals, where the staff and convalescent patients pulled it to pieces. The threads were made into swabs of various shapes and sizes; people thought nothing of rinsing a swab and using it on patient after patient. Wounds were left unstitched to prevent early suppuration and stuffed with a wound sponge or lint, none of it sterilized.

Frank Wilkeson, who served with the Union armies throughout the war, noticed that wounded soldiers nearly always tore their clothing away from their wounds, so as to assess them.[41] Many of them would smile and their faces would brighten as they realized a hit was not serious and that they could go home for a few months. Others, after a quick glance, would turn pale as they realized the truth that the wound was severe. Wilkeson is one of the few writers to record the actions of a man at the moment of wounding. During the battle of the Wilderness he saw a boy of about twenty skip and yell from a bullet through the thigh. He turned to limp to the rear and after a few steps kicked out his leg once or twice to test its working, regarded it attentively, flexed it again, and returned to the firing-line. A short time later the soldier dropped his rifle, clasped his left arm and exclaimed: 'I am hit again!' Tearing the sleeve off his shirt he saw that the wound was slight, so he tied his handkerchief around it and resumed his position. Wilkeson advised him not to push his luck and to go to the rear. As the soldier turned to answer him he staggered, fell, then regained his feet. 'A fountain of blood and teeth and bone and bits of tongue burst out of his mouth. He had been shot through the jaws; the lower one was broken and hung down . . . his open mouth was ragged and bloody and tongueless. He cast his rifle furiously on the ground and staggered off' – another impossible challenge to some surgeon already at the limit of his own endurance.

In the United States, as in Europe, disease was causing more casualties than wounds. Wounds came in daunting numbers during the big battles; sickness was more or less constant. Dysentery, for example, was endemic; it was believed that before the war ended most of the 2 million men who took part had suffered from it in one form or another; it killed 45,000 of them. Total Union deaths from disease were 183,287; 96,000 were killed in action.

Again, as in Europe, military doctors found almost insuperable the task of making officers understand that they had a duty towards maintaining health. It was not enough, the doctors stressed, for an officer to be a gallant leader with a thorough technical knowledge of his trade. He should know the fundamentals of hygiene, ventilation and cleanliness, he should ensure that his men did not drink contaminated water, that latrines were not dug near the cookhouse, that cooks should have clean hands. The typical reply from officers was that their business was to fight, not to keep a boarding-house.

General Jonathan Letterman, who organized the medical department of the army of the Potomac, thought that many medical officers themselves did not fully appreciate their duties and importance, and he sent out an illuminating report to his military doctors.

A corps of medical officers was not established solely for the purpose of attending the wounded and sick; the proper treatment of these sufferers is certainly a matter of very great importance and an imperative duty, but the duties of medical officers cover a more extended field. The leading idea which should be constantly kept in view is to strengthen the hands of the Commanding General by keeping his army in the most vigorous health, thus rendering it efficient for enduring fatigue and privation, and for fighting. The duties of such a corps are of vital importance to the success of an army, and commanders seldom appreciate the full effect of their proper fulfilment. Medical officers should possess a thorough knowledge of the powers and capabilities of the human system; the effects of food, raiment and climate, with all its multiplied vicissitudes; the influences for evil which surround an army, and the means necessary to combat them successfully. . . . When medical officers consider this subject, all their high, special, and important duties will naturally occur to them.[42]

If medicine and surgery had advanced little since the Crimea, hospitals had improved considerably, mostly because the entire control and administration of them was given to the army medical department; civilian authorities no longer had any control. Service doctors were to say that never before had the mortality among the wounded been so low, never had hospitals been so little crowded. Possibly this was an exaggerated idea of the improvement, but Deputy Surgeon General Charles Alexander Gordon, CB, of the British service, considered that the enlightened hospital policy of the US army had saved 100,000 lives.

Certainly in American hospitals soldiers were led to feel that they were relieved from the surveillance and strictness of barrack life. Everything was made subordinate to the care of the sick. Hospitals had their own flower and vegetable gardens and the soldier was nursed in an atmosphere of serenity. After discharge he might be sent to a convalescent home, where he would live in relative luxury.

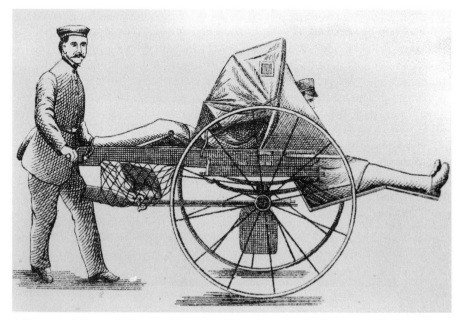

A Prussian field litter of the period 1860–70.

The Americans claimed too that the first regular tent field hospital* in history was organized during the battle of Shiloh, 6–7 April 1862. Dr B.J.D. Irwin, medical inspector of the 4th Division, army of the Ohio, had the abandoned tents of an infantry division made into a hospital, complete with operating theatre and dispensary for 300 patients. In the movements of the army following Shiloh and culminating in the siege of Corinth, Mississippi, the utility of large field hospitals was recognized and soon developed into a system. Surgeons saw that treatment of sick and wounded under canvas had many advantages over hospitals established in churches, houses and wooden and iron huts. The patients recovered more rapidly and were less susceptible to secondary infection, largely because of better ventilation and sanitation. Many much larger tent hospitals were used in the last two years of the war.

Most European armies sent medical as well as military observers to the American Civil War, and their observations tended to influence the medical practice of their respective countries. In association with the great Paris Exhibition of 1867 they certainly stimulated study of ambulance transport, for what surgeons had known for centuries was now accepted by others – that a wounded soldier's chances of survival decreased dramatically the longer his removal from the field was delayed. A committee of representatives from various societies for helping war-wounded brought together in Paris a large collection of conveyances, with prizes for the best hand-litters, wheeled litters and wagons; several governments exhibited their official form of ambulance. Some of the inventions were too frail for rough handling on the battlefield and others had structural defects, as did the wagon into which wounded men were slid into slots so confined that a stout soldier's stomach would press on the roof.[43]

The Prussians, in the war with Denmark in 1864 and in the brief war against Austria in 1866, were the first to use hand-wheeled litters. Early in the Danish war the Johanniter Order (Knights of St John) had some two-wheeled hand-litters made in Berlin. These carriages were constantly used, but their practical advantages were particularly noticed during the storming of the forts of Düppel. This was the first occasion on which wheeled carriages, moved by hand, were systematically employed during active operations.

In these wars, as in the Franco-Prussian War of 1870–1, the surgeons were often able to avoid amputations, and to resort to more intricate operations because of the rapid removal of wounded from the field to fixed hospitals. These hospitals had all the necessary equipment, but the surgeons were also influenced by the knowledge that they knew their patients could remain in hospital without the necessity for further removal until they were fit enough to travel without detriment to their wounds.

---

* Not strictly true. This was possibly the *largest* tent hospital, but the British had used tents in India in 1848 and the Prussians used them the same year.

Wounded could now be conveniently and comfortably transported by rail, but railways were a mixed blessing for military doctors. On the debit side was the ability of a general staff to concentrate great numbers of men for attack and defence. This meant, as doctors had already seen in the United States, that medical administration had to be prepared to cope with great numbers of wounded in a brief period. For the war with Austria the Prussians brought together, in three armies, 220,000 men to the Austrians' 215,000. These men took part in the battle of Königgratz (or Sadowa, as the Austrians called it) massed on the relatively short front of five miles. On the afternoon of 3 July, after great bloodshed, the Prussians turned the Austrian right flank and by four o'clock the Prussian line resembled a huge semicircle hemming in the masses of battered and broken Austrian troops. The nature of the ground prevented much use of cavalry, but on the line of retreat several sabre and lance conflicts occurred. By superior arms – the Prussians had the Dreyse needle-gun,★ the Austrians still used muzzle-loading muskets – by superior numbers and superior strategy, the Prussians won a resounding victory, but at a cost of 10,000 casualties. Austria lost 40,000 men, including 18,000 prisoners. For the doctors the one advantage of a short campaign – this one lasted seven weeks – was that disease was less likely to ravage an army. Some of the English physicians who went to the war to further their professional knowledge were disappointed that they could learn little about medical treatment, but the surgeons found their visit worth while. At this time the Garibaldi sonde – a musket-ball probe named after the Italian patriot for whose case it was invented by the French pathologist Nelaton – was a new surgical toy. By its aid it was easy to distinguish between a fractured bone and a bullet. A bullet buried four inches deep in the fleshy part of the thigh could be traced with the probe. A new American bullet-forceps was in use too, its peculiarity consisting in the sharply serrated blades crossing one another and not simply meeting as in other forceps; fragments of all shapes could be easily removed. The search after bullets was a matter of great interest to surgeons and their patients. Men would often claim emphatically that a ball had been extracted in the field when this was not so; the purpose of this assertion was to avoid the pain and discomfort of extraction. Dr Alexander Bruce, MB, FRCS, who spent some weeks visiting the military hospitals of Dresden, where many troops were treated, noted great excitement in some soldiers at the sight of a bullet removed from their bodies. An Italian soldier seized his bullet, bit it violently, and cursed it so furiously that it

---

★ The Dreyse was in use in Prussia in 1842, only four years after its invention. By 1859 only Sweden, Norway and France were also using breech-loaders on a small scale. The needle gun was so called because a long needle inside the bolt functioned as the modern striker. When the trigger was pressed the needle was driven by its spring, its point passed through the primer and hit the powder ahead. The subsequent explosion fired the bullet.

had to be taken from him to prevent his injuring himself. A usually phlegmatic Prussian soldier, seeing the ball which had been removed from his thigh, burst into tears and, shaking hands all round, divided his attention between blessing his audience and cursing his bullet. The men always kept the bullets as valuable relics, and would not have parted with them at any price.

It was Bruce who reported[44] the remarkable case of a soldier shot near the anus, the bullet passing the entire length of his penis to emerge at the end. The man died three weeks later from infiltration of urine. Bruce regretted that no post-mortem examination was made, but believed that the bullet had entered the bladder.

Bruce was interested in a particular suicide case since it illustrated the results produced by what he termed the 'favourite mode of suicide in vogue among the Prussian soldiers'. A Prussian soldier, a fine and very handsome man, 'shot himself through the eye after hearing that his wife and three children had died from cholera. The ordinary method of suicide, which he adopted, is as follows: The man loads his *zundnadelgewehr* [needle gun] in the usual way at the breech. He then drives down the barrel a small wad of cotton, pours water in until the barrel is about one-third full, and then drives in as far as the water a small cork or wad. Having prepared this enormous charge, this man must have looked down the barrel with his left eye, and pulled the trigger with his toe. Death would have been instantaneous.'

When France declared war on Prussia on 19 July 1870 most Frenchmen were wild with confidence. The French Army had a revolutionary breech-loading rifle, the Chassepot, with twice the range of the Prussian needle-rifle. It had the mitrailleuse, a machine-gun of twenty-five barrels, axis-grouped, which was sighted to 1,200 metres and could fire 125 rounds a minute. The French Army consisted of veterans who had fought in the previous decade in the Crimea, Italy and Algeria. But the French did not realize that the hallowed old combination of 'brilliant' leadership – usually intuitive – high morale and 'magnificent' cavalry charges was no match for a finely organized army superior in numbers and directed with deliberate competence. The Prussian planner, General Count von Moltke, reckoned correctly that the French would not be able to bring more than 250,000 men against his 381,000 – numbers were still increasing – and that because of their system of rail communications they would be compelled to assemble their forces about Metz and Strasbourg, separated by the Vosges Mountains. He planned a series of hard blows, with infantry and his devastating artillery, to shock the French into defeat. But such tactics result in heavy casualties, and even the Prussian medical services could not efficiently handle the casualties that occurred.

At the battle of Borny, 14 August, the Germans lost 5,000 and the French 3,800 in five hours. At the battles of Mars-la-Tour, Vionville and Rezonville, 16 August, the Germans lost 17,000, the French 16,954 in nine hours. At the end of this day heaps of dead and wounded lay everywhere.

At Mars-la-Tour, especially, the Prussians ran into a storm of fire they had never before experienced. It was an awful revelation of the power of the modern rifle. Of a total of ninety-five officers and 4,400 men who went into the fight, seventy-four officers and 2,425 men did not return – mown down in half an hour. A leading military historian of the time, Captain Fritz Hönig, who took part in the battle, said: 'I am not ashamed of owning that the French fire affected my nerves for months after. Troops that have survived an ordeal of this kind are demoralized for a considerable time. . . .' For doctors with foresight such a comment hinted at medical problems to come, for at this time little attention was paid to 'nerves'.

During the battle of Rezonville the famous *Todesritt* – the Death-ride – of the 16th Lancers and 7th Magdeburg Cuirassiers took place. This became to the German Army what the charge of the Light Brigade is to the British – and it was equally futile. Numbering about 600, the two regiments charged the French guns, cutting down or riding over every officer and man except one. They charged through another battery and now rode into French infantry, which broke. The survivors of the charge were in turn charged by two French cavalry brigades and rode back through fire from rifles, machine-guns and cannon. Only 90 lancers and 104 cuirassiers answered roll-call. The generals considered it a gallant charge; nobody asked the surgeons what they thought of the carnage.

But the casualties at Rezonville were light compared with those at Gravelotte and St Privat, 18 August, when the Germans lost 21,000 men and the French 12,273 in eight hours. At one period of this battle the Germans were exposed to a fearful fire, and were reported to have lost 5,000 men killed and wounded in fifteen minutes.

Even the toughest, fastest surgeon has limitations, and the medical officers in the field during and after these battles must have wondered if they could ever come to the end of the stream of wounded. But somehow they still found time for innovation, and it was during this war that the Prussians, for the first time on the battlefield, practised blood replacement by transfusion. Progress was slow, owing to clotting and to ignorance of blood grouping, for human blood is not universally compatible.*

In the besieged city of Metz the French medical services were caught without adequate supplies, and at the end of August *The Times* correspondent was reporting that for five weeks amputations had been performed without anaesthetic and the wounds dressed without antiseptic. There were then more than 19,000 sick and wounded, and 35,000 had died in the town alone during the siege. The prevailing diseases were variole (a type of pest), spotted typhus and dysentery. Scurvy had not become serious, though even the sick were getting their horse steaks and horse broths without salt. The discovery of a saline spring at St Julien was reported, but it was a ruse to encourage the army.

---

* The first transfusion of human blood was probably performed by J.K Blundell and L. Cline in 1818.

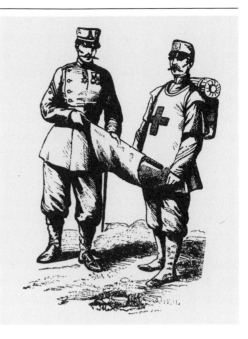

Invented by the Swiss Dr Landa, the *mandil di socorro* was a carrying apron used on the Continent between 1870 and 1885. The wounded man was supported against the chest of the rear bearer and his legs fitted through the slits, which had handles for the front bearer.

In 1870 the work of the Scot, Joseph Lister, in preventing sepsis was now beginning to have effect. Developing discoveries made by Louis Pasteur, Lister evolved his famous bandage, an eightfold layer of clean sterilized gauze saturated with carbolic acid, with a strip of mackintosh between the seventh and eighth layer to prevent bacteria from reaching the wound. An impermeable protective silk was placed between the skin and the bandage to protect the wound from the poisonous and corrosive effect of the carbolic acid. In 1867 Lister reported success in healing wounds without heavy suppuration. He also sprayed carbolic over the operating area to kill germs in the air.

The Germans went to war with the knowledge of Lister's antiseptic wound treatment – they were much more impressed with it than the English and French – but with no actual experience, and as a result Lister's theories were put into practice casually and inefficiently. Also, carbolic was scarce in the field hospitals. Not until the end of the campaign, with the Germans at the gates of Paris, did the British provide both sides with carbolic, mackintosh and silk. Little use was made of these supplies, for the stuffing of wounds with lint was simpler and easier. There was still no question of washing the hands before operating and disinfectants were merely a nuisance. The death quota of wounded was therefore still high, on an average 25 per cent, and, in the case of amputation, 40 to 50 per cent. One or two field hospitals, however, employed Lister's methods; the wounds were dressed with carbolic gauze and cleaned with antiseptic solutions. The cures in these hospitals so greatly exceeded the general level that the difference between the old and new treatment had the effect of a major experiment. Many German surgeons returned from the campaign convinced Lister partisans.

But other findings had even wider effects. The Franco-Prussian War converted every nation to the idea of metallic breech-loaders and, while doctors were appalled at the vast numbers of wounded these weapons produced, they recognized that the conical bullet of smaller calibre fired with greater velocity would tend to perforate the body and, if it did not hit a vital part, would leave nothing but a small track which would not suppurate but heal quickly. This was a decided improvement on the old lead ball, which smashed bone, bruised and lacerated viscera and carried before it portions of clothing and equipment.

Ambulance services were better organized than ever before, largely because of the influence of the Red Cross, but the symbol was abused. One of the first and most flagrant cases of abuse occurred in 1870, following the arrival at Le Havre of the so-called Irish Ambulance. The 300 Irishmen forming this unit were next heard of fighting as combatants in the defence of Châteaudun, against the Germans. It says much for the Red Cross that it was able to attract universal respect despite this and many other instances of abuse to gain military advantage.

Indeed ambulance services were better throughout Europe. The ambulance establishment of the Russian Army was more generous and probably more effective than those of the French and Prussian armies. A Russian ambulance group had 58 doctors, 8 other officers, 2,094 soldiers, 200 labourers, 150 4-horse wagons and 16 2-horse wagons. The Austrians had an efficient system of removal of wounded, with trained teams of three combing the battlefield and its surroundings. Spanish field ambulances were remarkably efficient, with *compagnies sanitaires*, whose members formed a cadre for the *compagnies de secours* in war. That is, these men were health and sanitation specialists in peace but ambulance men in war.

The three wars in which Prussia was involved, together with the American Civil War, placed great strain on military doctors, but administration, equipment and professional skills were superb compared with the means available to the surgeons who were courageous enough to take the field during the Russo-Turkish War of 1877.

CHAPTER SEVENTEEN

The Limits of a Surgeon's Endurance: a Navy/Army Contrast

It is impossible in a book of this length to deal with medical practice in every war of the nineteenth century; wars were raging in most parts of the globe – the Kaffir wars, the Maori wars, the Kandyan (Ceylon) war, the Burmese wars, the Afghan wars, three Chinese wars, the Sikh wars, the Egyptian and Sudan wars, the Serbo-Bulgarian war, the Spanish-American war, and so on. As always, disease on campaign or even during the peaceful periods of foreign service killed more men than enemy weapons. In India British doctors were continually fighting cholera, malaria, typhus and sunstroke, as were the French in North Africa. Often enough the regimental doctor was himself a victim of a disease. Few of the soldiers appreciated that the regimental MO was taking even greater risks with his life in tending sick men than when patching them up under fire. And they were under fire frequently. During the relief of Lucknow, 25 September 1857, Surgeon Joseph Gee treated many men wounded in a bayonet charge and had them evacuated. Later, trying to reach safety with the wounded men, Gee was surrounded and, though under constant fire, dressed other wounded men. He eventually succeeded in taking many wounded through crossfire to safety. The award of the Victoria Cross seemed reasonable enough.

Surgeons in British service, and, to a lesser extent in the French, were more likely to gain recognition than were others, but recognition was clearly unimportant to most military doctors. This was so in the case of the doctors who volunteered to help Serbian and Bulgarian wounded in 1876 and Turkish and Russian wounded in the war of 1877.

Working under the auspices of the National Society for the Aid of Sick and Wounded in War (later the British Red Cross Society), these doctors' only possible reward was professional satisfaction and they ran great risks to achieve even that.

In most of Eastern Europe there was virtually no army medical system, military officers cared nothing for casualties and the soldiers themselves were ignorant and superstitious. Even the Russians, who did have a system, found it inadequate under pressure.

At Alexinatz, Serbia, in 1876 a small team of surgeons under Dr Mackellar opened a hospital in the school, where they worked in constricted space by the light of candles fixed in pools of congealed grease on the floor. On a bad night an unbroken line of bearers would stretch down the main street into the open country. Many seriously wounded, left in the street, would have to wait from early morning to night for treatment and some, becoming desperate, would struggle out of their stretchers and crawl towards the school, only to bleed to death in the gutters. At times orderlies coming to fetch a patient for the surgeons would have to search for several minutes to find one still living. Frederic Villiers, in Serbia as an artist for the *Graphic*, fetched and carried for the surgeons or held the groping hand of some soldier on the operating table. One night, unable to tolerate the atmosphere of the operating room, he picked his way through a crowd of wounded, but at the street entrance a man plucked at his leg. As the man lifted his head Villiers saw that his face, crushed by a shell, was:

> . . . mere pulp and black as a Negro's with clotted gore. Staring appalled at this gruesome sight, he roused me by touching my boot and, slowly lifting his arm, pointed to the lower portion of his face. He repeated this action before I understood him; then I knelt by his side and poured some brandy from my flask down his throat. He could not express his thanks by word of mouth, but his eyelids trembled, and he lifted his arm again, bringing his hand gradually to the salute. The quiet patience of the soldier in this fearful plight will ever remain in my memory.[45]

Conditions the following year were worse. During the brutal conflicts between Russians and Turks men were being wounded in large numbers, yet at Yeni-Zaragh Dr Armand Leslie found only one Turkish field ambulance of a doctor and five dressers with no bandages and no courage – they bolted on the 31 July when they heard that the Russians were approaching. Leslie stayed to treat the wounded, who arrived on 8 August in batches of 200. As if spate of wounds was not bad enough, these men, so fierce in combat, moaned and whimpered like children when hurt. Leslie, however, found the smell worse than the sights and sounds. A little later Leslie discovered that he and Dr Francis Meyrick were the only surgeons with an army of 40,000. In trying to work too hard and too long Dr Meyrick, though a young man, collapsed from exhaustion and died. At Batoum Dr J.S. Young found 1,000 sick and wounded with only seven surgeons. Wounds were usually serious, for the Russians fired a heavy ball and internal bleeding and peritonitis were frequent. But the Turks stood chloroform well and their simple diet and sober habits gave wounds every chance to heal without serious complication. A difficulty was that without trained bearers the surgeons were receiving men who had no chance of survival while cases with good prospects were left on the field.

The rigours of this campaign, from the surgeon's point of view, were graphically described by Dr Harry Crookshank, writing to the Society from

Varna in October 1877. He had been ill for a fortnight with gastric fever and diarrhoea:

> . . . lying all day on a stretcher in a tent, covered with blankets, yet when not burning with fever, shivering with cold, nothing to eat but hard soldier's biscuits soaked in water and Australian mutton. . . . Then, in addition, every third day we would have to strike tents, march three or four hours, and then encamp again. I could do nothing but lie in the tent, and drink condensed milk in coldest stream water. I at last made up my mind to fall to the rear, when, on the morning of 21st September, heavy fighting began and continued till night. The whole of that night and the following day the wounded came pouring into our hospitals and tents in hundreds, and I was obliged to over-exert myself and help in the work, which so prostrated me, that next day I could not rise from the bed, so I determined to leave for Varna.

Dr Robert Pinkerton, serving at Orkhanie, reported the interesting case of a young soldier with eight wounds from one bullet. It had struck him on the middle of the right arm and passed through, causing a simple flesh wound; then it passed through the right breast below the nipple; then through the left breast and last of all passed through the left arm, fracturing the humerus. The man told Pinkerton he received the wound as he was leaning forward and just about to bring his rifle to the shoulder to fire. Another man was hit in the temple; the bullet penetrated deeply and caused protrusion of the eyeball, which had to be taken out.

Another man had the entire lower jaw, with the soft parts around and forming the floor of the mouth, carried away by a shell fragment. Although hideous looking, he recovered so rapidly that he was used as a hospital attendant. Generally speaking, wounds of the face, no matter how dangerous looking, heal quickly and well.

Pinkerton was one day confronted with three soldiers who had told their officers they had been wounded three days before in a skirmish with the Russians. The officers were suspicious and sent them to the hospital for examination. Pinkerton found one suffering from a very severe wound of the right elbow; the joint was shattered, and the soft parts immediately round it carried away. Another had a severe penetrating wound of the right hand. The third had the index finger of his right hand nearly blown off. The firearms had been discharged so close to the body as to scorch the surrounding parts and Pinkerton found grains of gunpowder embedded in the skin and tissues. The men with wounds of elbow joint and hand were in a deeply depressed state and their wounds looked unhealthy and dangerous. They were suffering from over fatigue and exposure, so Pinkerton was allowed to take them into the hospital under a guard, where they both died of blood poisoning. The third man was executed.

If a few Turks feared combat enough to mutilate themselves to avoid it, the great bulk of the Russians had a horror of surgery and preferred death to loss of an arm or leg. In Montenegro with the Russian Army, Dr John

Furley wanted to help a soldier with a broken thigh, but the man refused to accept treatment, insisted on being lifted into his saddle and, in agony, took himself off. 'If a man is wounded and can crawl he will hide himself away somewhere and leave his cure to God and native air,' Furley wrote.

Incredibly enough, many soldiers did not contract infection of their wounds or they survived infection. Antiseptic methods were by now in use in the Russian Army and one surgeon, Bergmann, produced figures[46] to illustrate the dramatic difference they could make.

	Deaths
Of 57 gunshot wounds of knee not treated antiseptically in the first instance	44.5 per cent
Of 15 gunshot wounds of knee-joint with fracture treated antiseptically primarily	6.6 per cent

The Crimean War had started reform of the British medical services, the Russo-Turkish War had much the same effect on the Russian system. It inspired a number of axioms from the great Russian military surgeon, Pirogoff, concerning war medicine and surgery. Chief of them are these:[47]

War is an epidemic of injuries.

Not medical or surgical treatment, but administration, plays the chief part in assistance rendered to the wounded and sick at the theatre of war.

Not quickly performed operations, but a properly organized and conservative treatment, is the chief object of surgical and administrative activity at the theatre of war.

A disorderly crowding together of wounded and sick at dressing stations and in hospitals is particularly to be avoided.

The severely wounded are to be removed as far as possible from the theatre of war.

Immediate removal of bullets, and the performance of primary operations, are not as necessary in present battles as was formerly ruled, and are rarely necessary if life is not in danger. Sieges are an exception to this rule.

The examination of fresh gunshot wounds with probe or finger, opening them further with instruments, and the removal of bone splinters are generally hurtful, and ought only, in exceptional cases, to be undertaken under surgical supervision.

Infection not only spreads by the air, which becomes a source of danger when large numbers of wounded are crowded together in closed rooms, but also by the surroundings of the wounded – linen, bedding, walls, floors, and above all by the attendants.

In treating gunshot wounds, the main points are – rest to the injured part, dressings which immobilize, dressings and suitable position, and also prevention of decomposition changes. Cold, antiphlogistics and low diet suit in exceptional cases; all lowering treatment is hurtful to the soldier, especially towards the end of a long war.

Pirogoff was evidently a student of Napoleon, for the phraseology and tone of his axioms are strikingly similar to Napoleon's famous military maxims. The surgeon's points, apparently profound at the time, are merely expressions of common sense. It is interesting that military surgeons were more amenable to common-sense suggestions than their civilian counterparts. Again and again it was the army or navy doctor who produced the breakthrough in medical knowledge; problems seemed to be solved under the stress of war.

Service medical officers too were masters of analytical reports and comparisons, rarely made for their own sake as similar civil reports tended to be, but in the hope that some doctor would be able to suggest remedies of system or treatment.

One such report[48] was made by Dr T.G. Balfour in comparing the health of British seamen and soldiers during the years 1859–68. His tables are very revealing as historical documents. I have taken those of the Home Station only, since it is perhaps not fully realized that at that time many servicemen suffered a variety of illnesses even in the relatively salubrious climate of the British Isles.

The average annual strength of the naval force, 214,640, on the Home Station during 1859–68 did not differ materially from that of the infantry regiments serving in the United Kingdom during the same period, 233,858.

Since sailors were much more liable by the nature of their duties to accidental injuries and to death from violence, frequently involving – as in the loss of a ship or the upsetting of a boat – considerable numbers of men, Dr Balfour deducted all such cases from the returns of both services before bringing into comparison the relative health of the men.

It is clear that admissions into hospital for diseases (exclusive of accidents and injuries) were proportionally higher among sailors, but that the deaths were 0.70, and discharge on account of disease, 2.28 per 1,000 higher among soldiers. The difference in the mortality rate is probably to a great extent accounted for by the difference of age in the two services. The proportion of boys was 10 per cent in the navy, and a little above 3 per cent in the infantry.

	naval force			infantry regiments		
aggregate strength 1859–68	214,640			233,858		
	admitted into hospital	died	discharged as invalids	admitted into hospital	died	discharged as invalids
total	222,541	1,810	5,855	194,048	1,860	6,106
deduct those from wounds and injuries	39,759	447	442	16,057	212	215
total from diseases	182,782	1,363	5,413	177,991	1,648	5,891
annual ratio per 1,000 of mean strength	852	6.35	25.22	761	7.05	27.50

	naval force		military force (cavalry)	
	exclusive of wounds and injuries ratio per 1,000 of mean strength			
	admitted to hospital	died	admitted to hospital	died
1830–36[49]	983	8.8	803	13.7
1859–68	852	6.35	761	7.05
difference	131	2.45	42	6.65

There is no way of making an accurate comparison of these results with those of some earlier period, since ships on the Home Station were previously grouped into two classes, the 'Home' and the 'Various'. The results of the Home were more favourable than the Various. The only data relating to troops of the line at home for earlier periods refer to the cavalry, among whom the admissions and deaths were generally lower than in the infantry. However, a comparison, even with these more favoured men, shows a significant reduction in both sickness and mortality.

aggregate strength	naval force 214,640				infantry regiments 233,858			
			ratio per 1,000				ratio per 1,000	
	admitted	died	admit	died	admit	died	admit	died
eruptive fevers	1,593	50	7.4	0.23	635	21	2.7	0.09
intermittent fever	1,677	2	7.8	0.01	1,229	4	5.2	0.02
remittent and continued fevers	2,970	119	13.8	0.55	4,481	118	19.2	0.50
dysentery and diarrhoea	7,463	17	34.8	0.08	2,995	14	12.8	0.06
cholera	37	9	0.2	0.04	9	7	0.04	0.03
sore throat	9,436	6	44.0	0.03	5,932	4	25.4	0.02
ophthalmia	2,064		12.1		5,478		23.4	
erysipelas [feverish skin disease]	702	18	3.3	0.08	453	20	1.9	0.08
rheumatism	13,278	8	61.9	0.04	5,300	8	22.7	0.03
syphilis	16,920	3	78.8	0.01	30,594	17	130.8	0.07
gonorrhoea	6,048		28.2		25,635		109.6	
stricture of urethra	717	6	3.4	0.03	578	4	2.5	0.02

Balfour's table showing hospital admissions and deaths from various diseases is profoundly interesting, not primarily because of the navy/army comparison, but because of the disease comparison which shows, for instance, rheumatism as the worst naval scourge and sore throat as the worst army one.

Eruptive fevers were twice as prevalent in the navy, probably because this service had more boys at that period of life when eruptive fevers are more common. Also, on board ship these sufferers would not have been separated from the fit. Measles was rife in the navy in 1860 and 1867, scarlet fever in 1861 and 1863, smallpox in 1860 and 1864. The incidence of dysentery and diarrhoea was higher in the navy because of poorer diet and exposure of sailors to wet and cold; for the same reason sore throat and rheumatism were more prevalent in the navy. Erysipelas probably came about because of poor ventilation aboard.

The venereal disease table produced by Balfour shows great disparity, which he accounted for by soldiers' greater opportunities to contract it.

Other tables showed that soldiers were more vulnerable to scrofula – an unhealthy constitutional condition with glandular swellings – and spitting of blood while sailors were more prone to delirium tremens, the effect of the rum to which so many reformers objected. Again, for reasons of less varied diet, sailors were considerably more prone to boils, abscesses and ulcers.

TUBERCULAR DISEASES

	naval force				infantry regiments			
			ratio per 1,000				ratio per 1,000	
	admit	died	admit	died	admit	died	admit	died
Scrofula [*characterized by degeneration of lymphatic glands*]	270	1	1.2		804	8	3.4	0.03
Phthisis [*consumption*] and haemoptysis [*spitting of blood*]	1,579	423	7.3	1.98	2,648	550	11.3	2.35

In this period too hygiene was becoming more of an integral part of army medical practice, at least in the British Army. The man most responsible for this was Edmund Parkes, a protégé of Florence Nightingale. Parkes was given charge of a hospital at Renkioi near the Dardanelles during the Crimean War in order to lighten the burden on the Scutari hospitals. Following ten years as Professor of Clinical Medicine at University College Hospital, London, he was appointed in 1860 to the Chair of Military Hygiene at the newly formed Army Medical School at Fort Pitt, Chatham. In this post he practically had to create the science he was to teach. During his term of office the design of barracks, hospitals and married quarters great improved – along the lines Dr James Barry had suggested – and the load of the soldier on the march was lightened significantly. Parkes's *Manual of Practical Hygiene*, first published in 1864, remained the standard work of military and civil practice for more than twenty years. On his death he was described by Baron Mundy, Professor of Military Hygiene in Vienna, as 'the founder and best teacher of military hygiene of our day, the friend and benefactor of every soldier'.

DISEASES OF THE NERVOUS SYSTEM

| | naval force | | | | infantry regiments | | | |
| | | | ratio per 1,000 | | | | ratio per 1,000 | |
	admit	died	admit	died	admit	died	admit	died
Delirium tremens	603	19	2.9	0.09	267	19	1.1	0.08
Epilepsy	800	12	3.7	0.06	636	8	2.17	0.30

| | naval force | | infantry regiments | |
	admitted	ratio per 1,000 admitted	admitted	ratio per 1,000 admitted
Boils and abscesses	32,715	152.4	15,485	66.2
Ulcers	14,612	68.1	7,311	31.3

But the way to sound hygiene and sanitation was another long hard road, and while medical officers were taught the principles of this subject they had not enough authority to put them into practice. Some generals were unbelievably wooden and uncooperative. In 1886 General Lord Wolseley described the sanitation officer as the most useless officer in the army and recommended any general saddled with such an 'encumbrance' to leave him at the base. Since Wolseley was for some years commander-in-chief of the British Army it was obvious that hygiene would not make startling progress.

CHAPTER EIGHTEEN

Development of the British Army Medical Service

A better army medical service began with the royal commission appointed in 1857 to inquire into barracks and hospitals. It made a number of suggestions, such as the formation of an army medical school, better pay for staff, the setting up of a hospital corps instead of the medical staff corps. It recommended too that medical officers be given authority to advise commanding officers on all matters relating to soldiers' health, including drill, diet and clothing.

The army medical school opened at Fort Pitt in 1860, and three years later moved to Netley, where it united with the Royal Victoria Hospital, on Southampton Water. This hospital was built at the express command of Queen Victoria, who laid its foundation stone in 1856. Ever since the beginning of the Crimean War, the Queen had fostered the relief of the sick and wounded, and throughout her reign she was keenly interested in military hospitals and in the training of nurses. In 1855 she frequently inspected the hospitals at Fort Pitt and Brompton, encouraging her broken servicemen. After one of her visits she wrote to Lord Panmure, the Secretary of War:

> The Queen is very anxious to bring before Lord Panmure the subject . . . of hospitals for our sick and wounded soldiers. This is absolutely necessary, and *now* is the moment to have them built, for no doubt there would be no difficulty in obtaining the money . . . from the strong feeling now existing in the public mind for improvements of all kinds connected with the Army and the well-being and comfort of the soldier.
>
> Nothing can exceed the attention paid to these poor men in barracks at Fort Pitt and Chatham . . . but the buildings are bad – the wards more like prisons than hospitals, with the windows so high that no one can look out of them; and the generality of the wards are small rooms, with hardly space for you to walk between the beds. There is no dining-room or hall, so the poor men must have their dinners in the same room in which they sleep, and in which some may be dying, and, at any rate, many suffering, whilst others are at their meals.

Netley, until its demolition in 1965, was part of the medical service's tradition, a tradition struggling to find expression in the 1860s.

The Army Hospital Corps had two functions: to provide orderlies for regimental, garrison and general hospitals – two or more of which were built – and stretcher-bearers in the field. The first commitment was soon reduced, for the corps' numbers were insufficient to staff the regimental hospitals; a combined system of hospital corps and regimental orderlies proved unsatisfactory and its duties were limited to general and field hospitals.

The headquarters and depot was at Chatham; this was moved to Netley at the same time as the school, and in 1875 it was transferred to Aldershot, the most important military centre in the country.

The Hospital Corps' ranks were filled by former members of the staff corps and soldier volunteers with over two years' service who were of 'regular, steady habits and good temper, and possessed of a kindly disposition', and had the ability to read and write well. They were, for the first time, on even status with the rest of the army, and ordinary military rank was conferred in place of the old grades. It was considered that its members had superior ability to the rest of the army, and they were expected to be better behaved. By a special order of the commander-in-chief, any orderly who was convicted of drunkenness had his conduct sheet marked. Legend has it that one combatant officer, whenever men of the AHC were brought before him, invariably said: 'Superior Corps, superior pay, superior punishment – 28 days' CB.'★

Better trained than their predecessors, these men showed bravery on the battlefield. Corps members were prominent at Rorke's Drift in the Zululand campaign of 1879, and also in 1881 against the Boers at Majuba, where Lance-Corporal J.J. Farmer won the Victoria Cross. But it was a corps without its own officers, and it lacked discipline, supervision and leadership.

There were a commanding officer and his assistant at the depot, but in the hospitals the men came under ensigns of regiments, who were appointed captains of orderlies and were later designated quartermasters. There was no possibility of maintaining efficiency and building up *esprit de corps*.

If the Army Hospital Corps was for twenty-six years a corps without officers, the army medical department had no subordinates. The royal warrant of 1858, which has been called the medical officers' 'Magna Carta', introduced the first elaborate code for the medical service as a whole, but still left it weak.

The medical department was hardly ever consulted on the higher levels of administration; until 1869 the director-general was not even attached to the military section of the War Office. Medical officers with units were still regimental officers, regarded solely as treaters of disease. The majority spent their entire service with their units and had no opportunity to improve their professional knowledge.

★ Confined to barracks.

However many units there were in a garrison, each had its own separate hospital establishment, buildings, officers, attendants, instructions and medicines. The responsibility for the correct working and the proper condition of these hospitals rested entirely with the commanding officer. The whole thing was absurdly inefficient and wasteful. In Germany the medical service was thoroughly efficient and in many ways exemplary; the system of regimental hospitals had long before been abandoned and the army now had the most perfect departmental system in Europe.[50] Just how efficient it was came out during Prussia's wars against Austria and France, and the obvious lessons were, this time, learnt, and the British Army Medical Service had its first fundamental change.

In 1873 all regimental hospitals, except those of the Guards and Household Cavalry, were abolished and replaced by garrison establishments, complete with chemical laboratories, libraries, museums and expert instruction. And all medical officers ceased to be regimental officers and came under the medical department.

Regiments and many senior officers violently opposed the new system, and to make the pill more palatable some concessions were made. Each regiment was permitted to retain the services of a particular MO for a term of years, different corps or units were allotted specific, separate wards in hospitals and their sick, as far as possible, were kept under the care of their own officers and orderlies. It was a quite needless rearguard action.

The new system now made it possible for the medical department to plan an organization in the field in case of war. This, frankly copied from the Prussian model, attached a medical officer to each battalion or equivalent unit, which was to provide sixteen stretcher-bearers, and founded the bearer company responsible for collecting all wounded on the battlefield and getting them to field hospitals.

The French had long had their *soldats infirmiers* – the battlefield bearers. Thoroughly trained at the Val de Grâce, the military medical college, by

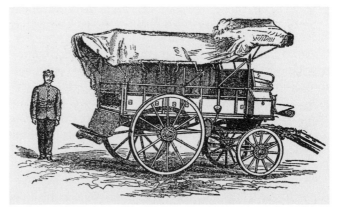

The ambulance wagon used in the British Army in about 1880.

the *médecin-en-chef* and his surgeons, these men were reliable assistants in field hospitals.

Bearer companies in the British Army date their origin from 1876, but the first bearer company employed in war was organized during the last phase of the Zulu War, 1879. Commanded by Surgeon-Major J. Hector, it did great service during the storming of Secocoeni's stronghold in 1879. In 1881 a bearer company was organized for war, complete in personnel and equipment. In this year too the Army Nursing Service was instituted.

Doctors were not averse to donning the mantle of Mars over the cape of Aesculapius. Surgeon-Major W.A. McKinnon, who would later be a director-general of the medical corps, serving in New Zealand in 1866, led a successful attack on a fortified position when regimental officers had become casualties. At Rorke's Drift, 1879, Surgeon J.H. Reynolds not only constantly tended wounded under fire but helped defend the hospital and won the VC.

A bearer company in the Suakin Expeditionary Force, 1882, went into action at the battle of Giniss, and joined in the pursuit of Osman Digna. In the Egyptian campaign of 1882, 163 medical officers and 820 other ranks of the Army Hospital Corps served eight field hospitals and two bearer companies. After the battle of Tel-el-Kebir the commander-in-chief, Wolseley, reported: 'I never saw men better cared for, and the removal of the wounded was very well done.'

Criticism of nursing in the field hospitals led in 1883 to a parliamentary commission, which came to the conclusion that inadequate nursing resulted from lack of control and supervision. It recommended, among other things, amalgamation of the army medical department and the Army Hospital Corps into a royal corps.

But what looked like a promising new birth was, in fact, abortive. The plan promulgated in September 1884 denied full military status to medical officers and soon after this even relative ranks – such as surgeon-major – were abolished. So much ill feeling developed between the medical profession and the War Office over this point and many others that practically all the medical schools refused to supply candidates for the army and soon even peace-time requirements could not be met. A twelve-year boycott was broken when the British Medical Association locked horns with the War Office and forced it to concede all the points at issue.

After this period of stagnation and dissatisfaction the army medical service was in a poor state. It had no dentists, ophthalmologists – no man in the army was allowed to wear spectacles – psychiatrists or anaesthetists. The general surgeons dealt with the specialized problems of ears, noses and throats. The Royal Army Medical Corps, when it came into being on 23 June 1898, had a lot of leeway to make up. Its motto, *In Arduis Fidelis*, was appropriate enough for a class of man who had endured so much adversity over the centuries.

The new corps saw its first active service that same year, at Omdurman. Sir Herbert Kitchener, the expedition commander, reported: 'The general medical arrangements were all that could be desired, and I believe that the minimum of pain and the maximum of comfort procurable on active service in this country were attained by the unremitting energy, the untiring zeal and devotion to duty by the entire medical staff.'

One of the medical staff was Lieutenant Colonel A.T. Sloggett, who was shot through the breast and lungs and reported dead in the casualty list. Later, on more detailed examination, it appeared just possible that life was not extinct. Sloggett's colleagues worked at reviving him. In three days the wound had closed, and in a month the patient had recovered. In 1901, during the South African War, Sloggett commanded a hospital at Deelfontein, and during the First World War was a notable administrator.

In view of the great challenges the medical services would face in 1899 and 1914 it was as well that they were finally on their feet and on a par with those of the European powers. At this beginning it would be useful to look back briefly at the accomplishments of some of the doctors who served the medical arm of the British forces. By no means comprehensive, it does give an idea of the vigour with which doctors pursued various aspects of military medicine. It is due to service medical officers that suitable barracks were erected, that a definite proportion of space per man was allotted; that in malarial districts upper-storied barracks were provided, that suitable rations in quality and variety were issued, that clothing was issued with regard to climate and nature of duties, that canteens were established as a check to drunkenness, that buildings suitable as hospitals were founded, that hospital diets made allowance for the requirements of the sick, that a restriction, as far as practicable, was placed upon the length of night duty, drills and exercises to which the troops were subjected. Recreation rooms, gymnasiums, temperance associations, savings banks and schools were first advocated by service doctors. There are other more specific accomplishments:

Medicine. To John Hunter is due the credit of having, by his experimental researches and investigations, done more to advance the art of healing than was probably achieved by any other man, though Thomas Sydenham, who fought with the Roundheads, is usually known as the 'father of British medicine'.*

Cholera. Girdlestone in India, Lind in England and Cleghorn in Minorca wrote on this great killer.

Typhus. The prevalence of typhus fever in armies was discussed by Pringle, Monro and McGrigor.

Diabetes. Rollo published a work in 1797.

---

* In the seventeenth century the practice of medicine was passing through a serious crisis, and it is to Sydenham, through his revival of the Hippocratic system, that modern medicine owes its origin.

Beri-beri. This disease, which afflicted troops in Ceylon, was first described scientifically by Marshall, and later by Ballingall and Malcolmson.

Malta Fever. In 1863 Marston published a report on Malta fever as a disease distinct from enteric fever, with which it had previously been confused. Bruce, posted to Malta in 1884, isolated from the spleens of nineteen out of twenty fatal cases the organism of the Malta fever infection which is now known as *Brucella melitensis.* This was a brilliant piece of research, but not until 1904 was Bruce able to show how the disease was acquired by man. The source was in goat's milk.

Yellow Fever. The greater part of literature on this subject comes from army and navy officers. Early authors were Cleghorn and Irvine; Bancroft wrote on the disease in 1807, Pym 1815 and 1848. Fellows produced a report on epidemic form of the disease in Spain, 1802. Chisholm, Lemprière, Gilchrist and Smith also wrote on it.

Remittent or Paludal Fever. Pringle, McGrigor, Jackson, Henderson (3rd Light Dragoons) and Mouatt all supplied information.

Dysentery and Hepatitis. Pringle, Fergusson, Veitch, Forbes and Somers, all men of high reputation, brought about improvements in treatment. Pringle was the first to use the Mexican drug ipecacuanha. Chisholm and Marshall wrote of the disease and Fergusson in the West Indies noticed that there was a regular increase of hepatitis after soldiers had received their pay. Murray, in India, was probably the first to test the advantages of puncturing and exploring the viscus in cases of abscess.

Inflammation. Thomson published a valuable work on this subject. Hunter elucidated the process of adhesion, a doctrine described by John Bell as having done more for surgery than any other general observation, not excepting the circulation of the blood. Guthrie first treated erysipelas by means of free incisions.

Syphilis. Clowes, in the sixteenth century, recommended mercury to be used in the treatment of this disease. Wiseman advocated the same views. Hunter instituted a theory and laid down a method of treatment for the disease, neither of which was superseded for nearly a century. Hennen believed that different forms of ulcer might follow from one infection – a question which attracted the attention of Franklin and McGrigor, who ordered a series of statistics to test the theory.

Ophthalmia. McGrigor described the history of this disease in Egypt. In 1820 Veitch (52nd Regiment) published a work on the disease, which he considered contagious, a view supported by Peach, surgeon of the same battalion, by

Forbes, surgeon of the Royals, and by Marshall: Hennen described the way in which soldiers induced the disease, especially after the passing of Windham's Act, which allowed pensions to men disabled by ophthalmia. Guthrie wrote extensively on this and all other species of ocular disease.

Malaria. The work of officers of the Indian Army was important, though a young French Army doctor, Laveran, was the first, in 1880, to describe the malarial parasite. Ross, in 1897, demonstrated that a female anopheles mosquito had become infected from a patient with malaria. He won the Nobel Prize in 1902. Another army contributor to malarial research was S.P. James. Malaria had always been the major health problem in India.

Aneurism. Hunter brought about the first real improvement in treatment – the application of the ligature to the affected vessel at a healthy part and nearer to the centre of the circulation than the dilatation itself. Hennen wrote on the manner of treating aneurism and Tuffnell advocated treatment of aneurism by compression.

Tetanus. Badenoch (59th Regiment) described the disease as seen in Java in 1811; and McLaggan, Guthrie, Hennen and McGrigor published works on the subject.

Ulcers. Home was among the earliest authors who stated principles for treatment of ulcers. Marshall wrote a description of the various forms among troops in Ceylon; and Ballingall gave accounts of them in Java and Rangoon.

Guinea Worm. The literature of this disease is almost entirely due to army surgeons, chiefly Chisholm, McGrigor and Bruce (88th Regiment).

Physiology of the Stomach. Modern knowledge is largely due to sustained observations by the American army surgeon Beaumont, 1795–1853, on the gastric ulcer which resulted from a musket wound suffered by the Canadian half-breed, Alexis St Martin.

Pathology. The whole science of pathology owes much to Aitken, who was appointed Professor of Pathology at the Army Medical School in 1860.

Drunkenness. Scarcely a medical officer of the eighteenth and nineteenth centuries failed to deplore drunkenness and to urge its repression. Those who submitted proposals to check it include Blane, Trotter, Lind, Lemprière, Gordon, Jackson and Marshall.

Change of Air. The advantages from change of climate were long recognized by army surgeons. In 1794 Rollo pointed out that fever cases often relapsed because they could not convalesce in healthy localities. Lemprière gave many examples of the advantages of moving troops from infected localities. In 1811 Wright recommended that the soldiers who were still suffering from the fever of Walcheren should be sent to Malta or other warm climates. His proposals were adopted with good results.

Soldiers' Wives and Children. Hamilton was the first to advocate the cause of soldiers' wives and children. He urged the necessity as well as the policy of treating them well.

Wounds. Clowes was among the earliest English authors on wounds 'made with gunshot, sword, halberde, pike, launce or such other'. Gale introduced a styptic powder. John Bell gave instructions on treatment of wounds of the intestines and suggested various sutures to induce adhesion of cut surfaces. 'A man should not of necessity be cut because he had the misfortune to be shot,' he wrote. Boyle (62nd Foot) published some illustrative cases of the same treatment. Thomson, with John Bell, advanced the method of treating gunshot wounds of the chest. He published an account of fourteen cases of gunshot wound of the bladder, and gave rules for treating such injuries. Wiseman, 'the father of British surgery', discussed whether gunshot wounds were or were not poisonous. Hunter taught that, in certain cases, 'balls when obliged to be left, seldom or ever did any harm when at rest, and not in a vital part'; and Guthrie pointed out that in such cases a membranous sac formed around the missile. Guthrie was the first to show that wounds of the diaphragm do not close, and to lay down definite rules regarding trephining in cases of injuries of the skull. He taught the principles of treating penetrating wounds of the chest. Hennen was another notable author on these subjects. Rose (Coldstream Guards) published an account of the injuries sustained by men of his regiment at the battle of Toulouse, 1813. Longmore, Professor of Military Surgery at the Army Medical School, 1860, is sometimes spoken of as the father of modern war surgery and during his thirty-one years' tenure he had great influence on the treatment of wounds.

Amputation. Gale, writing in 1563, deplored the horrible method then in use of performing amputations, observing that 'the heated irons so feared the people with the horror of cauterization that many of them rather would die with the member on than abide the terrible fire by means whereof many people perished'. The first improvement suggested seems to have come from Woodall, who recommended that the operation should be performed through a joint, since this caused less surgical shock and did not expose flesh and blood vessels to the same extent. Wiseman, and after him Hanby, advocated primary operation after wounds, as against the delayed; views in which they were later supported by Hume, Hennen, Thomson, Guthrie and Ballingall. Hunter advocated excision of the joints in certain cases as a substitute for the larger operation. Guthrie, while he proved the advantages as a rule of the primary operation in cases of gunshot wounds, advocated delay in certain cases for a few hours to enable a patient to rally from the shock of the first injury. Ballingall, in his work on military surgery, discussed the relative merits of primary and secondary amputation, and those of circular or flap operation.

Ligature of Arteries. The Frenchman, Paré, was the first surgeon who systematically employed ligatures for arteries, and who gave definite instructions for their application. Early in the seventeenth century he was followed in this practice by Woodall, who recommended use of the needle and ligature for occlusion of vessels after amputation. Monro urged the necessity of taking up the arteries with as few as possible of the surrounding tissues after amputation, and condemned the system of placing a compress between one side of the vessel and the noose of the thread. John Bell demonstrated the possibility of the limb being nourished by cross-connecting vessels after its larger arteries had been tied.

Post-mortem examinations were practised in the army by Cleghorn before they were so in civil practice. Brocklesby, Pringle and Home all advocated this method of investigating the action of disease.

Plan of the Medical Arrangements of an English Army Corps (overleaf)

This diagram shows every Regiment, Battalion, and Battery in an Army Corps, as also the number of units in each Division (seven Battalions of Infantry, one Regiment of Cavalry, three Batteries of Artillery, one Company Sappers, two Bearer Companies, and Four Field Hospitals.

In the rear of each unit is the Battalion, Battery, or Regimental Surgeon with the Regimental Bearers, two to four men per Company. The dotted lines show the path of the wounded to the two Bearer Companies of the Medical Staff Corps, with each Division, which must not be confounded with the *Regimental* Bearers working under the Battalion Surgeons (Bearer Company, four officers, fifty-seven men, MSC).

Behind the two Bearer Companies are the four Field Hospitals of each Division, each Hospital equipped for 100 Beds, and manned by the Medical Staff Corps (five officers and thirty-four men each). These Hospitals are supplied with Transport, and march with the Army.

In their rear, on the road leading to the front, is the Advanced Medical Store Depot of the Army Corps, supplying medicines to the front.

The winding road is the Line of Communications, which may be from 100 to 200 miles long, and which extends from the Base of operations to the Army in front. Along it are placed at the various *Etappen* posts the eight Stationary Hospitals of the

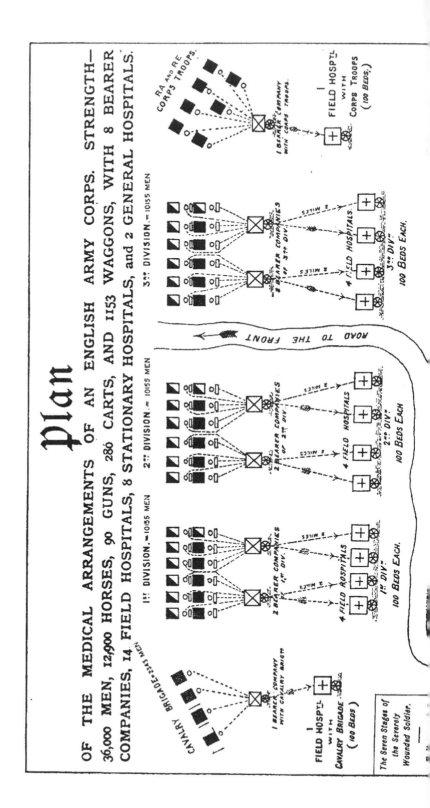

Plan

OF THE MEDICAL ARRANGEMENTS OF AN ENGLISH ARMY CORPS. STRENGTH— 36,000 MEN, 12,900 HORSES, 90 GUNS, 286 CARTS, AND 1153 WAGGONS, WITH 8 BEARER COMPANIES, 14 FIELD HOSPITALS, 8 STATIONARY HOSPITALS, and 2 GENERAL HOSPITALS.

The Seven Stages of the Severely Wounded Soldier.

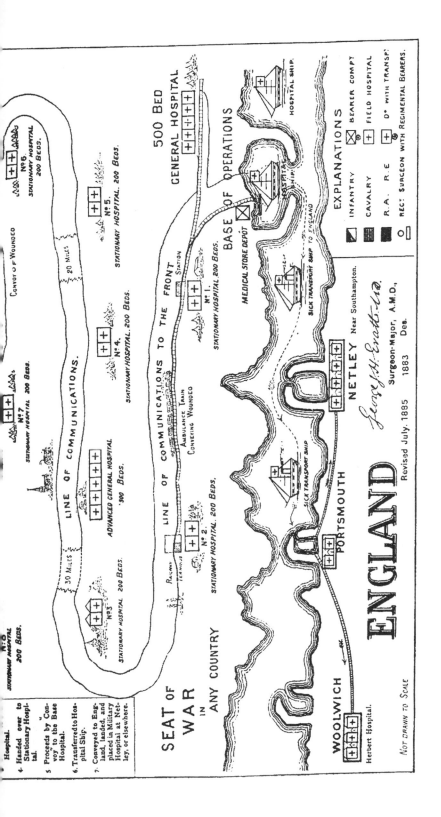

Line of Communications, each accommodating 200 wounded, and each manned by ten officers and sixty-five men of the MSC. The sick and wounded returning from the front are conveyed by 'Sick Convoy' either in waggons, ambulance trains, or by steamer from stage to stage until the Base is reached.

The winding road is so drawn to save paper. One of the General Hospitals (500 beds) is placed at the Base of operations, and is called the Base Hospital; the second General Hospital may be placed where most needed. (General Hospital 21 officers and 123 men, MSC).

The Ships are the Hospital Ships at the Base of operations, and the Sick Transport Ships conveying the wounded and sick from the Base to Netley, Portsmouth and Woolwich. (Hospital Ship 200 beds, 8 officers, 42 men, MSC).

The Volunteer Forces need one Bearer Company, and one Field Hospital for each Regimental District. These units to be made up of Volunteer Medical Staff Corps Officers and Men, in addition to all existing regimental aid.

GEORGE J.H. EVATT, MD, *Surgeon-Major, Army Medical Staff.*

Woolwich, August, 1885.

Total Medical Staff Corps with Army Corps

262	Medical Officers.
34	Quarter-Masters.
2041	Men, counting Batmen but excluding Regimental Bearers.
1	Surgeon-General P.M.O. Army Corps.
1	Surgeon-General P.M.O. Communications.
1	Deputy Surgeon-General, as Sanitary Officer.
1	Deputy-Surgeon-General, P.M.O. each Division.
1	D.S.G. as P.M.O. Base; 1 D.S.G. each General Hospital.

CHAPTER NINETEEN

The Boer War and a Harsh Lesson

The Boer or South African War of 1899–1902 was a more distressing war for physicians than surgeons, for the British Army still would not accept the necessity for good hygiene and sanitation.

Though only 22,000 troops were treated by the RAMC for wounds, injuries and accidents through the thirty months of operations, twenty times that number were admitted to hospital with disease; 74,000 suffered from enteric and dysentery alone – both preventable diseases. Over 8,000 died from enteric. The degree to which such inroads into manpower influenced the conduct and duration of the campaign is inestimable.

Few doctors could have been surprised by any of this. The post of sanitation officer had been abolished against their advice, the regimental officers still regarded as beneath their interest all matters concerning the health of their men. When they did condescend to consider health they at once delegated the matter to a sergeant. The troops were not given even a smattering of knowledge about personal hygiene, such as washing of the hands or eating utensils. Facilities for purifying water were practically non-existent, and camps which came up to a regimental sergeant-major's standards were often, from a doctor's standpoint, dangerously unclean.

Fever broke out early in the war as the thirsty troops drank freely from the muddy, germ-ridden Modder River – it had 'mair of a bite', a Scottish soldier said – from polluted supplies in besieged Ladysmith, and it took on the proportions of an epidemic when the army halted for six weeks in Bloemfontein, capital of Orange Free State, in the spring of 1900. At one period there were as many as 5,000 cases at a time in the town's hospitals, and forty deaths a day.

Typhoid was another scourge, a disease far more dangerous than Boer bullets, against which Surgeon Sir William Leishman waged a successful campaign. Conditions were generally difficult for surgeons; they were pestered by flies in a dust-laden atmosphere, water was often scarce and supplies, because of the great distances, irregular.

The soldiers would have ignored lice as cheerfully as they ignored the foulness of water, but lice are difficult to ignore, and it became customary for regiments, on halting, to strip and pick off the *anoplura*. As a private said to Surgeon Shipley:[51] 'We strips and we picks 'em off and places 'em in the sun, and it kind o' breaks the little beggars' 'earts.' Unfortunately soldiers could not be dissuaded from scratching or from touching their eyes after insect bites, and this led to more infection.

A private soldier, A.F. Corbett,[52] who fell a victim to enteric on the march to Johannesburg, left an account of his evacuation to hospital at Springfontein. About two dozen were packed in open coal-trucks, but they were beyond caring, and all desperately in need of something to drink. At Springfontein several men died and were buried there. The survivors were issued with a tin of condensed milk between eight.

> On arriving at our next station we were encamped in small marquees, about ten in each. We lost quite a number of men at this hospital, one or another being carried out each morning. . . . I happened to be blessed with a good sense of humour, always joking no matter what happened . . . always saying to myself, 'Thank goodness it is no worse.' One morning another poor fellow in the next bed said, 'You'll be the next.' I turned by head to him and replied, 'Not while you're there, Jock,' and sure enough he turned slightly green in the night and would not stay in bed, so the orderlies tied him to the bed with sheets. But he had gone in the morning. . . .

The inroads made by disease can be clearly seen against the statistics of efforts to fight it. The medical department mobilized 151 staff and regimental units, 19 bearer companies, 28 field hospitals, 5 stationary hospitals, 16 general hospitals, 3 hospital trains, 2 hospital ships, 3 advance depots and 2 base depots of medical stores, as well as many units raised locally in South Africa. More than 21,000 hospital beds were in use, apart from accommodation in the field hospitals. By the end of the war the RAMC had had 8,500 men through its ranks plus 800 trained nurses of the Army Nursing Service.

If the picture of disease was depressingly familiar, that of wound treatment was impressively different, partly because of the 'first field dressing' each soldier now carried. A small package, it contained two sterile dressings in waterproof covers, each consisting of a gauze pad stitched to a bandage together with a safety pin. The idea originated with the Prussians and was officially introduced into the British service in 1884, though there is reference to the dressing before that time. A soldier was supposed to be able to apply a dressing to himself if not too badly wounded, or to a comrade.*

In one analytical series of 214 cases of chest wounds only 30 died – a mortality rate of 14 per cent. In the contemporary Spanish-American and Manchurian wars the same low rate applied, despite treatment inferior to

---

* The author used these dressings several times on other soldiers during the 1939–45 war. In some cases they certainly kept infection from wounds.

that given British troops. The cause for the more favourable issue of war wounds of this period has been attributed to the practice of antiseptic treatment of wounds. George Gask, however, believed that the improvement was due to the character of the weapon – the powerful Mauser rifle – that inflicted the wounds, rather than to the method of dressing applied.[53]

The Mauser, at a distance of 5 yards, was capable of driving a bullet 55 inches into a log of pinewood. In one patient Surgeon G.H. Makins traced the path of a Mauser bullet from its entry at the occipital protuberance. It traversed the muscles of the neck, passed through the thoracic cavity, fractured the third and fourth and grooved the seventh and eighth dorsal vertebrae, grooved the seventh and eighth and fractured the ninth and tenth ribs, traversed the muscles of the back and finally lodged against the hip bone – 25 inches in all.

The same conditions – high muzzle velocity, small bore, cone-shaped bullet – responsible for the length and directness of the tracks, accounted for the frequently multiple character of the wounds implicating either the limbs or viscera – lung, stomach, liver; neck, thorax, abdomen, pelvis, thigh. Also for the frequent infliction of two or more separate tracks by the same bullet – arm and forearm with the elbow in the flexed position; both legs, or both legs, penis and scrotum; leg, thigh and abdomen, with a flexed knee; arm and trunk. It was remarkable how often the same bullet would wound two or more separate men, not infrequently wounding lightly the first man and inflicting a fatal injury on the second. The bullet's small calibre allowed the neatest and most exact multiple injuries. A soldier who was crawling on all fours was hit on the flexed middle digit of the hand. The bullet entered at the base of the nail, first emerged at the junction of the finger bones, re-entered between the wrist and hand, and finally emerged from the back of the wrist. An old type ball would simply have smashed his hand.

In marked contrast to earlier wars, bullets rarely carried foreign bodies into the wounds, though Surgeon Makins saw several instances in which portions of cigarette cases and in one instance small pieces of glass from a pocket mirror were carried in without any obvious ill effect. Clothing was not often carried in, the khaki being clearly perforated, but the thick woollen kilts of the Highlanders, and thick flannel shirts, occasionally furnished fragments. The frequency with which portions of kilt were introduced was the strongest surgical objection to its retention as part of uniform on active service.

The Boer War provided some remarkable instances of psychological disturbance. A patient wounded over the cervical spine, and who suffered later with a slight degree of spinal concussion, emitted an involuntary shriek like that of a wounded hare on being struck. Another, after receiving a Martini rifle wound of the chest, lost all sense of his surroundings for several hours and spent a long time trying to write on a white stone lying near him on the veldt. Suddenly realizing his position he was baffled in trying to account for his actions.

Reactions varied from battle to battle. After the battles of Belmont and Graspan the patients reached hospital in high spirits, minimized their injuries and wanted to return to the front, while after the battle of Magersfontein the men were depressed and miserable, shock was more pronounced, and their sufferings were undoubtedly greater.

A striking instance of the entire absence of initial pain was shown by a man shot through the buttock, the bullet then traversing the abdomen. This soldier remained unaware that he had been hit until on undressing he found blood in his trousers and exclaimed: 'Why, I have got this bloody dysentery!' But his internal injuries were severe enough to lead to death thirty-six hours later.

Retained bullets sometimes caused surprises. One man had a retained bullet in the pelvis. During the voyage home he had an attack of retention of urine and a catheter would not pass. He was placed in a warm bath and shortly after he passed a Mauser bullet through the urinary duct, and thus saved himself a bladder probe through the penis.

Some wound cases puzzled surgeons, even in collaboration. A soldier was wounded at Paardeberg by a bullet which entered the inner side of the leg and emerged about two inches above the cleft of the knee on the outer side. Dressings were applied, and a week later the man arrived at base hospital with little apparent trouble in the knee joint. He was put to bed and warned against movement but on the second day walked to the latrine. When bending his knee to sit he had an agonizing pain in the joint and had to call for help. He was carried back to bed in a collapsed condition. The knee commenced to swell; there was rise of temperature and great pain, together with extreme restlessness. Major Burton, after consulting Surgeon Makins, incised the knee-joint bilaterally. No improvement followed, and a week later Major Burton amputated through the thigh. An attack of secondary haemorrhage a few days later combined with septic infection ended the soldier's life. The surgeons could not be sure what caused this death.

Other men survived for some time after appalling wounds. A Highlander, lying to fire at Rooiport, was hit in the skull by a ricocheting bullet fired from 1,000 yards. The wound was large enough for the surgeon to put three fingers into a mass of pulped brain and brain matter, and bone fragments were found in the external wound. The bullet passed on through the base of the skull and eventually lodged after causing more damage. Semi-conscious, he was carried off the field, the wound was cleaned and the bone fragments removed. Then he spent three days in a wagon *en route* to hospital; the wound became infected and the soldier died on the fourteenth day from general septicaemia.

Another Highlander was hit by a shell fragment which perforated his top lip by an irregular aperture and struck his upper set of false teeth in such a way as to turn the posterior edge of the plate towards the tongue, which was cut in half transversely through its base. The soldier, still able to speak distinctly, said that the plate had been driven down his throat, but nothing was palpable either in the throat or on external examination of the neck. On the second day swelling of the neck developed, especially on the left side, and signs of laryngeal obstruction became prominent. The surgeon administered chloroform, but when he put his finger into the cavity at the back of the throat the man's respiration failed and a hasty tracheotomy had to be performed. No foreign body was palpable with the finger in the pharynx. Tracheitis and septic pneumonia developed, and the man died of acute septicaemia thirty-six hours later. Death occurred just as the division received marching orders, and no post-mortem examination was made.

Wounds of the scrotum were not uncommon in South Africa, especially in connection with perforation of the upper thigh. Makins saw wounds of the testicles on several occasions, but in only one was castration necessary. He was told of one case in which destruction of a testicle was followed by an attack of melancholia, culminating in the soldier's suicide. Wounds of the penis also occurred, but as a rule were unimportant, surgically anyway.

The medical service was severely criticized in Britain, and after the war a royal commission examined these criticisms. It was obvious from all evidence that mistakes had been made, but Lord Roberts and Lord Kitchener, both of whom had been commanders-in-chief, pointed out that the medical service was not inefficient; it had been saddled with greater handicaps than it could cope with in its embryo shape. The commission concluded that 'in no campaign have the sick and wounded been so well looked after as they have been in this'. The many foreign observers who roamed the campaign areas apparently thought so, for many aspects of British practice were transplanted to other armies. In the Russo-Japanese War of 1904–5, for example, bacteriology and hygiene were taken seriously, with the result that the Russians, while losing 34,000 men killed in action, had only 9,000 die from disease.

The RAMC had suffered its own casualties: 21 officers, 293 others. The corps won 6 VCs, 12 CBs, 27 CMGs, 27 DSOs, and 38 DCMs. Only the Royal Artillery could claim a greater number of distinctions.

A surgeon-captain, Arthur Martin-Leake, then serving with the South African Constabulary, a military unit, won a Victoria Cross for gallantry on 8 February 1902.* He went out to the firing line to dress the wounds of a soldier under heavy fire from about forty Boers only a hundred yards away. Then, tending a badly wounded officer, he was himself shot three times, in right arm and left thigh.

---

* Kitchener, to whom the original recommendation was made, was disinclined to endorse it, as Martin-Leake had done nothing more than his 'manifest duty'. Martin-Leake was awarded a second VC for gallantry on 19 October 1914; later he died of wounds. Two of the only three double VCs were won by medical officers; the other was Captain N.G. Chavasse, RAMC (see p. 165).

The Boer War had, like the continental wars, involved large numbers of men, and it was all the more obvious that if this trend continued the medical services would need to be prepared for it. Much of the success of the efforts to bring about this preparation was due to General Sir Alfred Keogh, director-general 1905–10, and to the support he had from Lord Haldane, the War Secretary. The medical school was transferred from Netley to London, where it was reopened as the Royal Army Medical College. A school of sanitation was opened at Aldershot in 1906 to train regimental officers and NCOs who formed the nucleus of hygiene detachments within their units; this was the first formal move of the British Army towards hygiene. Regular courses of instruction were given at all the major military establishments and the subject became part of officers' examinations. By 1914 the British Army was better equipped than any other in knowledge of field sanitary science. Intensive research was carried out into water filters, and water-carts with sterilizing apparatus were built. In a War Office reorganization in 1904 the director-general was given status only one step below the adjutant-general, which meant that doctors could now make themselves heard in military planning. The old Army Nursing Service became, after 1902, Queen Alexandra's Imperial Nursing Service and had its duties rationalized.

In 1906, on doctors' suggestions, the Field Ambulance was instituted. Combining the functions of the bearer company and the field hospital, it was divided into bearer and tent divisions. This was followed by the clearing hospital, the forerunner of the casualty clearing-station and the pivot on which turned the removal of sick and wounded. It received casualties from the field ambulance units and distributed them to other Royal Ambulance Corps units in the rear. All this reorganization was supported by the formation of various reserves and volunteer units. The whole radical reorganization shaped the RAMC into a formidable medical force. It was late in arriving compared with the German, Swiss, Austrian and French medical services; in some respects even the Russian service had been more developed. But it was to become the most efficient of them all.

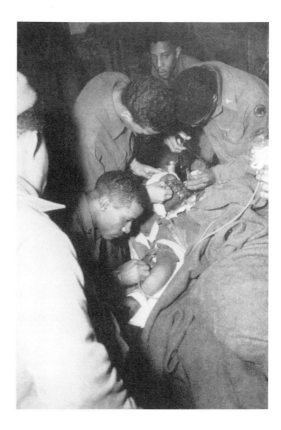

An officer wounded in Italy, 1943, receives treatment from the medics of the Black segregated 92nd Infantry Division. (US Signal Corps)

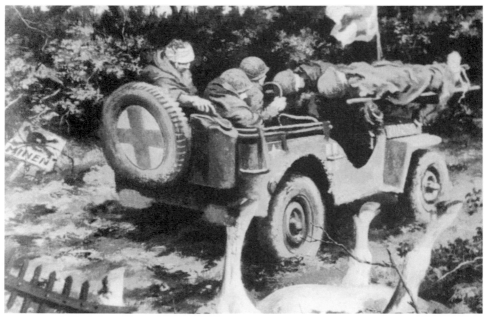

Wounded are driven to safety through a minefield. (US Signal Corps photograph of a painting by Lawrence Beall Smith)

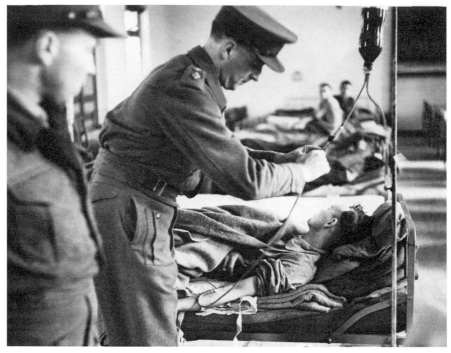

A blood transfusion for a soldier whose leg has been amputated, France 1944. (RAMC)

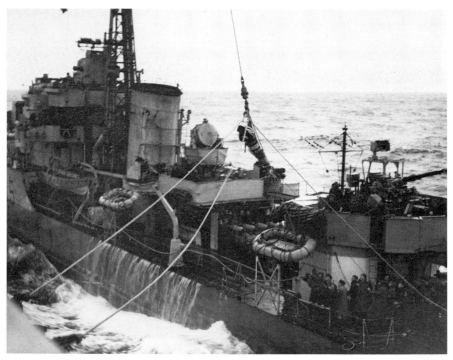

The hazardous task of getting a patient safely lifted to a hospital ship is finally accomplished. (Royal Navy photograph)

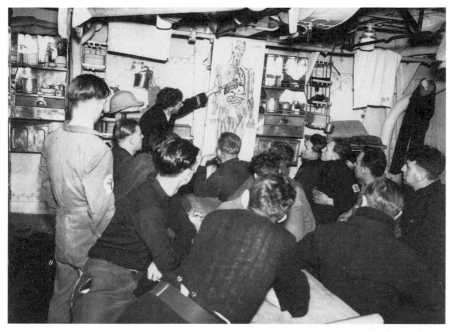

During a convoy to Russia a surgeon lieutenant gives a lecture on first aid in the torpedomen's mess deck, which was used as a sick bay during an emergency. (Royal Navy)

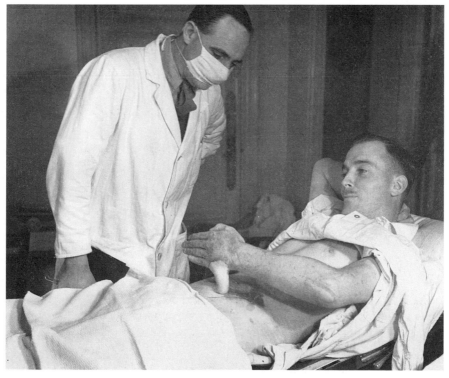

Skin grafting after a wound was a slow and delicate operation. This man, wounded during the Second World War, is having skin grafted from his abdomen to his wrist.

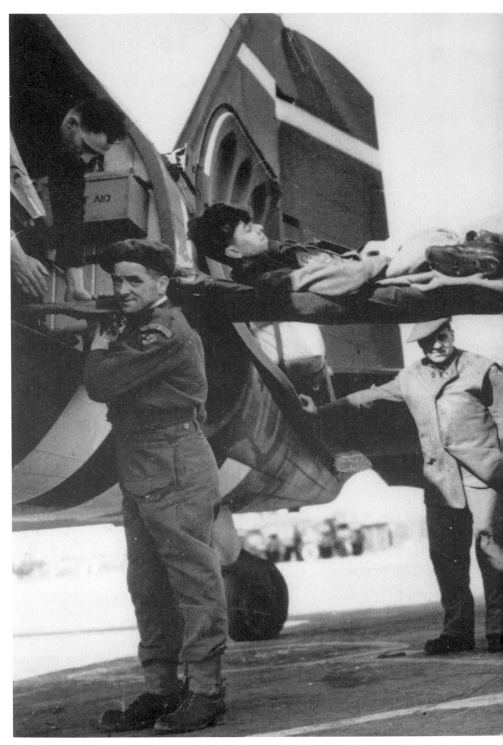
A soldier wounded in France, 1944, is unloaded from an RAF Transport Command Dakota at

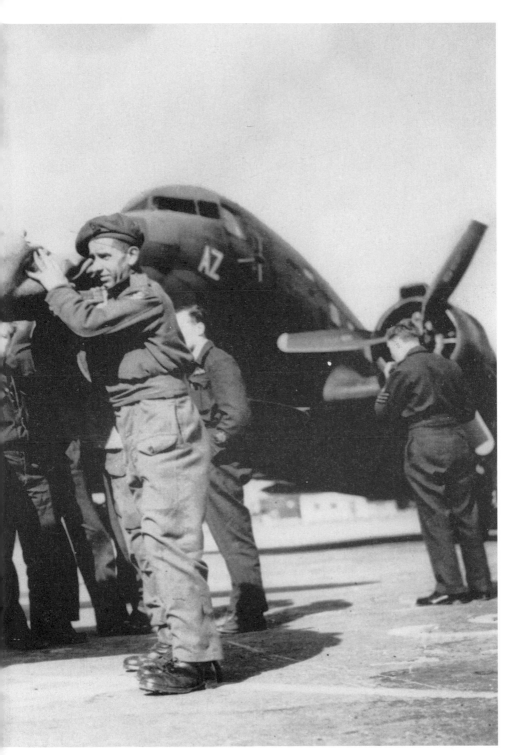

an airfield in England. The casualty's boots came with him. (RAF)

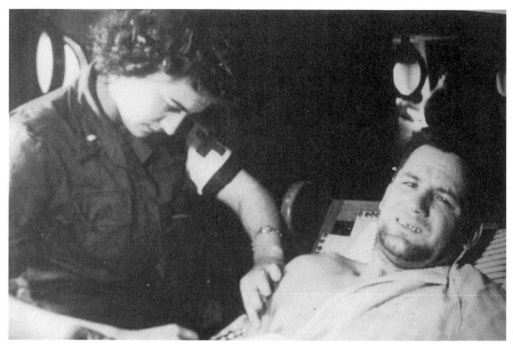
An American nurse administers life-saving penicillin to a soldier who is being evacuated by sea from the fighting in Normandy to a hospital in Britain, summer 1944. (US Signal Corps)

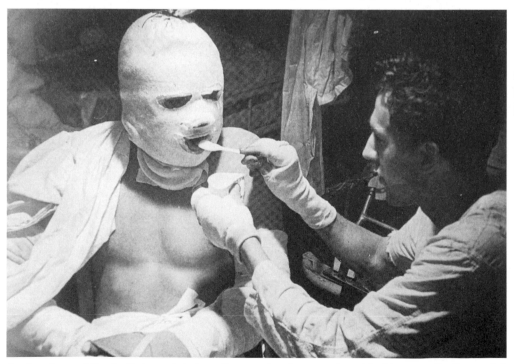
An American soldier, badly burned during a Japanese kamikaze attack on his ship in the Pacific, needed medical help to perform every function, 1944. (US Navy)

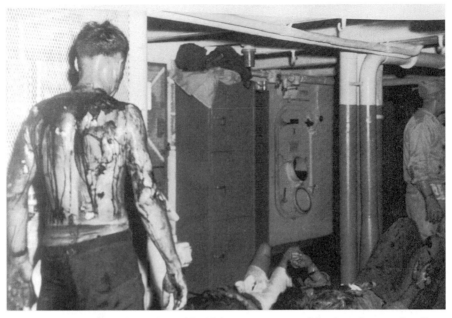

A burned and bleeding sailor walks to his ship's treatment centre following a Japanese kamikaze attack off the Philippines, 1944. (US Navy)

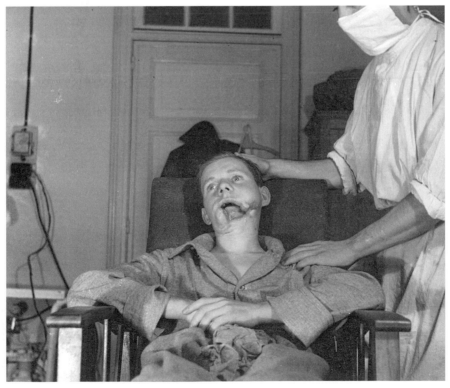

A German prisoner of war with a large part of his mandible blown away, France 1944. He received the same expert attention as that given to British soldiers. (Imperial War Museum)

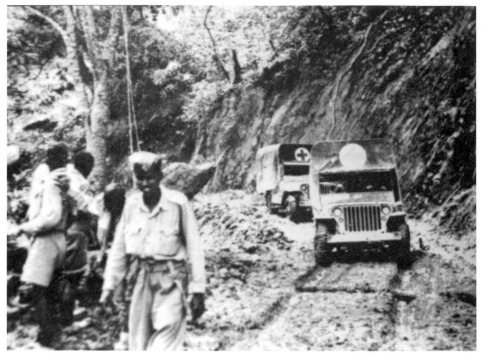

A Jeep ambulance convoy brings wounded back to hospitals in Burma, 1944. Some did not survive the gruelling evacuation process. (US Army)

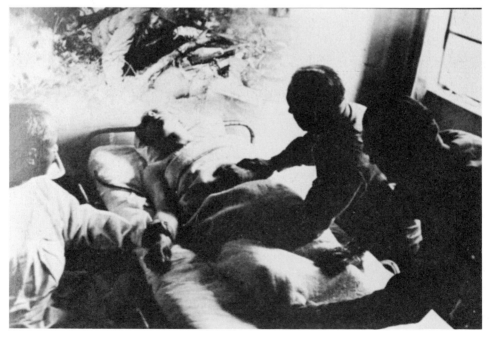

A rear hospital of the US Army Medical Corps. The doctors are dealing with an extreme case of battle fatigue from the fighting in Germany, 1945. Treatment included sedation with sodium amytal stimulation with insulin and light hypnosis, with scenes of combat screened on the wall. (US Army)

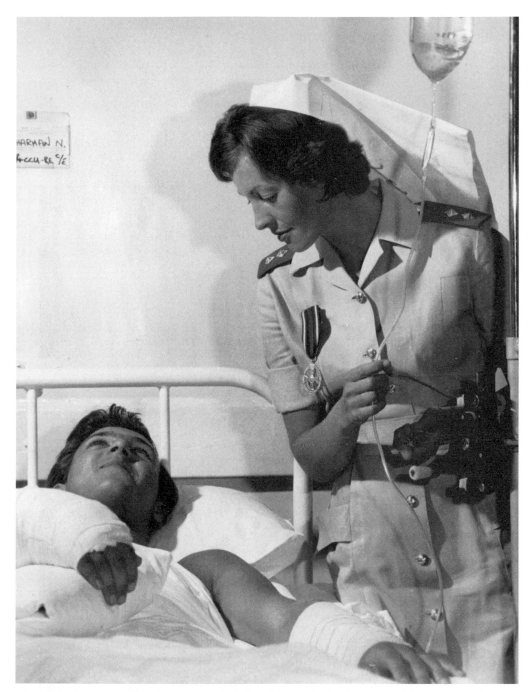

Lieutenant Margaret Ford of Queen Alexandra's Royal Army Nursing Service administers a saline drip to a patient in Cyprus, 1966.

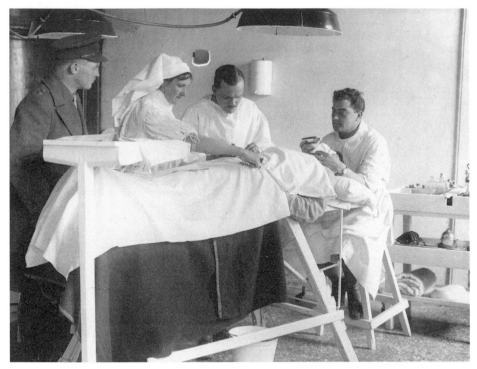

Lieutenant Margaret Ford administers to a patient in 1966. (Army)

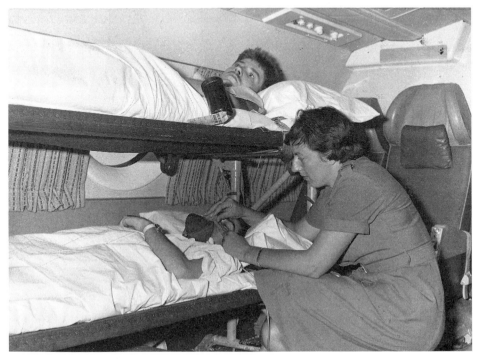

An RAF nursing sister gives a patient oxygen during a flight from North Africa to Britain. (RAF)

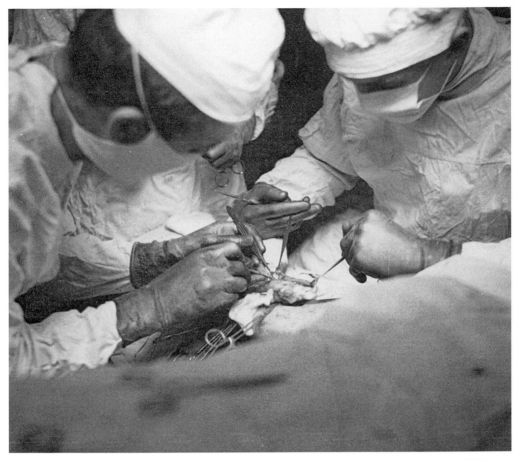

Two British Army sureons, Major Clarkson and Captain Laurie, carry out a delicate operation. (RAMC)

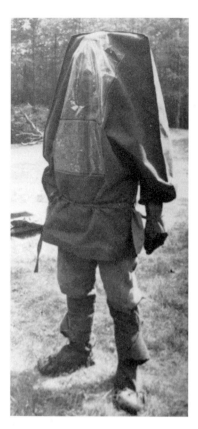

An NBC casualty bag specially designed for walking wounded. Actually, it is a half-bag.

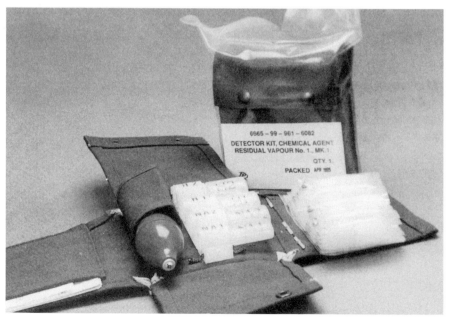

Modern soldiers carry much more than a wound dressing. This British self-detector kit for chemical warfare is attached to a soldier's belt.

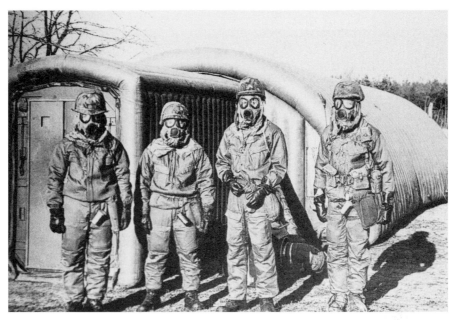

American Army medics prepared to treat NBC casualties. Behind them is an inflatable hospital with an air-conditioning system.

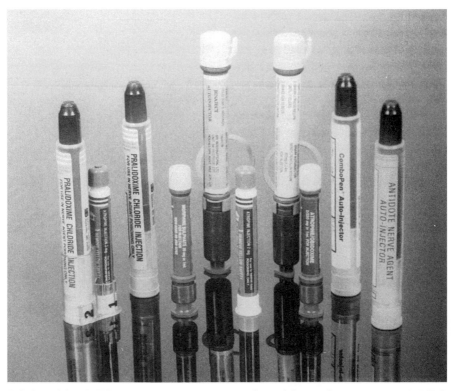

Britain and its NATO allies possess a wide range of auto-injectors for troops to use in NBC conditions.

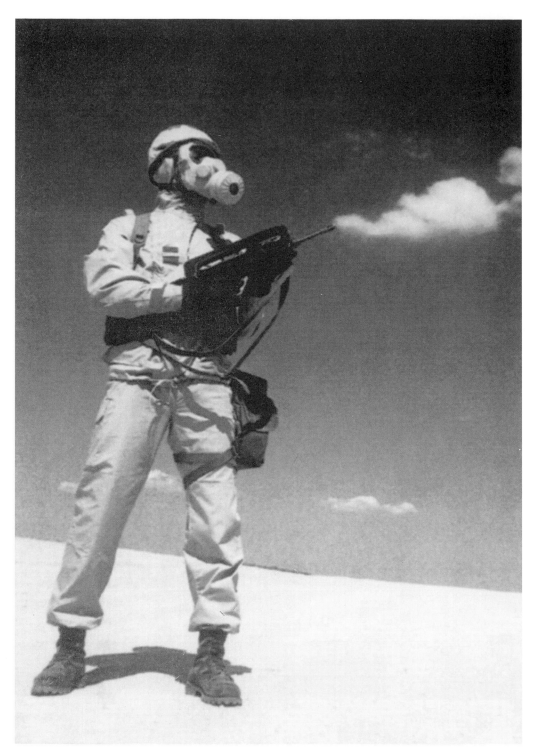

An NBC suit for the Tropics. This design is for the French Army but other armies have similar suits.

CHAPTER TWENTY

First World War and the Challenge to Medicine

At the beginning of the First World War surgeons started with the assumption that the wounds would be more or less of the same character as during the Boer War and that the conflict would be a relatively humane one. In view of the vast size of armies and the more lethal qualities of weapons and missiles – and there was no secret about this – it is difficult to understand the misconception. Probably the medical staffs' early assessment of the severity of the war was, like that of the various general staffs, coloured by the conviction that the war would also be short. Those doctors who were serving when the first convoys of wounded arrived at the British, French or German hospitals were dismayed and startled. Nearly all wounds were severe, lacerated and were suppurating. Later, as the war of movement deteriorated into trench warfare, wounds from bomb and shell became common. Surgeons had to recast their ideas of treatment and the whole character of medical administration had to be remodelled.

Surgeons accustomed to single-wounding were, despite their professional calm, horrified when confronted with a soldier with multiple wounds. A man might have chest, head, spine and abdomen wounds; the same shell fragment might traverse the abdomen and the chest, and these abdominal-chest wounds formed a dangerous and difficult class to deal with. If the intestines were perforated these had to be sutured to save life, and one had to weigh the advisability of operating on both the abdomen and the chest through separate incisions. Medical and surgical progress was painfully slow and neither steady nor continuous, with disproportionate ebb and flow.

To survey the medical aspect of this great conflict in relatively digested form it is best to see it first statistically and generally and then from the viewpoint of the surgeon, nurse and patient. Obviously, with millions of men killed and wounded, the treatment here must be selective.

Before the war doctors were taught to use a method of casualty estimation propounded by the Austrian general, Cron, whose formula was based on a study of casualties in European warfare before his time. Unreliable though it was, Cron's formula did provide a better-than-nothing basis.

Cron estimated that only three-fifths of the total force would be engaged in actual fighting, the remaining two-fifths consisting of reserves and ancillary services in the rear. A study of the order of battle and the disposition of the fighting units would show whether this figure of three-fifths was to be altered or not. Cron then estimated that those engaged would suffer 10 per cent casualties, so that the final conclusion was that the total number of casualties would be 10 per cent of three-fifths of the strength, or 6 per cent.

Both *Field Service Regulations* and *R.A.M.C. Training* stated that 'an attack on an enemy possessing little or no artillery should not result in more than 5 per cent casualties, while an attack on a highly trained force, equipped with the latest modern weapons and holding a fortified position, may cause an attacking force to lose 40 to 50 per cent of its strength'.

Experience in the great battles in France showed that in the first 48 hours the wounded to be evacuated amounted to 20 per cent of the troops engaged; by the end of the first week the wounded evacuated was 40 per cent of the troops actually engaged.★

The casualties for four famous battles were:

Somme	17.1 per cent
Arras	7.8 per cent
Messines	5.7 per cent
Ypres	7.5 per cent
average	9.5 per cent.

Cron's formula was not very wide of the mark.
More specifically:

CASUALTIES IN MAJOR BATTLES OF THE FIRST WORLD WAR

battle	date	approx. strength	casualties	percentage
Mons, 1914	23–24 Aug	40,000	3,784	9.46
Mons Retreat, 1914	22–28 Aug	100,000	14,409	14.40
Loos, 1915	25 Sept–18 Oct	260,000	37,802	14.50
Cambrai, 1917	20–28 Nov	160,000	23,057	14.41
	30 Nov	180,000	18,584	10.32
German Offensive, 1918	21 Mar–8 Apr	471,000	128,893	27.36
Somme, 1916	1 July	420,000	31,581	7.50
	2 July	390,000	12,753	3.50
	3 July	378,000	10,000	2.60
Ypres (Passchendaele) 1917	31 July–6 Aug	238,000	34,184	14.30

★ An American comparison: Love, in *War Casualties*, states that in 98.8 of the divisional combat-days the loss was 50 per 1,000 or less of division strength, and in 1.2 per cent it was greater. Since a casualty-day of approximately 6 per cent occurred not infrequently in divisions in severe combat, Love advised commanders to make provision for a 6 per cent casualty-day for infantry divisions in severe combat.

The actual casualty ratio per 1,000 per annum in France was:

1914 battle casualties	448.23
non-battle casualties	356.15
Total	804.38
1915 battle casualties	472.61
non-battle casualties	875.28
Total	1,347.89
1916 battle casualties	487.39
non-battle casualties	481.60
Total	968.99
1917 battle casualties	381.05
non-battle casualties	529.37
Total	910.42
1918 battle casualties	440.47
non-battle casualties	595.16
Total	1,035.63

These figures show the great wastage during a year's campaign, but many men returned to duty.

The percentage of deaths among those admitted to medical units for 1914 to 1918 was 7.61 per cent of wounded and 0.91 per cent of the sick. Around 82 per cent of those who were wounded and 93 per cent of those who were sick returned to some form of duty. Those evacuated to the UK amounted to 40 per cent of the total. The final disposal of those admitted (with approximate percentages) was:

disposal	wounded	sick or injured	of total strength
Returned to duty in front line			
a From front line medical units	7	21	18
b From hospital or convalescent depot	57	63	60
Returned to duty on line of communications,			
garrison or sedentary occupation	18	9	12
Died	7	1	3
Discharged from the Service as invalids	8	4	5
Disposal otherwise, but not stated	3	2	2

The medical service, among its other functions, was a great agency of reinforcements; approximately 78 per cent of all sick and wounded returned to duty in the front line. During the dangerous days of the German breakthrough, March 1918, the convalescent homes in France discharged 300,000 men back to front-line duty.

Lieutenant Colonel T.B. Nicholls of the RAMC produced a summary of casualty statistics and evolved formulae for calculating certain numbers.[54]

The statistics:
Wounded. Cron's estimate: 10 per cent of three-fifths of the force, i.e. 6 per cent.
British Field Service Regulations estimate: 5 to 10 per cent.
Attacking fortified position: 40 to 50 per cent.
In a certain battle: 20 per cent in first 48 hours, 40 per cent by the end of first week.
Average per division in four battles: 9.5 per cent.
Approximate average for all important battles: 9.62 per cent.
Gas casualties: 20 per cent of total.
Neurological casualties: 0.25 per cent of total.
Venereal rate: average constant sick, 6 per cent per annum.
Average daily sick admissions 0.3 per cent of strength.

The formula:
i To find remaining on seventh day:
$$n = x \times y - (0.4x).$$
ii To find remaining on twenty-first day:
$$n = x \times y - (6x + 0.5xz).$$
iii To find remaining on any day after twenty-first:
$$n = x \times y - (5.6x + 0.9xz).$$

Where:
x = daily admissions.
y = number of days from commencement of admissions.
z = number of days past twentieth day.
n = number of remaining, which it is desired to find.

It can be seen that during the First World War casualties, relative to the vast numbers of men employed, were not excessive – but they were in themselves very large figures indeed. Some battles, such as the protracted agony of Verdun, 1916, produced greater casualties; between them the French and Germans had nearly 1 million killed and wounded. Such numbers imposed great strain on medical services.

Initially transport was also under great strain. When the war broke out in August 1914 most of the transport was horse-drawn and there were no motor ambulance convoys.* The organization was based on a chain of evacuation in

---

* In Britain, motor ambulances were first used during the 1911 army manoeuvres and doctors repeatedly stressed that they should be quickly brought into general use. The Army Council decided that there was already an unwieldy amount of mechanical transport in the field and that the evacuation of casualties from field ambulance to clearing hospital could be handled by using local transport and the empty supply and ammunition lorries returning from the front. The arrangement broke down at the first practical test.

which the sick and wounded were passed through a series of posts – the regimental aid post, the collecting post, the advanced and main dressing stations, the casualty clearing station – until finally they reached the large general hospitals where the specialist departments were largely concentrated. Fairly soon, however, clearing stations, originally designed merely as sorting stations, expanded into the forward areas to take, in some cases, up to 1,000 patients, provided with nursing sisters and all specialist facilities. In the British service most of the radical organization was due to General Sir Alfred Keogh and Sir Arthur Sloggett; they saw the RAMC expand from less than 20,000 in 1914 to 13,000 officers and 154,000 other ranks.

Because of the surgeons' assumption that practice would be similar to that of the Boer War it was considered, for instance, that the best treatment for chest wounds would be to leave them alone unless an empyema (a collection of pus) should form, in which case a drainage operation would be performed. The belief that operative measures were unnecessary is probably the main reason for the lack of surgical assistance provided for men suffering from chest wounds, but several other factors had an influence. The main one was the fear which persisted for a long time that handling a wounded lung might restart bleeding and that a wide opening of the chest and subsequent sepsis might cause death.

Also, owing to military exigencies in the early days of the war, the medical arrangements would not allow anything like active surgery being performed close to the front line. The wounded men had to be evacuated to hospitals at the base, where often they arrived too late for anything but conservative treatment. In the belief that active surgical treatment would be harmful rather than beneficial, a statement of advisable methods of procedure was drawn up for doctors and published in 1915. A typical passage:

> No doubt many men shot through the chest die in a few minutes, but of those who live long enough to reach a field ambulance or a clearing station the great majority recover. . . . The most important treatment of all is absolute rest in the recumbent or semi-recumbent position. . . . If the opening in the chest be large so that air passes in and out during respiration the skin around should be painted with iodine and the opening of the wound firmly closed with antiseptic gauze covered by strapping. . . . A third of a grain of morphine should be given subcutaneously as soon as possible. . . . The presence of haemothorax is rather to be taken as an indication for non-interference. . . .

This approach tended to ignore the very high mortality in the field. The British made no field survey, but a German doctor, Sauerbruch, gives records showing that of 300 dead examined in the field 112, or 37 per cent, were wounded in the chest.*

---

* Loffler examined 469 dead in the German-Danish war of 1864 and found 29 per cent dead of chest wounds. In the New Zealand War of 1863 there was 50 per cent mortality.

In the British field ambulances the mortality rate was 7 per cent and in the casualty clearing stations 15.9 per cent. At base hospital the figure was constant at 6 per cent.

Not until the end of 1916, when the fighting on the Somme was dying down, did surgeons have opportunity to investigate cases and think about treatment. By this time vast improvements in medical services had taken place. Hospitals well staffed with capable nurses, equipped with excellent operating theatres and fine instruments, had been established close to the front line. Wounded were now often received a few hours after injury. Surgeons had facilities for making post-mortem examinations, and physicians, pathologists and radiologists were available for teamwork treatment and investigation.

Wounds inflicted could broadly be divided into three classes: those caused by rifle or machine-gun bullet; shrapnel balls or portions of shell; bomb or grenade. The proportion of each class varied with the type of action. In open and moving actions wounds by rifle bullets preponderated; in trench warfare the number of those caused by fragments of shell was much greater. Wounds due to shrapnel balls were few, and late in the war almost disappeared. Wounds caused by fragments of shell were least favourable, for the jagged fragments made large holes, splintered bones, lacerated tissues and often carried with them fragments of germ-laden cloth or equipment.

If this threefold classification seems to ignore bayonet and bludgeon wounds it is because most surgeons of all armies saw little evidence of hand-to-hand fighting. Indeed for centuries surgeons have discounted the idea that large numbers of soldiers have been wounded by the bayonet. Certainly bayonet charges made by determined troops, such as the Australians and New Zealanders, often put the enemy to flight without hand-to-hand fighting ensuing. However, I think surgeons may be mistaken in their assumption that few wounds are made with the bayonet. Such an assumption ignores the frequent and early fatality of bayonet wounds; a man with a bayonet wound in the throat, stomach or chest does not live long enough to reach the surgeon. Again, a bayonet wound is often a secondary one. That is, soldiers attacking forward after firing at an enemy often kill with the bayonet disabled troops who are nevertheless still firing their rifles or machine-guns. I can only say from experience in the Second World War that bayonet fighting occurs more frequently than most surgeons believe, although few soldiers would engage in it if they still had a bullet in their firearms. Similarly many soldiers making trench raids in the First World War were armed with clubs and bludgeons of the most vicious type. A man smashed over the head with one would hardly be worth carrying to the surgeon.

Regardless of possible ignorance about close-quarter combat, the doctors realized before long that something infinitely worse than ever before experienced was happening to soldiers, that men's bodies were being called upon to endure not only grievous injuries from pieces of metal, but great strain from the incredibly heavy and sustained bombardments, from living for long periods in cold and mud, from poisonous gas – and much else. The war was being fought largely over farmland, thus the ground was heavily infected with bacteria and contamination of wounds was probable. Practically all wounds were infected from the outset, through the skin, clothing, missiles or soil; many of the wounded lay in the open for hours or days before aid could be rendered, and were suffering from shock, exhaustion and loss of blood. They were terribly vulnerable to tetanus, sepsis from staphylococci or the more deadly streptococcus and, above all, the dreaded gangrene, which could spread rapidly, converting the muscles and tissues into a sodden mass of putrefying flesh distended with stinking gases.

It was soon found that the ordinary first-aid routine at dressing-stations and other surgical units behind the front lines failed to prevent subsequent sepsis; the wounded arrived at the base hospitals with sepsis well established, abscesses and not infrequently general blood poisoning. It was realized that full operative treatment in well-equipped hospitals within twelve to twenty-four hours of the infliction of a wound, and before sepsis had been established, was of primary importance. Through the advice of Sir Anthony Bowlby (St Bartholomew's Hospital) and Sir G. Makins (St Thomas's), consulting surgeons to the army, so experienced from the Boer War, mobile casualty clearing stations, equipped for every operative necessity, were established within easy reach of the battle-front. To these, after first aid, the wounded were brought by ambulance; they were resuscitated by warmth, or blood transfusion.

The correct treatment of a contaminated wound to prevent infection and suppuration was a mechanical cleansing carried out a few hours after the injury, before organisms had time to grow and infect. This was attained by excision of the damaged and devitalized tissues and removal of foreign bodies, followed by early closure of the wound either by primary or delayed suture. The establishment of this principle was, in George Gask's opinion,[55] the greatest contribution to military surgery made during the First World War. It resulted from the relatively new mastery of anatomy, physiology and pathology and was equally applicable to any part of the body – to wounds of the soft parts, head, abdomen or chest.

Within twenty-four hours men so treated at a field hospital were sent to a base hospital in well-equipped hospital trains for any further procedures that might be necessary. These measures led to a great decrease in the incidence of sepsis and in the prolonged suppuration and pain and misery of an exhausting illness. The introduction of the Thomas splint (named after the surgeon-inventor) for fractured legs was another great advance. With this appliance fractures could be put in good position, with perfect rest, and safety in travelling.

Before the First World War surgeons tended to use some form of pressure chamber or intratracheal insufflation apparatus when it became necessary to open the pleural cavity. It was evident that such an apparatus was impracticable in the field and a few trials with the ordinary anaesthetics proved that, under the conditions, a patient could be anaesthetized and one pleural cavity could be opened widely without any grave danger. Patients with thoracic wounds bore operation well and took an anaesthetic satisfactorily, and pressure chambers were unnecessary. Surgeons such as Gask preferred chloroform; the French used ether and the Americans gas and oxygen. Many British surgeons used local anaesthetics. The other great fear – that handling a wounded lung might restart serious bleeding – also vanished, for it was found that manipulation of the lung was easy, was not attended by a serious fall of blood pressure and did not cause bleeding.

An initial crisis was an outbreak of tetanus. In the early days of the war the known incidence was 1.47 per 1,000 wounded, but it really exceeded this figure. In September 1914 it was 8.8 per 1,000. Mortality was high during 1914–15: 78 per cent. Sir David Bruce was asked to do something about this danger, and so effectively did he work with anti-toxins that in 1919 the mortality had dropped to 15 per cent.*

Shellshock was something else doctors had to learn to handle. Medically true shellshock is both mental and physical in origin. It is caused by being close to a bursting shell of high calibre. The soldier is practically always blown over by the blast of the shell, is buried by the debris and deafened by the explosion. A temporary vacuum is formed around him, which is rapidly filled by a great rush of air, causing a transitory increase of atmospheric pressure. The brain is a delicate structure, surrounded by cerebro-spinal fluid which protects it from outside influences. Any sudden severe change in the atmospheric pressure causes a disturbance in the cerebro-spinal fluid, and may produce an injury to the underlying cerebral tissue. Shellshock is a distressing complaint. A man of intellect and vitality, quick in decision, a pleasant companion, a trusted friend and an efficient soldier becomes a different person, with twitching hands, apathetic eye and full of curious indecision. Most cases are curable, but the condition is apt to recur when the individual is subjected to a similar shock.

Many officers and men were invalided home from shellshock; such men were, as a rule, not neurotic. The majority in the First World War were men who had done their duty, often in the face of almost certain death, and many won decorations for bravery. Some doctors believed that the more highly educated a man was, the more vulnerable he was to shellshock. This was not really the case but it was true thar a man who had grown up in 'soft' conditions was more likely to suffer shellshock than one who had endured continual privations as a young man. Because many men who had a pampered

---

* In the Italian campaign of 1943–4, 96,164 UK and Commonwealth soldiers suffered wounds. Only 31 of these developed tetanus, and 22 of them recovered.

upbringing were also well educated, doctors drew a false conclusion about the relationship of education to shellshock. Very large numbers of poorly educated men were also affected by the condition.†

New and dangerous complaints were trench foot and trench fever. Trench foot was caused through men having to remain for long periods knee deep in water until the feet turned into a mass of chilblains. Sometimes gangrene set in. It was a curse in all armies and on most fronts; many troops on Gallipoli lost their feet to amputations. At the time of the attacks on the formidable Hohenzollern Redoubt, France, British troops were holding trenches in foul weather, standing waist high in liquid mud. Sometimes men slipped under the mud in their exhausted sleep and their bodies would be dug out next day. The food was sodden and the men kept themselves alive on rum, the officers on whisky. A captain visited a friend one night to see if he had anything to eat. The friend had not and complained that he and his men were living in horrible trenches.

'Come and see mine,' the captain said, and showed his friend a place where three men were sitting in mud nearly to their armpits, huddled together, moaning in their sleep. Later, in the early morning, he found them sunk a little deeper and woke them and got them out, and set a fresh man to each, to shake them, rub them and put them up in the dry, outside the trench, till the morning mists had cleared and they had to get into it again. It was not really surprising that men suffered from trench feet.

Trench fever, which laid large numbers of men *hors de combat* for a long time, at first baffled the most erudite physicians; it had both influenza and typhoid characteristics. Finally the Trench Fever Committee, under the enterprising Sir David Bruce, traced it to the louse, which was attacked by disinfectant centres, bath units and laundries.

In the ninth month of the war doctors were confronted with a new type of casualty – the soldier wounded by gas. Chlorine, which the Germans liberated from cylinders in the front near Ypres, swept in clouds onto trenches held by British, Canadian and French native troops. They had no protection against gas and many were killed outright; they were probably luckier than those who lingered in great agony. Later, even more dangerous gases, such as phosgene and mustard gas, were fired in shells. Mustard gas was an evil thing, blistering the skin and, in some cases, stripping a man's entire body of skin.* Within sixty hours of the first gas attack doctors had made available 90,000 crude improvised masks of cotton waste in muslin containers and, within a month, 2 million of them. The medical services of

---

† Shellshock should not be confused with the condition called by Huot of the French Medical Service 'le cafard', which is merely a nervous debility that attacks men after long spells in the trenches under arduous conditions.

* An Australian soldier, Trooper Rolph, lived for five years in a warm-water bath after losing his entire skin.

Britain and France set up a gas centre for each division, a gas casualty clearing station in each army area and base hospitals specializing in gas treatment. Since two could play at the same game and, since the prevailing winds blew *towards* the Germans, they too had many gas casualties. British gas casualties amounted to 185,000 of which 9,000 were fatal.

The scourges of earlier campaigns – enteric, plague, smallpox, cholera, typhus – were no great problem during the First World War, except in a few isolated areas. But dysentery and diarrhoea caused a lot of trouble, notably in the Near East. On Gallipoli, 1915, almost every soldier was attacked, so that the RAMC dealt with 85,000 cases of disease in addition to the 115,000 battle casualties. In Lower Mesopotamia heat and insanitary camps led to much dysentery, malaria and heat stroke. During the siege of Kut, 1915–16, the average daily number of men under treatment – in a force of only 14,500 – was 1,351. The Turkish enemy suffered as much. In Macedonia, British, French, Serbian and Greek troops suffered from malaria. The British had 6 million cases of sickness, the French 5 million, the Germans 7 million and the Russians a roughly estimated 11 million. The great difference from earlier wars was that, comparatively, so few men died of illness.

CHAPTER TWENTY-ONE

Surgeons in the Field

To the doctors in administrative posts, and even to those at base, what happened on a grand scale and to the soldier in the line was inevitably largely academic. To the surgeon in the field each wounded man, battered, dirty, bewildered, was very much a human problem. The author makes no apology for the harrowing nature of some of the following incidents; it is as well that everybody should know how vilely the human body is treated in war and what the nursing surgeon, nursing sister, bearer and orderly are called upon to do in treating it.

Philip Gibbs, watching human wreckage coming down from the salient of Loos in December 1915, from the chalkpits of Hulluch and the mud of the Hohenzollern Redoubt, which had been partly gained by a battle which did not succeed, succinctly described the receding human tide of battle. At the casualty clearing station – the town hall of Lillers – he saw 'men with chunks of steel in their lungs and bowels vomiting great gobs of blood, men with legs and arms torn from their trunks, men without noses, and their brains throbbing through open scalps, men without faces. . . .'[56]

Gibbs also told the story of the young soldier who went in the first rush into Mametz Wood, 1 July 1916, but was left behind in a dugout when the troops retreated before a violent counter-attack. Some German soldiers passed this hole and threw a bomb down on the off-chance that an English soldier might be there. It wounded the lonely boy in the dark corner. He lay there a day listening to the crash of shells through the trees and not daring to come out. In the night he heard English voices and shouted loudly. But as the English soldiers passed they threw a bomb into the dugout and the boy was wounded again. He lay there another day; the gun-fire began all over again, and lasted until the Germans came back. Another German soldier saw the hole and threw a bomb down, as a safe thing to do, and the boy received his third wound. He lay in the darkness one more day, not expecting to live, but still alive. When the English came, finally capturing the wood, one of them, thinking Germans might be hiding in the dugout, threw a bomb down – and the boy was wounded for the fourth time. But this time his cries were heard. The surgeons had a lot of trouble with his wounds but he survived.

Yet there were moments of humour on the battlefield. On one occasion Surgeon Geoffrey Sparrow, serving with the Royal Naval Division in France, crawled out to see a wounded man lying in the open. He found him nursing a badly fractured jaw and suffering from numerous other wounds. He did not complain of his pain, the shell-fire or cold; he did not even ask if the wound was likely to be fatal. His only question was: 'Is my false teeth all right, sir? I paid two-thirteen-nine for them at Goldstein's just afore war.' The surgeon's assurance that his lower denture was intact had a remarkably sedative effect on the man and undoubtedly increased his chances of recovery.[57]

There was so much to be done, and so many soldiers for whom surgery could do so little – the abdominal cases that died so soon, the brain cases that took so long to die. And of all the dreadful wounds in war the lacerating brain wound was the most harrowing; restless, noisy, delirious, the victim struggling with the orderlies, babbling incoherently about private matters, crying for water and yet spitting it out when brought. Morphia was useless and only chloroform would put the brain to sleep, for an hour or two, until the morphia acted. During the First World War British surgeons were never short of morphia or of chloroform and for that they were grateful.

A doctor's day could be terribly full of tragedy. Captain Harold Dearden one evening confided laconically to his diary[58] that a sister had called him at 3.30 a.m. to see a man with a bullet in the spine, and who was very bad. Dearden found him vomiting blood, with a temperature of 103, his pulse very rapid and too feeble to count – obviously dying. The soldier was quite lucid and said he felt a good deal better than he did when he came in, which military doctors know is very common before death. About an hour later, while Dearden was holding him sideways to vomit, the man just flopped through his hands with the blood still running down his face and died. Dearden went afterwards to give an intravenous injection of ether for an anaesthetic to a French Canadian, whose legs were badly shattered by shell-fire and needed double amputation. Orderlies were scarce, so Dearden lent a hand to lift him from his bed on to the stretcher. He was in great pain in any position and movement only aggravated it. He was also terribly nervous and had completely lost self-control. He did not want to be moved at all and kept calling out: 'I can't bear any more, you'll only hurt me!' When they did lift him he screamed: 'I knew you would, I knew you would! Oh! Oh!' he kept this up all the way into the theatre and until he was under the anaesthetic. 'He was a smallish man to begin with; and when he had his two legs off at the thigh he looked like a tortured child somehow – so little, almost inhuman.'

Another morning Dearden was called at four by the night sister to look at a tetanus man who had spasms, his jaw tight shut and looking like 'a horrible wooden image with that same fixed grin they all get'. He was in terrible pain and kept asking: 'How long will this last for, Doctor?' Dearden, knowing it was hopeless, said: 'Oh not long now, boy; this first stage is always the worst; when you get over this, you'll be as right as rain.' He sent the sister for chloroform and kept the soldier under until nine o'clock, when he died.

Dearden wrote of a boy whose leg he had hoped to save, but which he was forced to amputate just above the knee. 'The lad was very good when I told him I thought he'd better have it off, but he looked straight ahead of him and said nothing – just looked, with his poor thin nostrils working like a rabbit's, and shooting a dry, dirty tongue out every few seconds to moisten his gluey lips. I don't think he heard many of the lies I told him about men who could do everything with an artificial leg that they could ever do before, but there is really nothing else you can say.'

Telling lies cheerfully is a basic part of a field surgeon's intellectual equipment. Dearden had a young soldier with two feet off and dying, though he was quite conscious. Dearden patched him up, got him on a stretcher, gave him a cigarette and left him, when he called the doctor back, saying something which he couldn't catch, for his lips and face were cut and bleeding. He wiped the boy's mouth, and the soldier said clearly and quietly: 'shall I live, sir?' 'Live!' Dearden said. 'Good Lord, yes – you'll be as right as rain when you're properly dressed and looked after.' 'Thank you, sir,' he said, and went on smoking his cigarette. He died as they were getting him on the ambulance.

One doctor had a patient aged about thirty-three with the entire front wall of his abdomen blown away, so that dressing him was a matter largely of keeping his intestines out of the bed. He was dying fast and simply lay and vomited with that 'easy grace that all peritonitis cases get, and his face with his pain, the shock, and the morphia he has had is just a writhing, twisting sheet of sweating grey linen'. The doctor was writing this description on a chair in the garden before lunch, and he could hear another man groaning He had half his buttocks blown away, and though he had had morphia he groaned and groaned. He would stop if somebody would sit and talk to him, but recommenced immediately he was left.

The type of case most requiring assistance was the man with a large open wound, with fracture of the ribs and a retained missile. George Gask did his first big thoracic operation of the war at the end of 1916, the patient being a young Australian doctor, admitted with a large open wound of the lower thorax and a retained missile. Gask chloroformed the patient, opened the wound, excised four inches of broken rib and using a rib-spreader opened the pleural cavity wide. In the cavity of the pleura he found a shrapnel ball, a bit of rib and a large piece of khaki tunic. Removing them, he cut off the jagged ends of rib, cleaned the pleura cavity of blood and closed the chest in layers. The patient recovered well after only a short convalescence, rejoined his field ambulance unit and was awarded the DSO for gallantry. Gask and others examined the patient in 1917 and in 1918 and found the cure to be sound and permanent. This successful case made a deep impression on many surgeons and revealed the possibilities of thoracic surgery in the field. In several instances missiles were extracted from the heart, chiefly by French surgeons, with subsequent recovery of the patient.

Doctors had crises every day. One MO was trying to save a man who had practically the whole of his upper right arm blown away, leaving a wound from his shoulder to half an inch from his elbow – a great gaping channel oozing pus. As suppuration increased his vessels began to rot and bleed, and finally he had a very heavy haemorrhage which nearly killed him. Fortunately the doctor happened to be in the ward just when it came on. As soon as the sister took off his dressings a great jet of blood shot out across the floor and the doctor had to catch hold of the artery with his fingers and hang on while another MO, sent for in a hurry, anaesthetized the man on the bed. They tied the vessel properly, but loss of blood left him pulseless and blanched, and it was obvious that he could never fight against his sepsis in that state. The doctors got a man who was slightly wounded and would otherwise return to the trenches again next day to consent to be bled – on condition of being sent to 'Blighty' as a reward. The transfusion was astonishing. The patient, 'a bleached, pulseless, whining coward, who screamed and shed tears at the sight of a hypodermic needle and had never smiled for days', became a new man. His colour came back, he began to take an optimistic interest in what was going on – all within ten minutes. The surgeon had never seen anything which impressed him more. 'It proves how all our emotions are products of our metabolism; and how a saint might very well be turned into a crusty old cynic by a short course of dyspepsia!'

Military doctors have always been impatient with men who show fear disproportionate to their wounds, perhaps because they also have profound respect for the severely wounded man who makes light of his hurts. Dearden wrote in his diary of a sixteen-year-old from Scarborough, with a badly smashed knee that would possibly have to be amputated. This boy screamed loudly whenever the wound was being dressed, 'being a poor, wizened, red-headed little coward at the best of times'. Nevertheless Dearden sat and held his hand and covered his eyes with cotton wool while the wound was being dressed, counter balancing this gesture of sympathy by threatening to hit the boy in the stomach every time he shouted. He told him that he was no Yorkshireman and that as a Lancashire man himself he was ashamed of him. After this the boy endured his pain silently, though he cried a lot, scared more by the sight of the hole in his leg with tubes sticking out of it than by the pain.

Some men were incredibly brave. A French doctor told the story of an officer wounded in fighting at Compiègne in 1917.[59] Gangrene had set in and both legs, an arm and the fingers of the other hand were amputated. To an orderly detailed to watch him the officer said: 'I'm sure you need not pull me up so high in the bed now – I'm ever so much shorter.' On the night he died he told the surgeon: 'If only you had not cut off both my hands I could have shown you my favourite game of patience.'

Sometimes even a doctor could not tell without examination whether a man was wounded, and this could lead to pathetic situations. During the fight for the Bourlon Line, near the Hindenburg Line, in 1918 Dearden, having lost many stretcher-bearers, grabbed some German prisoners to help carry wounded. One man did not want to carry, and the doctor hit him over the head to persuade him. Back at the regimental aid post the German sat down on the dugout steps, and every time Dearden approached him he would pluck him by the coat and say something. Then a shell pitched close and blew the roof off the dugout entrance. Dearden was frightened by the explosion, but the German sat unmoved. Investigating, the doctor saw that he was holding his trousers together with one hand, and when he pulled the hand away the entire contents of his belly spilled out over his knees. Dearden tucked them in again, covered him up and gave him two grains of morphia to suck. It was the best he could do for the man. As if that episode were not distressing enough, half an hour later he saw a German with both legs blown off pulling himself along the road on his chest and elbows. Just outside the church a machine-gun bullet hit him in the neck and he died instantly.

Surgeons were not often uncertain, indeed after a time they developed an intuition about wounds and disabilities. But the men in the ranks were frequently abysmally ignorant. Their lack of even basic knowledge about the functioning of the human body or about first-aid led to many deaths. Private George Swindell, 77th Field Ambulance, saw ignorance lead to a particularly pathetic incident.[60] He and other bearers were detailed to carry out of the lines a young soldier with a severe abdominal wound. To have the barest chance of survival he had to be in hospital by nightfall; it was then midday. The MO injected morphia, warned the bearers not to jolt the patient and on no account to let him have any water. His lips could be wiped with a wet rag, but this was all. Drinking would kill him. The bearers started – two carrying, one shielding the man from the hot sun, the other wiping his hands and forehead with a damp rag. When the effects of the drug wore off the soldier became restive and cried for water and when the bearers would merely wet his lips he cursed them for murderers. After a long, arduous portage the bearers were walking past some houses, congratulating themselves on having got the man out alive when several infantrymen came out of a house.

Hearing the patient raving for water they shouted at the bearers and even threatened them. 'Give the poor devil some water!' they yelled. Swindell, all 5 feet 2½ inches of him, went over to them and told them to shut up.

Some artillery men now appeared, and a sergeant, before the bearers could stop him, thrust a water bottle into the wounded man's hands. In seconds he was guzzling the water. The bearers hurried the patient to the MO at the hospital, who opened his bandages and said angrily: 'You've killed this man! You know you have no right to give abdominal wounded water!'

The bearers brought out stretchers only with great difficulty and under great danger. Carrying a stretcher along a trench was safer than being in the open but more difficult, for the men would have to lift it shoulder high to pass some sharper, narrower angle, and every few yards they would slide and stumble on the slippery and uneven trench boards. Sometimes they would have to rush past a spot which the enemy machine-gunners could enfilade; other spots were notorious for rats. The bearers of the 2/4th London Field Ambulance talked for a long time afterwards about one young soldier they brought out of the line. With three comrades he had been caught in a shell explosion which had killed the others an left him insane. He was quiet and amenable in the bearers' hands, but implored them constantly to allow him to go out and gather wild flowers in memory of his friends.

Swindell brought out a man of the Cheshire Regiment with more than 200 small wounds, all in the front of his body. The MO was puzzled because he and Swindell had not found one serious wound, yet the man was almost unconscious. He told Swindell to lift the man's head while he looked for wounds on his shoulders. Swindell found a piece of shell about three inches long protruding from the back of the soldier's head. Two officers worked for some time to extract the piece of jagged metal, deeply embedded in the bone. The force of a shell explosion caused astonishing injuries. After a bombardment near La Clytte in May 1918 Swindell and other men of his field ambulance unit entered the remains of a Nissen hut shelled by the Germans to find a man sitting with his back to the wall, 'as pale as death', but alive enough to ask for a smoke. He had been standing up when the shell – a 5.9 – burst only five feet from him. He had two terrible injuries – his legs were turned round and round. "Just as if you were wringing out a flannel' – as Swindell put it. The bones and flesh were pulverized by the explosion and the legs were summarily amputated at a first-aid post.

The official designation of 'first-aid post' give a misleadingly reassuring picture, for it was often no more than two medical orderlies crouching in a shell-hole or behind a pile of sandbags with a stretcher beside them. At best it was a low-ceilinged shelter in a dugout with stretchers along the walls, with, in the centre, just enough room for the doctor and his assistant and a table. In the heat of an action their clothing would be, quite literally, saturated with blood. There would be no time to dispose of bloody bandages, which would form in a heap on the floor.

The horrors of the first-aid post were standard – men holding their intestines in both hands, broken bones tearing the flesh, arteries spurting blood, bared brains, maimed hands, empty eye sockets, pierced chests, skin hanging down in tatters from the burned face, missing lower jaws. . . .

In the French service morphine, often in short supply, was given only to the seriously wounded on the operating table. For lack of insecticide the doctor constantly had to brush away flies gorged on decomposed flesh; the only light was provided by acetylene lamps, flashlights or candles, and sometimes it was necessary to work in the dark, with doctors groping to wind or unwind a bandage.

During the battle of Verdun, with casualties arriving constantly at the field operating depots, the overworked surgeons had to make rapid, arbitrary decisions about which men to take for treatment; there was no use in wasting time and medical equipment in hopeless cases. There was not even time for pity. The surgeon would indicate that a particular case was rejected and the orderlies would carry him from the operating cellar and put him down in the open behind cover, where other orderlies were permanently posted to fight off the rats. Despite the dying state of these men some, when shells fell near, would try to get up to find better cover.

These men died where they lay, but every established hospital had its 'Death and Glory' ward for terminal cases – the men who had no chance of survival. Bearer Swindell worked in such a ward for several days and, though no poet, saw facets of it that might startle others, yet his view, not written for literary effect, has a strange validity. He wrote of the terminal ward:

> This one was the most tragic, the most wonderful, the most beautiful; every feature of life rushed before one here. The tragedy was the death of youth, the wonder was that men could face such shocks and live, the beauty was the nurses; from bed to bed they would go, one of them in particular being the very incarnation on earth of an angel. She sent men on their last journey with a flicker of a smile . . . their gaunt and furrowed faces, lined and aged with pain and suffering. . . . Sixteen hours a day in that ward were enough to break the spirit of war in any man and we had days of it. The one thing that stays in my memory is the passing of these men, never a cry against their fate, taking it with the rest of their wounds. . . .

Swindell, paying tribute to two of his officers, Captains Charles and Alderson, regarded them as 'wonderful surgeons or butchers'. In came a patient, off went his bandages. 'Poor devil,' the surgeon would say, 'gangrene has set in; he must have it off half way up the thigh.' They worked on the principle, followed by the surgeons of the Peninsular War, that once gangrene had gained hold to cut a limb just above the rot would be a waste of time since another operation would certainly be necessary. Swindell saw arms and legs come off without the doctors showing any hesitation. Swindell found out what happened to these limbs when one morning he and a mate were detailed to operate the incinerator.

To stay sane amid the carnage surgeons had to view their work impersonally. Some became eccentric, some developed a callous veneer, some did not even allow themselves to think. The doctor colonel commanding the hospital at Corbie, Somme, in mid-1916 cheerfully labelled his hospital the 'butcher's shop', for it really was just that, and joking about it was this surgeon's defence mechanism. 'Come and have a look at my cases,' he invited Philip Gibbs one July day.[61] 'They're the worst possible – stomach wounds, compound fractures and all that. We lop off limbs all day long and all night!'

A new batch of cases had just arrived and was laid in rows on the floorboards. The colonel bent down to some and drew back their blankets to feel a pulse. The men were all plastered with grey clay, sometimes mixed with thick clots of blood. 'That fellow won't last long,' said the MO, rising from a stretcher. 'hardly a heart-beat left in him. Sure to die on the operating table – if he gets as far as that. . . .' From another bundle under a blanket came an agonizing wail.

In a ward Gibbs saw one man with both legs amputated to the thigh and both his arms to the shoulder-blades. 'Remarkable man,' said the MO 'His vitality is so tremendous that he is putting up a terrific fight.'

Gibbs spoke to a man with one leg and one arm gone and the other leg going; it was uncovered and supported on a board hung from the ceiling. Taking Gibbs for a surgeon, he pleaded to have his leg saved, but as they moved on the MO said casually: 'Bound to come off – gangrene.' He indicated a boy sitting up in bed, smiling at the nurse who felt his pulse. 'Looks fairly fit after the knife, doesn't he? But we shall have to cut higher up. Gangrene again. I'm afraid he'll be dead before tomorrow.' And as Gibbs left the hospital the cheerful colonel shouted: 'Come in again, any time!' He was staying sane.

In the hospitals, as in the field, there was occasional humour. One night a doctor on ward rounds saw a patient come towards him holding a blood-stained handkerchief to his ear. 'I reckon it was my gal's fault, sir,' he said. 'Last Thursday was my birthday and my young woman – meanin' kindly of course – sent me a bottle of sweet-smellin' 'air oil. Of course it ain't no good to us out here, let alone addin' to the weight of yer pack, but I didn't like to chuck the stuff away, seein' as 'ow she'd sent it, so I give my 'air and 'ead a tidy dose of it last night and woke up to find a blankety rat asittin' on me shoulder and alickin' of it orf, and when I moved me 'ead why 'e bit me through the ear.'

Next of kin were sometimes taken to France to visit badly wounded men, a practice humanitarian in some ways, but ill-advised in others. Doctors sometimes felt that the distress caused to the relatives of the stricken man was much greater than any comfort they could bring to him. The mother and sister of a soldier were with him in his dying hours.[62] An amputation case, conscious and feeling little pain, he kept rocking his head from side to side and saying to the surgeon: 'I'm all right now, sir. Just give me something to do, anything you like sir, I'm all right now, sir.'

His pulse was too feeble to be counted, his face was chalky and 'the red oozing stump of his leg sticks straight up into the air like some horrible thing in Chinese lacquer'. The doctor sent his sister out, for her crying was disturbing the other men, but his mother stayed on, trying to give her son water out of a feeding cup. Every time he swung his head the spout struck his projecting teeth and water splashed over his chin and neck. He knew nothing of this and at least it was something for the mother to do. The doctor knew the soldier would stop before the mother tired. In circumstances such as this a doctor felt that relatives were much better kept away from the scene.

In their own hospitals surgeons' authority was unquestioned; those in prison camps have always had to work under great and sometimes insuperable difficulties. In a prison camp near Paderborn, Germany, in 1916 Captain R.V. Dolbey of the RAMC found sanitary conditions appalling, with sewage percolating into the water of a stream which was the sole supply for washing clothes, food bowls and for ablutions. The camp was swept by almost every infectious disease – scarlet fever, pneumonia, typhoid, dysentery, cerebro-spinal-meningitis, mumps, measles. . . .[63]

There was a large number of surgical cases, the most urgent being nerve injuries with consequent paralysis of muscles. The British doctors could not persuade the German surgeon to treat them properly or permit the British to undertake the necessary massage or electrical treatment. Nor could the men be sent to the big hospital in Paderborn. The camp hospital had six rooms, each sufficient for a maximum of twenty patients. Into every one were crowded at least seventy men suffering from a variety of infectious diseases. The sick and wounded lay on palliasses on double-decked iron beds. Acute pneumonia cases and cases of pulmonary tuberculosis lay, side by side, in soiled clothing and coughed in each other's faces.

The hospital had no toilets and no bedpans. Sick men had to go fifty yards in the coldest weather to the latrines. The one clinical thermometer in the camp was passed indiscriminately from mouth to mouth without disinfection.

In the First World War surgeons themselves faced many more dangers than ever before, with the possible exception of the ship's surgeon in the days of muzzle-to-muzzle fights. With the longer range of artillery, hospitals were often under fire. More than this, the regimental surgeon had to expose himself time and again in his efforts to treat wounded men. Some surgeons, their orderlies and bearers went far beyond the bounds of normal duty. The most notable was certainly Captain Noel Chavasse of the RAMC, serving with the Liverpool Regiment.

At Guillemont, France, in August 1916, Chavasse's battalion took part in an attack and he tended the wounded in the open all day, frequently in view of the enemy; that night he spent four hours searching for wounded in front of the enemy's lines. Next day he took one bearer with him to the advanced trenches, and under shell-fire carried an urgent case 500 yards to safety, being wounded in the side by a shell splinter. That night he led a party of twenty volunteer bearers, rescued three wounded men from a shell-hole only twenty-five yards from the German trenches, buried the bodies of two officers and collected many identity discs. The Germans threw bombs and fired machine-guns at him, but Chavasse was not further wounded. He saved the lives of twenty wounded men, apart from treating the many others who passed through his hands. His reward was the Victoria Cross.

In September 1917 Chavasse went out to rescue a wounded soldier and, while carrying him to the dressing-station, was himself wounded, but for two days not only continued to work at his post but frequently went out to search for and attend to the wounded who were lying in no man's land. Practically without food during these two days, exhausted and faint, Chavasse nevertheless helped to carry in a number of men. In saving lives he lost his own – dying of his wounds and winning the VC a second time.

Of the eight doctors who won the Victoria Cross during the First World War four were killed in action. One of those who survived, Lieutenant George Allan, serving near Fauquissart on 25 September 1915, collected and treated in the open, and under shell-fire, more than 300 men. Even after one shell had stunned his only assistant and killed several of his patients, and a second shell had half buried him with debris, Allan continued to work single-handed.

It would be pointless to draw comparisons between the British service and those of the other belligerent nations. By this time administration and treatment were more or less uniform among the Western Powers. The picture in Russia and Turkey was decidedly inferior, and many soldiers, wounded and sick, simply died without any treatment, there being insufficient trained people to provide it. Despite these regional failings it is true, as the Austrian Zinsser said in 1935, that: 'Nobody won the last war but the medical services. The increase in knowledge was the sole determinable gain for mankind in a devastating catastrophe.'

CHAPTER TWENTY-TWO

What the Sisters Saw

Long before the First World War nursing had developed into a genuine profession – though it might more aptly be called a vocation. The usually willing but often crude and amoral women of the eighteenth century, frequently co-opted into nursing from the ranks of the camp followers, had been replaced in the Crimea by a mixed force of dedicated professionals, enthusiastic amateurs and nuns who were more concerned with the soldier's spirit than with his body. By 1914 nursing services were staffed by thoroughly trained, highly efficient women, many of them young. The difference these women made to military medical practice cannot even be estimated. Their imperturbable competence, their feminine serenity, their astonishing mixture of firmness and gentleness, their apparent tirelessness – all had a profound psychological effect on sick and wounded soldiers. Conversely the sufferings of the servicemen had a deep but usually less obvious effect on the nursing sisters.

Their observations provide a different perspective on the human material on which they helped the surgeons to work. Self-effacing, always at the doctor's elbow, they had to know almost intuitively the personality of each surgeon and physician, to divine what he would expect of them, to anticipate his instructions. They had somehow to preserve a professional detachment, yet be a combination of mother, sister, wife and sweetheart to the battered and wasted men they nursed.

Sister K.E. Luard, who served in a hospital train, with a field ambulance and in a base hospital, spent three years in charge of a casualty clearing-station (CCS) at Lillers. Here she saw as much drama as anybody during the war, and fortunately kept a diary of her most vivid experiences and impressions.[64]

On 21 October 1915 she arrived at the infants' school – part of her CCS – just in time to see a delirious boy, with a bad head wound causing a large brain hernia, tear off his dressings and throw a handful of his brains on the floor. This was literally true – and the soldier was talking all the time the sisters re-dressed the hole in his head and picked up the handful of brains. The boy was quiet for a little while, then became delirious and did not recover.

On 6 November a little night sister pulled a man round who was at the point of death with bronchitis and acute Bright's disease. The doctor suggested a vapour bath; the sister found a primus, some tubing, a kettle and cradles, and got it going. She later repeated the treatment and in the morning the man was speaking and swallowing, and back to earth again, though only just.

In March 1915 one of Sister Luard's patients was the glass-eyed Corporal W.R. Cotter of The Buffs, who was admitted with his leg bombed off. Noted for his bravery and for lone scouting at night for enemy snipers, Cotter was induced to relate his latest exploit. He had been leading a bombing attack at the Hohenzollern Redout, took his men up a wrong turning, and came on to 'thousands of Germans'. He somehow got his men away again but minus his leg. 'It was dark, and I didn't know me leg was gone – so I kep' on throwing the bombs and little Wood he kep' by me and took out the pins for me.' At last Private Wood got Cotter into a dug-out in a crater and stayed with him all night.

On 14 March General Gough, the corps commander, and two other generals arrived to see Cotter and tell him he was recommended for the VC Later that day the corporal had a severe haemorrhage and so nearly died that the surgeons dared not give him an anaesthetic to take off his gangrenous leg through the knee. Cotter was unconscious anyway. The sisters slaved at him all the evening, but he died at 8 p.m.

The sisters' calmness was often a façade to cover deep emotion. On the night of 31 May 1915 a patient whom the sisters of Sister Luard's CCS knew as 'Jack' was dying, paralysed from a wound in the spine. He did not know what was the matter with him and could not feel anything; he simply went on smiling and making polite little jokes 'and thanking and apologizing until we could all cry'. Another patient, Reggie, was worse that night, holding out his hand and asking: 'Will you come and sit by me for a little while and hold my hand – it encourages me.' Another soldier who had lost one eye and could not see out of the other was also feeling bad and wanting a sister to sit and talk with him. But one of the difficulties of the First World War was that nurses were usually too busy to sit and talk.

Certain situations were so pathetic they could hardly fail to be distressing. A boy of seventeen, badly wounded in the chest, was brought, blue and gasping, into Sister Luard's CCS on 24 May 1916. While she was washing him next morning, he said, speaking in gasps: 'I fought I was too big to be walkin' about the street wivout joinin' . . . I fought a lot of fings when that shell hit me. I fought about . . . goin over the water again . . . and I fought about seein' Mother – and I fought about dyin'. Will they let her come and see me quick when I get to a hospital in London? I fink I'll write to her this afternoon.' Later, with great difficulty, he gave the sister his mother's address. He died at five o'clock. To Sister Luard his gasping recital of his 'foughts' was the 'most upsetting thing that has happened of all the upsetting things'.

Another sister saw a colleague break down while working in a field hospital in Malines. Two Belgian soldiers had just been carried in, one shot through the buttocks, the other with his arm hanging by a thread of flesh from the shoulder. Despite a tourniquet the wound was bleeding constantly.

The man had been shot through the diaphragm too and his face was livid and twisted with pain. An English surgeon injected saline. 'Once he looked me full in the eyes,' the nurse wrote later, 'and I think the pity in my eyes answered him.' The patient was struggling wildly – unusually for such wounds – and the sister holding him down was sobbing, so the other took her place. She had one arm and one side, a priest held the other side and two Belgian women stroked the victim's face. He shouted and writhed, raised himself and blood gushed from his mouth. . . .

Sometimes the decision about amputation was left to the patient – if he were in a condition to make a decision. When one leg had already been amputated and the decision to be made was whether to have the other off or die the problem was not as academic as might appear. Sisters were accustomed to debating the point, for a man at first might be set on dying, perhaps he could not face his wife with both legs gone. They would tell him what his wife would say and try to convince him that life was still worth living.

But it was not always worth living in France. On 23 September 1916 Sister Luard wrote: 'There is a man in with both eyes and the top of his nose scooped out by a bit of shell. When I was cleaning him up he told me he was forty-nine, but he'd given his age in as thirty-eight to join the army. Then he said, without any sort of comment: "I think I've lost my eyesight," as if it had been his rifle or his boots.' He died.

There was also the soldier with his right arm in fragments, a penetrating chest-wound and a piece of shrapnel in his abdomen. He said he was 'a bit uncomfortable, but nothing to talk about!' He reached the sisters in the preparation ward pulseless, with instructions on his label to 'generally counteract shock'. After six hours they had him fit for operation. The surgeons amputated his arm and dug the metal out of his inside. He died, but many soldiers, given up as hopeless, sat up a week later and asked for a boiled egg. Sister Luard had a soldier patient whose 'inside was dragged up a bit' by a piece of shell in his pericardium, the covering of the heart, into which the piece of metal disappeared. The surgeon followed its passage three inches with his finger and then thought he had better leave well alone and stitched the wound. The soldier left on the ambulance train a few days later, smoking, with the hole and the metal still in his heart.

Sometimes sisters would cure a soldier given up by even the most optimistic surgeons. One of the most remarkable of these cases was a Belgian – 'Harry' to the sisters – in a Malines hospital staffed by English nurses. He was brought in with a gaping head wound and his body thin and so wasted that a sister could encircle his ankle with finger and thumb. His mouth was full of solid food – he was unable to swallow – and on his back was a gangrenous sore. The doctors examined him, shrugged and walked out. Then the sisters had to fight red tape when a Belgian officer and two men arrived to take him to a Belgian hospital – the move would have killed him. For many weeks this man was kept alive by the dedication of Sister

Jordan. He needed more constant – and unpleasant – care than any other case in the hospital, but gradually the sister brought Harry back to life. Interest and intelligence came into his eyes, the sore grew cleaner, and after a time he even sat up. After several months, without any treatment or even a subsequent examination by the doctors (so the sisters said) he was sent to England to convalesce. Somebody promised solemnly to let them know where he was sent, but sisters are accustomed to broken promises.[65]

Mairi Chisholm and Elsie Knocker – who became famous as 'the two of Pervyse' – had experiences that would have shocked surgeons. These two women – Mairi was only nineteen when she went to France – ran a first-aid post close to the front line. One afternoon in March 1917 two men were brought into the post too far gone for anything to be done. They were bad head cases and the brains were protruding. Immediately they were dead the nurses put them in the back yard, with shells coming in all the time. They helped to search through the clothes of the dead men, one a boy of nineteen who had been in the trenches only two days. As Mairi was searching through the pockets of a big overcoat she came across brains, evidently blown there by the force of the explosion. 'A very curious incident,' she called it.

During the Somme battles Alexandrina Marsden, nursing in a French hospital at Soissons, helped at several operations without anaesthetic.[66] I have already mentioned that the French were sometimes short of morphia. This victim had to be gagged and held down by orderlies, so that the surgeon needed half an hour to complete the arm amputation operation. Then he was exhausted and Sister Marsden was dripping with perspiration and feeling ill. Some of the patients who underwent operations without anaesthetic in her hospital were surprisingly docile. One man, operated on for a hernia, suffered such severe shock from the pain of the first incision by the surgeon's knife that his body became almost numb; he relaxed immediately, as though in a trance, and thereafter felt practically nothing.

This sister assisted during the operation on a French soldier who, through an explosion, had lost most of his lower parts, including a section of his stomach. He was patched up and restored to some sort of life.

Keeping the theatre hygienic was a constant problem. A tent with a mud floor invited germs – and so did the operating table. For a time the staff had to make do with a large deal kitchen table which required continual and careful scrubbing. another difficulty was lack of strong disinfectants. After one operation, Sister Marsden instructed a French nurse to scrub the table with soda. She returned to the theatre to find the girl squirting a siphon of soda-water – instead of caustic soda – over the table.

The poor standard of training among French nurses was a talking-point among their English counterparts, but it was probably higher than in Russia, where even trained sisters were continually doing things that horrified the English sisters serving there. They gave strong narcotic or stimulating drugs indiscriminately, such as morphine, codeine, camphor or ether without a doctor's orders. When untrained sisters and inexperienced dressers did this, which constantly happened, the results could be deplorable. Violetta Thurstan, in Russia in 1915, saw a dresser give a strong hypodermic stimulant to a man with a serious haemorrhage.[67] The bleeding vessel was deep and difficult to find, and the haemorrhage was so severe after the stimulant that for days the man's life was in danger from extreme exhaustion due to loss of blood. Sister Thurstan also heard a sister, whose only training was a two months' war course, say she had given a certain man ten injections of camphor within an hour because he was so collapsed, but she had not told the doctor she had done this nor had she let him know his patient was so much worse until he was at the point of death.

It would be repetitive to dwell on ward experiences of nursing sisters in the Second World War, but those of Geneviève de Galard during the French campaign in Indo-China, 1954, must find a place because they represent the exactions of nursing in jungle wars. Sister de Galard became famous as the only nurse in Dien-Bien-Phu when besieged by the Vietminh, though she was only one of several outstanding nurses of the campaign. The medical problems were serious and the labours of the few surgeons unceasing; Sister de Galard's work is perhaps best described as unpleasant.[68] At least twice a day it was her task to change the dressings on six abdominal cases who had colostomies; her hands were immersed in bundles of gauze soiled with faeces, yet she always did this with a smile or a joke. Then she washed her hands, rinsed them in spirit and went on to the next case, perhaps to renew the dressings on Sergeant Heinz, who had three stumps – both arms and a leg were missing. As a lot of dirt had got into the wounds in the first place and the antiseptics were not always effective, the stumps had not healed. At first each dressing produced a crisis in Heinz and for hours afterwards he lay in a coma, overcome with the pain. Half an hour had to be taken over each stump, very slowly unsticking the old dressing and putting on the new one with extreme care and patience. Sister de Galard was the only person to achieve this without making Heinz cry out.

Another soldier, Müller, had a compound fracture high in the left thigh and an enormous wound in the buttocks and loins on which plaster could not be used. With a fracture of this kind the normal procedure would be to put a splint along the tibia and adjust a metal ring round it from which is suspended a weight of up to forty pounds. This forces the ends of the bones into position and reduces the pain, which is always acute when a fracture is not held rigid. The wounded man would be placed on a large bed with straps and a system of cords and pulleys enabling him to be raised, providing access to the wound underneath and making the dressing of it comparatively simple. But such a bed and apparatus of pulleys could not be fitted into the rough shelter – even had the equipment been available.

An attempt was made to achieve the necessary traction by winding bands of adhesive plaster round the leg, but the constant sweat had made this come unstuck. Müller was fitted with a large splint which had to stop exactly at the point of break – at the top of the thigh where it joined the pelvis. It was necessary to turn him on his side to reach the wound underneath, an operation which forced howls of pain from him. It took two hours to renew the dressing, with Müller asking for a rest every five minutes. He had a cardiac stimulant injected and a little fruit juice to drink. It required all Sister de Galard's patience to bring this exhausting task to a satisfactory conclusion.

Another of her patients was Courtade. A bullet had hit his spinal cord and produced paralysis in both legs. He was lying in a shelter bed which the sister had to pass by ten or fifteen times a day. It was: 'Geneviève, help me to move my right foot – I can feel pins and needles coming on.' – 'Geneviève, put a little cotton wool under my knee, it's hurting.' – 'Geneviève, there's an insect under my right calf, I'm sure there is, do look.' – 'Geneviève, I'm thirsty . . . I can't sleep. . . .'

Serene and smiling, Geneviève would move the foot which refused to move, slip some cotton wool under the knee, rub the lifeless calf with a little spirit, give the soldier something to drink or fetch him a tablet. . . .

In 1854 a nurse's duties were mainly mechanical and manual; in 1954 they had become intellectual. Geneviève de Galard – or any other nursing sister – could have received at her aid post a wounded man on whose uniform would be pinned the label: 'Compound fractures of both legs caused by a grenade, anti-tet-tox, morphis, half a mill. units of penicillin.'

She would have to know not to touch the dressing, for undoing the dressing of a shattered leg is dangerous and can produce a fatal secondary shock. The doctor might order an injection of Phenergan-Dolosal and ask for two pints of blood. He would have to work quickly when the sister told him that blood pressure was down to 62. Opening the vein at the ankle, with such a wound, would be impossible, but he could probably do so at the elbow. The sister would now have two bottles of plasma flowing, a needle in each arm, but not too quickly in case the heart should be damaged.

She or the doctor would put other needles into the undamaged thighs of the patient – Coramine, Syncortyl, K-thrombyl, anti-gangrene serum, more penicillin. Blood pressure might rise, only to fall to the irreducible minimum of 40. The doctor would order two drops of warmed blood a second, and half a dose of Phenergan-Dolosal. As blood pressure rose the sister would be told to get out two more flasks of blood – and on its introduction pressure would rise still further. The doctor would nod now to the sister to cut the bandages. 'No arterial blood,' she would say, 'no lesion of the large vessels.'

The team, with infinite care, would make a more permanent dressing and then fasten a splint; pressure would be stabilized by injections of glucose saline and occasionally a little cardiac stimulant. Camphor solution or strychnine might be used, and to prevent infection developing there would be a final injection of penicillin and streptomycin.

Intellectual, empirical, practical.

Major Grauwin, who performed hundreds of operations under dreadful conditions – great heat, dirt, flies, lack of essential equipment and drugs and under constant enemy attack from close range – considered Sister de Galard the most indispensable member of his willing and competent staff. Most field doctors take nursing sisters so much for granted that they are unlikely to express either fluent or fulsome opinions about them, but it is quite certain that they would not like to go to war without them.

CHAPTER TWENTY-THREE

Second World War and Doctors in the Desert

The Second World War did not burst on the world's military medical services with the same horrifying impact as had the First World War, for during the period 1919–39 doctors had evolved many new methods of treatment. The British service was fortunate, paradoxically, in being engaged in many campaigns through which new ideas became new practice. It seems not to be realized that the RAMC provided the only organized medical service in north Russia during the anti-Bolshevik campaigns, 1919–21. The surgeons treated not only the sick and wounded of the Allied contingents – British, Italian, Serbian, French and White Russian – but the Russians themselves. The RAMC men also organized and trained a Russian army medical service and set up a school of army sanitation in Archangel. This was an arduous campaign for doctors and their assistants as troops were scattered over hundreds of miles in small garrisons and outposts. A journey of three days from front line to main dressing-station was frequent until railway coaches were converted into mobile main dressing-stations and operating centres. Specialists were flown in to treat casualties that could not, without harm be taken a long distance out. The doctors had laboratories, dental surgeries and ophthalmic centres, to which men would be brought by reindeer, pony or dog sledges or, in summer, by hospital barges along the great rivers.

In Kurdistan other troops were evacuated in mule cacolets down mountain tracks but they might be *en route* for ten days or more. The French were still using cacolets in Algiers and Morocco and British and French doctors wanted some more rapid evacuation. In 1919 a De Havilland, adapted to take just one stretcher and an attendant, was used experimentally in Somaliland. In 1920 the French produced an aircraft designed for ambulance work, and soon British designers had evolved another such plane, but neither was successful and troop-carriers were modified to carry stretchers. The first serious attempt at evacuating casualties was made in Iraq in April 1923 when about 200 cases of diarrhoea and dysentery among a column of British troops operating in northern Kurdistan were flown to Baghdad, a mileage of 9,615 being completed in 129 hours' flying time. In Palestine and Iraq between 1925 and 1936, 1,783 soldier patients were evacuated by air, with surgeons sometimes giving treatment in flight.

The British medical service after 1919 was so energetic and achieving so much in research that it led the world in army medical work; it was as if all the efforts of the pioneers were coming to fruition. In 1919, for instance, directorates of pathology, under Sir William Leishman, and hygiene, Sir William Horrocks, were set up. The Army Dental Corps was established in January 1921 and was to do much valuable work in jaw surgery. For the first time doctors were asked to make purely scientific assessments in military clothing, rations, equipment, accommodation and ventilation.

Doctors now had better terms of service, so that good brains were attracted into the army. Equally as important, men were now being trained as radiographers, physiotherapists, laboratory assistants and dispensers.

Just before the Second World War the army formed its own blood transfusion service, with a blood bank at Bristol. The United States Army had led the world in this field, using blood transfusions on a large scale in the latter days of the First World War. Transfusion was used again on some scale during the Spanish Civil War, 1936–9.

Another great aid for the field doctors was the evolution of the sulphonamide drugs, first introduced in Germany in 1935. They greatly reduced the incidence of septic infection, notably in wound treatment, pneumonia and cerebrospinal fever. By 1939 these drugs were sophisticated and were to save many lives in war. Indeed by 1939 so many drugs and treatments had been proved and improved that the servicemen of the war about to come had a much higher chance of surviving wounds and illness than any soldiers before. Of course the treatments applied as much to the sailor and to the new type of warrior, the airman, as to the soldier. Each, in one way or another, was more vulnerable than the others; the airman, for instance, was more likely to suffer serious burns – but generally the dangers were common to all. Burns were more frequent than before among soldiers and sailors; in some campaigns the proportion was one in ten.

For Britain the conflict lasted longer than for anybody else – 71 months; but military casualties (as distinct from civilian ones) were much lighter than those of the First World War. They amounted to: killed in battle or died of wounds, 104,076; wounded, 239,437. The RAMC treated 5 million cases in all. Wounds were difficult, having been made more complex by air bombing, machine warfare generally and greater use of mines and flame-throwers. Nevertheless techniques were so developed that even abdominal wounds were healed in over 50 per cent of cases; during the First World War three in four died. These figures do not tell the whole story. Many more desperate cases reached the operating table than in the First World War because of the presence of transfusion services and field surgical units. There is still, however, no easy way of saving a man with several abdominal wounds; he has to be worked for and fought for.

Mortality from thoracic injuries had been 54 per cent; now it was 5.7 per cent. Amputations dropped from 70 to 20 per cent and mortality dropped remarkably. Damaged eyes had been lost in 67 per cent of cases; in the Second World War the figure was down to 37 per cent.

With vast numbers of men involved in war the medical services grew correspondingly in size. The combined British service had 1,180 units, including 148 field and general hospitals and 50 field surgical units; the Germans had 1,200 units, including 80 casualty clearing-stations and 200 field ambulance units; the Russians, by 1945, 1,500 medical units; and the Americans, in the same year, 2,200 medical units. All these reflected the revolutionized philosophy about military casualties.

In the Second World War the strategic aspects of healing almost took precedence over humanitarian aspects. Neither the German nor the Red Army could have afforded such fearful losses if a high percentage of the wounded had not been returned to the ranks. The four chief reasons for the high rate of survival and return to service were the use of penicillin, the sulphonamide and other drugs against infection in wounds, the use of the closed plaster treatment of compound fractures, blood transfusion, and the new ways of organizing the medical services so that casualties could be given treatment in the shortest possible time.

The whole approach to field surgery – and I use this in its broadest sense to include the sea and air – was as much a science as was the treatment of a particular type of wound or disease. Much of this science was compressed into the doctor's *Field Surgery Pocket Book*. He was, for instance, given an outline about the 'wounding agents'. This outline should be starkly significant to the general reader.

1. Rifle and machine-gun bullets.
2. Jagged fragments of shell, bomb, mortar and mine, accounting for 70 to 80 per cent of all wounds.
3. Minute fragments and razor-blade-like flakes of metal.
4. Bayonet, dagger and knife.
5. Blast – air, water.
6. Crushes, blows, falls from a height.

1. Bullets being of high velocity, are likely to pass right through the body, from front to back, from side to side, or obliquely, depending upon the line of fire and the position of the man. They cause small entry and larger exit wounds and usually produce multiple injuries within.
2. Fragments from shell, bomb, mortar and mine are of lower velocity and tend to become embedded in muscle, bone, solid viscus, or to lie free within the abdominal cavity or some hollow viscus like the bladder. The wound of entry is larger than that of the bullet, and irregular in outline. A man may be hit by several such pieces and sustain generalized wounds.
3. Minute fragments and thin flakes of metal are important because they may leave no more than what appears to be a mere scratch or abrasion on the surface, yet the internal injury may be severe and multiple. It stresses the need to examine the whole of the body surface and to keep any such case complaining of symptoms under observation.

4. The wounds caused by these sharp cutting weapons speak for themselves.
5. The blast of bombs, bursting in air, and depth-charges in water, may inflict severe intro-abdominal injuries in men nearby without there being any external signs.
6. Crushes from falling debris, being buried by collapsing earthworks, or falling from a height as from a parachute wrongly manoeuvred, may all result in injuries to intro-abdominal organs, and such cases should be kept under observation.

Percentages of wounds can be further refined:

Mortar bombs and HE* shell fragments	60 per cent
Machine-gun bullets	15 per cent
Rifle bullets	10 per cent
Others	
Land mines	
Grenades	
Booby traps	15 per cent
Anti-tank shell	
Aerial bombs	
Types of Wound	
The types of wounds are generally these:	
Limb wounds, including fractures	80 per cent
Chest wounds	8–10 per cent
Abdominal wounds	?–4 per cent
Head wounds	2–4 per cent
Others	2–8 per cent

Wounds are frequently multiple, requiring several operations on the same patient.

In the Second World War the field surgeon's life did not begin and end with his amputation or appendicectomy. He had to train his orderlies, for without competent assistants his work was more difficult and sometimes wasted. He had to be able to find his specified site by map reference, set up and take down his tent, know how best to load his gear, know enough of army system to be aware of his geographical place in that system. He had records to keep and stocks to watch.

Field surgery as practised in the Second World War was highly educational and developmental for the surgeon. It sharpened his surgeon's judgment and strengthened his self-reliance – he could rarely call for a second opinion.

---

* Wounds caused by high explosive shell fragments are commonly miscalled shrapnel wounds. Shrapnel was rarely used in the Second World War.

Because each day he must check those patients he retains he learns much about post-operative treatment. He learns to take and make notes clearly and concisely so that the next doctor in the chain of evacuation can pick up the threads of treatment. In the field too the surgeon learns more in a single campaign about the risk of infection than he would learn in years of civil practice.

In British service, where possible, it was a rule that surgeons were not kept in the field longer than twelve months before being returned to a base hospital. There were sound reasons for this. Surgeons are only human, and the strain of working for very long hours in the stench of blood and powerful smells of anaesthetics and disinfectants, of constantly seeing blood-stained and mud-stained clothing and dressings and exhausted, worried men, of making one amputation after another or sewing up intestines – all this is a great strain. Inevitably too there is a tendency for a tired man to lower his standards of asepsis and even perhaps those of surgery. It is no longer possible for a surgeon to be continually at work in the field for as long as Guthrie or Larrey. In admiration of these two men it would be easy to suggest that perhaps surgeons, like soldiers, are not as resilient as those of earlier years. Indeed there *could* be some truth in this. But, more practically, modern military surgeons are under greater mental stress from the threat of bombing, from the rapid movement of armies and from the extremely high standards of surgical work expected. Again, Guthrie and Larrey did not expect relief; their modern counterparts do expect it. Psychologically this makes a big difference.

Except in emergencies few novices were at work in field surgery during the Second World War. No newcomer treated fresh casualties without an apprenticeship of periods in a base hospital in the fighting zone and at a staging post in the chain of evacuation. A surgeon needed such an introduction to field surgery if he were not to make mistakes when he himself took a surgical team into the field.

Brigadier Charles Donald, OBE, ChM, FRCS, deputy director of medical services to the British Eighth Army, has pointed out that a surgeon needs character, physical fitness and adaptability as well as skill.[69]

There are required a zest and a capacity to go on doing a good job for many consecutive hours, perhaps for several consecutive days, to be up and about at all hours, to take the rough with the smooth, to think in terms not only of technique but of humanity, to perform the little kindnesses as well as the big operations.

In a war which ranged over the globe, involved half its nations in scores of campaigns and was fought in every kind of terrain and climate, it is obviously impossible to deal with all aspects of military medical practice. I intend to deal with the campaigns in Africa, Sicily and Italy, with brief references to other theatres, as the best way of giving some idea of the problems facing the surgeon and his helpers.

Clinical needs will always clash with martial necessities. The medical services' ideal would be to have an array of holding medical units close to the front line. Naturally military commanders are more interested in fighting units and cannot allow their battle areas to be cluttered with non-combatant units. Compromise was unavoidable during the campaigns of movement between 1939 and 1945. Only the really serious cases could be held close to the line, for to move them at all would be to kill them. The proportion of casualties kept where operated on did not exceed 5 per cent. The others were started along the chain of evacuation. This meant that doctors and their helpers had to use fine judgment in deciding on holding or forwarding. All along this chain the RAMC staff had to watch the condition of the evacuees, noting the pressure of plaster casts, being vigilant about secondary haemorrhages and in changing dressings.

Because of the need for a patient to travel it was rare, after the first year or so of the war, for suture to be made immediately after excision, except of course for head and abdominal wounds or when the surgeon could be sure of retaining a patient until it was time for stitches to be removed. Surgery of the abdomen benefited particularly by continuous gastric suction coupled with continuous drip infusion. This was largely due to the surgeons of the Middle East campaign under their mentor, Sir Heneage Ogilvie.*

The chain of evacuation (see overleaf for diagram) would vary, but in North Africa the casualty's progress was something like this:[70]

50 miles to his own regimental aid post (RAP) (Going bad.)
25 miles to brigade advanced dressing station (ADS) (Going bad.)
30 miles to advanced main dressing station (AMDS) (Going very bad.)
30 miles to staging post. (Going almost impossible.)
50 miles to main dressing station (MDS) (Going almost impossible.)
60 miles to railhead. (Per motor ambulance convoy.)
80 miles to CCS (Per hospital train.)
150 miles back to general hospital. (Per hospital train.)

The phrase 'going almost impossible' meant that ambulances were frequently slowed to a few miles an hour, or stopped altogether. Ambulance drivers had to find their way along lines of communication which might stretch for 2,000 miles, with very few clear markings at any point and only elementary tracks to follow. The driver had to think about his patients as well as his route, and had to be careful to find as smooth a track as possible.

Because the essence of desert war is mobility, surgery, like the fighting men and their supplies, had also to be put on wheels. This was done by giving the light sections of some casualty clearing-stations their own transport and by the formation of small mobile field surgical teams, consisting of surgeon,

---

* Baron Larrey had used the indwelling stomach tube 150 years previously to feed a soldier whose jaw had been shattered.

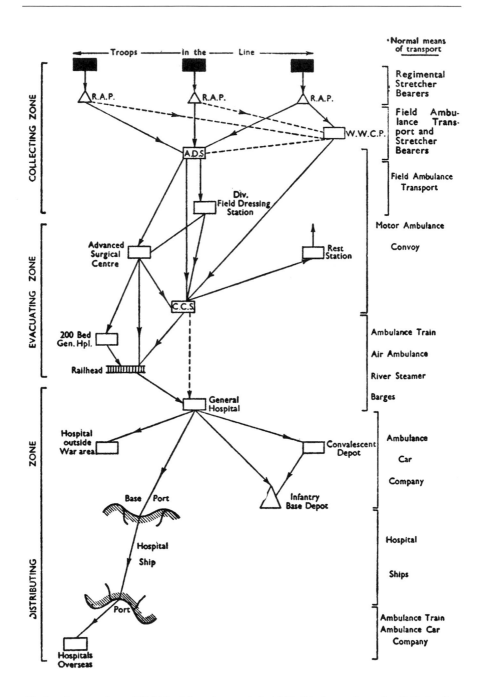

Chain of evacuation of British sick and wounded, 1919–45, shown from the field (top) to home (bottom).

anaesthetist, a few trained orderlies, a car and a lorry. They could keep up with the fighting and provide surgery to casualties whose further journey to the CCS would be dangerous. These field surgical units, which could carry out a hundred operations from their own supplies, were something new on the battlefield, as were field transfusion units, mobile neurosurgical units, mobile maxillo-facial surgical teams, field water-purification, hygiene and sanitation units. The military medical services of the world were now acting quite aggressively, going forward to meet casualties and to prevent disease rather than being content to cure them when they came.

The CCS was the key unit of field surgery. Reinforced by field surgical units, it could have several operating teams to take their spells of duty and remain fresh. Because of the sisters on its establishment it offered high standards of nursing. It had good lighting, X-rays and good tents and it could provide better diet.

The static periods in North Africa gave opportunity to prepare for the big battles – Alamein, Mareth, Wadi Akarit – when heavy casualties could be expected. In between times there were pursuits, with minor actions. For the set piece battles casualty clearing stations concentrated fifteen to thirty miles from the front line; in front of them were the field surgical teams and some main dressing-stations. After a breakthrough the MDS moved forward with their field ambulances and the CCS moved one by one, until they stretched out as a chain of daily staging posts back to base. The wounded were passed back along this chain.

The Russians were proud of having much the same system, although their chain of evacuation was usually shorter since their base hospitals were closer to the front. After immediate first-aid treatment a casualty would be 'classified' and sent to one of half a dozen specialized field surgical units, each handling a specific type of injury. There would seem to be a danger of over-specialization, but the Russians claim that a man with several wounds was not first treated for the abdominal ones and then, say, sent elsewhere for his head wounds. The weakness of the system was that the person making the initial classification, possibly in the dark and under fire, would often not fully understand the casualty's major trouble and might send him to the wrong specialist unit. By not splinting fractures but by putting them into plaster casts at once and by giving many wounds only superficial treatment before passing the patient back, the Russians believed that they substantially reduced the high potential mortality. As in previous wars, the Russian soldiers were certainly hardy and many survived as much because of their robust constitution as because of skilled treatment.

In the British campaigns the medical administrator and the doctor had the same problem, looked at from different ways. The administrator had the worry of the long road evacuation and the diversion of CCS and field ambulances to act as staging posts. To the surgeon all this meant that his patients would undergo an added strain which it was essential to ease for the badly wounded.

The desert campaign was essentially a tented one for CCS and field ambulances; suitable buildings were rare and operating vehicles were discarded because of their cramped conditions. But tents had their difficulties – no floors, difficulty in maintaining an equable temperature; lighting, flyproofing, sandproofing. Flies and sand were the greatest troubles, while having to disperse tents because of danger from possible bombing was most inconvenient; no surgeon wanted his pre-operative and post-operative tents too far from the theatre. Ideally the general hospitals should have been able to follow the other medical units closely, but speed of the campaign made this impossible – a general hospital set up near Benghazi was soon 800 miles behind.

Surgeons and their assistants had bizarre experiences and dangerous adventures in the desert war. One doctor and his orderlies were overrun by Germans. The British counter-attacked successfully and found the surgeon again. 'You still here?' they said. The surgeon was too busy for conversation.

The Germans attacked successfully a second time, and again the British counter-attacked. 'You *still* here?' they said. It happened four times; even Field-Marshal Rommel called in. 'No one seems to take any notice of the regular visiting hours,' the doctor said sourly. Or so the story goes.

On 12 December 1940 in the battle of Sidi Barrani, Lieutenant J.M. Muir was MO to the first battalion of the Argyll and Sutherland Highlanders. Wounded about 7 a.m. by a shell splinter, he insisted on being propped up beside his vehicle, and so that his senses might remain clear refused an injection of morphine. Though dangerously wounded and suffering intense pain from severe wounds in the pelvis and in the shoulder, for eight hours he gave directions to his stretcher-bearers on how to deal with the wounded as they reached the RAP. He remained at his post until the last wounded man had been evacuated, and only then did he consent to be placed in the ambulance himself. He won the DSO.

On 24 November 1941 the dressing station at Gasr-el-Abid was attacked and occupied by the enemy. During the attack, when his tent was riddled with machine-gun fire, Corporal S.W. Scannell did his best to make his patients safe and continued to treat and encourage them. During the next nine hours he carried out treatment, though repeatedly fired on by enemy sentries whenever he left the tent for essential requirements. Due to his bravery and care all the patients survived, and Scannell won the MM.

On the night of 15 January 1943, during the attacks on Wadi Chfef, Private William Shedden was in charge of a squad of stretcher-bearers attached to one of the forward companies. The attack led into a deep enemy minefield south of the wadi, heavily sown with anti-personnel mines which caused casualties. Despite the danger of setting off more mines he led his squad into the minefield and evacuated fifteen casualties of sappers, tanks and infantry. As they were going in for the last casualty a mine exploded, killing his younger brother, who was one of the squad, and injuring the other two stretcher-bearers. Shedden was dazed by the blast and the realization that his brother had been killed, but attended the casualties as they lay in the minefield and evacuated all of them to the RAP. He was awarded the MM.

The anti-personnel mine made its appearance in great numbers in North Africa and produced wounds which worried the surgeons. Roughly the size of a 2-lb jam jar and actuated by being trodden on, this mine sprang five or six feet into the air, exploded and scattered about 300 metal balls. Wounds were nearly always multiple, though their severity was later excelled by the multiple wounds of the six-barrelled German mortars. Shock from such wounds is severe and one or more of the wounds is apt to be serious, a penetrating abdominal injury for instance. The surgeon was constantly having to ask himself, as he dealt with one wound after another, how much the patient could stand.

The first parachute surgical unit went into action in North Africa. The surgeon and anaesthetist and their orderlies dropped with their equipment, including an operating table, instruments, dressings, plaster of Paris, blood plasma, sterilizer, anaesthetic equipment, drugs, medical comforts and a bedpan. Only the barest essentials in their most compressed form could be taken. Beds, blankets and an operating theatre had to be improvised on descent.

Major C.G. Rob, MC., the surgeon, performed 136 operations on Allied troops or prisoners with only four deaths, and nine operations on civilians. Twenty-five per cent of the troops were discharged to duty within six weeks. The surgical centre also handled cases who were too far gone for treatment or not in immediate need of it. Altogether 238 cases were admitted to the dressing station and only 17 died, including 11 who were in such a bad way that they died almost immediately on admission. Major Rob attributed this low mortality to the operations being performed in an average time of 10½ hours after injury. Blood for transfusions was obtained from the parachutists themselves who had been blood-grouped beforehand.

CHAPTER TWENTY-FOUR

Sicily, Italy, North-West Europe: Jungles and Guerrillas

The mobile field surgical units and light sections of the CCS fitted into the early part of the Sicilian campaign, 1943, landing at different points with field ambulances and immediately dealing with the most serious casualties. Some of these early units had to wade ashore with their panniers. Fighting conditions in Sicily were severe, with high temperatures and humidity and even more flies than in North Africa; the soldiers' resistance was lowered by the strain they endured. The surgical units kept up with the troops, but casualties often needed more sleep than surgery. Many of those with abdominal wounds, who would have lived in the drier, cleaner desert, expired listlessly on the second or third day after operation.

Getting to Syracuse, the main medical base, was a further ordeal on rough, winding roads with demolished bridges – and malaria had now become a problem. The general hospitals were under such pressure for beds that men who should normally have been kept in them had to be evacuated by hospital ship and plane.

Surgeons mostly worked now in buildings – schools, monasteries, churches, houses – generally unclean to begin with. There were the usual improvisations to cope with – taps without water, drains which did not and non-existent lavatories.

Hospitals were sometimes difficult to locate. The American war correspondent Ernie Pyle,* who had fallen ill, was sent off in an ambulance to find a certain clearing station, but the crew could not locate it and drove, said Pyle, half way across Sicily before giving up and starting back on a seventy-five mile agonizing drive over dusty gravel roads. They found the clearing station set up within four miles of where they had started from.

Ernie Pyle saw many soldiers die in Sicily and movingly reported one tragedy:[71]

---

* He was killed covering the Okinawa invasion in 1945.

Dying men were brought into our tent, men whose death rattle silenced the conversation and made all of us thoughtful. When a man was almost gone the surgeons would put a piece of gauze over his face. He could breathe through it but we couldn't see his face well.

Twice within five minutes chaplains came running. One of those occasions haunted me for hours. The wounded man was still semiconscious. The chaplain knelt down beside him and two wardboys squatted nearby. The chaplain said: 'John, I'm going to say a prayer for you.'

Somehow this stark announcement hit me like a hammer. He didn't say: 'I'm going to pray for you to get well', he just said he was going to say a prayer, and it was obvious to me that he meant the final prayer. It was as though he had said: 'Brother, you may not know it, but your goose is cooked.' Anyhow, he voiced the prayer, and the weak, gasping man tried vainly to repeat the words after him. When he had finished, the chaplain added: 'John, you're doing fine, you're doing fine.' Then he rose and dashed off on some other call, and the wardboys went about their duties.

The dying man was left utterly alone, just lying there on his litter on the ground, lying in an aisle, because the tent was full. Of course it couldn't be otherwise, but the aloneness of that man as he went through the last few minutes of his life was what tormented me.

American practice was a little different from the British. Some divisions had two clearing stations, and ordinarily only one would work at a time while the other rested; the second would then leapfrog the first, set up its tents and begin to receive patients. In emergencies both would work at once. Clearing stations were really small hospitals, with five doctors, a dentist, a chaplain and sixty men, with six large tents and few smaller ones. A clearing station could strike camp, move and set up again in a remarkably short time, in Sicily some were required to do this three times a day.

Pyle's nomination for the man with the most nerve in Sicily was a soldier with two holes in his back so big Pyle could have put his hand in either one. As the surgeons worked on him he lay on his stomach and talked volubly. 'I killed five of the sonsabitches with a hand grenade just before they got me,' he said. 'What made me so damn mad was that I was just out of reach of my rifle and couldn't crawl over to it, or I'da got five more of them. Jeez, I'm hungry! I ain't had nothing to eat since yesterday morning.'

In Sicily, as on any front, each day produced its quota of freak wounds and hairbreadth escapes. American surgeons picked out more than 200 pieces of metal from one man. There was hardly a square inch of him that was not touched, but none made a vital hit, and the soldier lived. Another soldier had a small hole in the front of his leg just below the hip. It did not look serious, but beneath the wound the leg bone was shattered and arteries were severed, and the surgeons had difficulty closing the arteries so he would not bleed to death.

One man had caught a small shell fragment in the wrist. It had entered at a shallow angle, passed up the arm to the elbow and remained there. The skin was not even broken at the elbow, but over the spot where the fragment stopped was a blister as big as a pigeon's egg – raised by the heat of the metal.

Following the invasion of Italy by the Eighth Army, at Reggio, 3 September 1943, there was another forward-moving operation for the medical units; eventually a chain of staging posts reached 300 miles back to the Straits of Messina. In the December cold, rain, snow and mud made conditions difficult, and casualties were got back for treatment only by the devotion of the ambulance men, who often had to manhandle stretchers over rough country. In contested landings, as at Anzio and Salerno, medical posts had to dig in and sandbag, and while patients were received promptly after wounding, post-operative care was difficult to provide, with frightful, almost continuous, noise and a rain of metal from shells, bombs and anti-aircraft fire. Wounds, with the armies in semi-static, Flanders-like positions, were commonly multiple and severe from mortar-fire.

As elsewhere, the detached field surgical units (FSUs) caught the imagination of the administrators and almost inevitably there was a tendency to exploit them beyond wise limits. That is, they were moved too frequently, they were sometimes too far forward and therefore within range of the enemy's guns and within the noise area of their own guns. This was adverse for surgeon and patient. The field ambulances liked to have the FSUs attached; it meant that temporarily they were more than staging posts, that they were provided with cases of great clinical interest and that their nursing orderlies received valuable education.

Education under battle conditions was apt to be advanced and arduous. One orderly was with a unit surrounded for eight days during the bloody battles for the dominating hill of Monte Cassino in February 1944. This man, with nothing more than scissors and small knives, undertook surgery, and surgeons who later saw his work noted that it was competent. Generally surgical practice became even more efficient in Italy when reserve surgical teams were formed. Drawn from base hospitals, these teams were a version of the Americans' two-team leapfrog system; they took over the equipment of the original surgical team and gave its members a spell.

The development of forward specialized work is one of the most interesting aspects in the war's surgical history. Mobile ophthalmic units, long needed in forward areas, saved the eyesight of many soldiers. Forward orthopaedic units were also established and patients could be held for two or three months so that traction devices need not be disturbed. At the time of Alamein a neurological unit existed in Cairo and later, when the army had moved 800 miles forward, a second unit was established. In Italy, in November–December 1943, it had much work following the heavy fighting on the Trigno and Sangro rivers. The maxillo-facial unit also went forward, and in the end the three units were grouped together. An advanced maxillo-facial team was vital if the fractured-jaw patient was to have early and adequate fixation – the dental surgeon's business. A surgeon with plastic training also went forward and was involved in many aspects of facial surgery – jaw drainage, removal of foreign bodies, closure of deep layers of cheek wounds, the accurate suture of lips, immediate replacement of displaced fractured nasal bones, cheek bones, and the repair of torn eyelids. Without such help the patients would have had to wait at least three days before they could reach an advanced base hospital.

One aspect of field surgery different in type and quantity in the Second World War from any previous war was that the surgeons, when not busy with their own casualties, found much work in treating the local population, many of whom were badly injured by mines and booby traps. In Italy particularly the surgeons patched up children who had been damaged by booby-trapped fountain pens or watches.

The extent of the doctors' British military casualties can be seen from figures. Killed or died of wounds, 23,263; wounded, 63,212; non-battle casualties varied from 633 per thousand troops in 1943 to 482 per thousand in 1945.

So much had been learned, transmitted and codified in the earlier campaigns that the medical organization of the North-West Europe campaign of 1944–5 was the most efficient of any war in history. Sickness among troops was half the First World War ratio, despite adverse conditions. The troops were in contact with many diseases among liberated political prisoners and servicemen and among the starving refugees, but only twenty-five troops contracted typhus and none died of it. Dysentery and venereal disease were the most common complaints. The overall recovery rate was 94 per cent, a remarkably high figure to which hygiene, swift evacuation and new techniques contributed.

The advent of penicillin had been one of the great events of the war. Discovered by Sir Alexander Fleming in the 1920s, it passed almost unnoticed and its exploitation as a therapeutic agent began only in 1940. First used in warfare in Egypt in 1942, it assumed an ever-increasing importance in North Africa, Sicily, Italy and the Pacific. Injected into veins or muscles in liquid form or applied directly to the wound in powder form, penicillin kills large numbers of bacteria in a few hours. It saved 12 to 15 per cent of cases which would previously have been fatal or would have needed amputations, and halved the time needed in hospital.

Good surgery coupled with penicillin produced the following figures for primary healing of limb wounds at the battles of the Senio River and the Po Valley towards the end of the Italian campaign:

	100–90 per cent healing	89–50 per cent healing	under 50 per cent healing
With fracture (298)	240	49	9
	(81 per cent)	(16 per cent)	(3 per cent)
Without fracture (1,555)	1,380	152	23
	(88 per cent)	(9 per cent)	(3 per cent)

The results at one hospital reserved for delayed primary suture of limb wounds were even better; 90 per cent healing was obtained in 98 per cent of 624 patients with flesh wounds. The great curse of the chronically infected wound had virtually disappeared from the battlefield.

Another medical success was mepacrine. Until the Second World War quinine was the only drug regularly prescribed in the tropics to prevent or reduce the effects of malaria. As the Far East war developed it was seen that malaria was a major menace and that existing measures to protect the soldier against it were inadequate. For several reasons quinine was likely to be scarce. The medical services recommended that one tablet of mepacrine be taken daily by each soldier. When the incidence of the disease did not fall as anticipated a series of urgent experiments carried out at Cairns, Queensland, proved that by taking this dose of mepacrine regularly the soldier could not possibly develop symptoms of malaria, no matter how many times bitten by infective mosquitoes. It was now possible to defeat the disease in the highly malarious jungles of Burma and New Guinea. The responsibility for taking the anti-malaria drug became that of the individual officer and soldier, and with punishment for failure to do so the incidence of malaria fell to negligible proportions.

Malaria was responsible for 80 per cent of all admissions to hospital in Burma, and during the first Arakan campaign, 1943, it laid low 120 men for each battle casualty. By 1945, due to mepacrine, the rate was six to one battle casualty and 90 per cent of affected men were fit for duty after three weeks' treatment.

Despite an overall improvement in sanitation, bacillary dysentery continued to remain a primary cause of manpower wastage until the introduction of sulphaguanidine treatment in the Middle East by Boyd and Fairley in 1940. In full doses this drug quickly controlled the symptoms of acute dysentery and brought about a rapid cure. Dyspepsia was one of the main causes of sickness; in a large hospital between 15 and 20 per cent of patients suffered from it. Probably the patient was suffering from it in civil life but ignored it or could nurse it. Healthy men who showed dyspeptic symptoms were usually suffering merely from a change of environment and diet.

It must be said that without the transfusion service and the transfusion officer in the field neither the physicians nor the surgeons could have achieved their significant successes. At the blood supply depot at Bristol a trained staff of over 300 received the blood collected from voluntary donors by mobile army medical teams. Here blood and plasma were prepared for transport and storage and medical officers were sent abroad to organize the collection, preparation and storage of blood in the field.

During the battle of Alamein, October 1942, 7,393 casualties were admitted to the main dressing-stations. One in ten of these had to be transfused to save their lives, and on the average three bottles were required for each casualty transfused. At Agheila, 1943, 1,393 wounded were admitted and one in six had to be transfused.

One in thirty of the first 300 men to land on the Sicilian beaches on 10 July 1943 was an RAMC man, carrying on his back a tall, round tin containing a pint of liquid plasma and a transfusion set. Casualties soon began to come to the improvised first-aid post. Some men had suffered damage to arteries, or had had their legs fractured by machine-gun bullets. Within an hour serious casualties of this kind were receiving transfusions. Meanwhile sixty men of a field service unit had landed more elaborate equipment from a special boat. An hour later a really large dump of medical stores had reached the shore. Among these stores were 300 bottles of plasma. They were followed by a field transfusion unit and a casualty clearing station; and off-shore lay a hospital ship with 200 pints of blood held in reserve. As the advance continued the RAMC men kept well up with the foremost parties. Wherever resistance was met they looked round for shelter – perhaps a half-ruined cottage or an overhanging rock – and established a first-aid post ready for action, saving life in the midst of death and destruction.

Many wounded men were saved on the Normandy beaches who would have died in similar conditions in the First World War. One of the chief reasons for the low death-rate among casualties was that the men in the landing-craft, the ships, the transport planes and the gliders took blood with them. Strapped into the equipment of the medical units of the paratroops and all other assault units were bottles of the blood product, plasma, and transfusion sets, in waterproof boxes. Transfusion officers with the assault troops carried waterproofed instruments and dressings, so that, without waiting for their special lorries to be beached, they could set to work dripping life-blood into wounded men.

Soon after the transfusion teams had waded ashore came field transfusion unit lorries, equipped with refrigerators with 1,100 pints of fresh, whole blood. Blood plasma was also carried in other military vehicles – slung on the underside in containers which in the ordinary way hold trench mortar shells; four bottles and two transfusion sets took the place of three shells.*

A Highlander who had been lying in a field for three days with a shell splinter in his chest before the stretcher-bearers found him was pulseless when admitted to an advanced dressing station. At first the doctor despaired of his life. A transfusion officer decided to give him a transfusion. After he had been given four pints of blood he revived and started to relate his experiences. A lance-bombardier who had had both legs shattered by an 88-mm shell was given a transfusion within fifteen minutes of becoming a casualty.

As the troops fought their way inland supplies of blood and blood products followed them. More plasma, in wicker baskets, was dropped by parachute to airborne troops and isolated units. No force was ever better equipped for transfusion or for other medical services than the Army of

---

* It should be noted that the primary importance of plasma, the colourless, coagulable part of blood in which the corpuscles float, was that it can be given to any man, regardless of his blood group. However, the quantity which can be safely given is limited.

Liberation. The methods of carrying the blood and transfusion sets were improved and elaborated as the result of experience gained in the Sicilian, Salerno and Anzio landings. Sergeant Blake, a sapper aged thirty, had the experience of watching his leg travelling many yards through the air. He was admitted to an advanced dressing-station, given morphia and a pint of plasma. Only four hours later they got him to the main dressing-station. He would never have got there but for the plasma. He was given two pints of blood and then operated on; during the operation, a long one, another three pints of blood had to be used.

Transfusion saved lives in the air services too. Squadron-Leader Jim Duncan was wounded over Berlin in 1943, but managed to bring his bomber limping back. He ordered his crew to bale out over Norfolk. Then, almost fainting, he guided the bomber back towards his airfield, and crashed through a hedge a few hundred yards away. The leaking engines caught fire, and Squadron-Leader Duncan received that terrible new injury, that burn of hands and face, which comes from the intense heat of high octane petrol, far worse than any ordinary burn which doctors had had to deal with before. Air Force burn left Duncan practically without a face, though his eyeballs were safe.

A man suffering from Air Force burn has only one chance – immediate blood transfusion. Burns quickly affect the blood stream. There is no bleeding away of the whole blood as when an artery is severed, but the circulatory system becomes leaky and the blood plasma seeps away rapidly, some into the injured tissues, some to other parts of the body, because the blood vessels are no longer able to hold their contents. The result is delayed or secondary shock, collapse of the heart, and death some hours after the burn.

Squadron Leader Duncan lay on his hospital bed wounded, burned and unconscious. The moment he arrived at the hospital a movable blood transfusion set was wheeled up to his side, the needle was pressed into the vein in his arm and the plasma began to drip. He was taken to the operating theatre, his wound cleaned and dressed, the fractured limb closed up in an immovable plaster case, the burned flesh cut away from his face and hands, always with the drip, drip of the transfusion set.

Meanwhile his own plasma was leaking out and hour after hour more plasma had to be dripped into him to keep him alive. Slowly the gain of blood increased until he began to pull round. Then followed long weeks of healing. At last he was strong enough to stand his second ordeal, the protracted operation of plastic surgery by means of which he was given new eyelids, new lips, new cheeks, a new nose. In this second ordeal, blood transfusion contributed largely to success. This man, strong as he was normally, could hardly have borne as he did flesh re-modelling had not blood been readily available.

There was a fear that surgeons were perhaps delaying too long in the hope or expectation that transfusion would greatly improve the patient. At such times, especially when the transfusion officer believed that further transfusion was unlikely to be helpful, he had to say so. Transfusion was used even more in the American service than in the British.

Though more sophisticated blood-transfusion techniques helped plastic surgery, it was dedicated talent which made the latter so important during the Second World War. There seems to be a misconception that plastic surgery had its beginnings during this war; in fact, during the pre-Christian era when Hindu husbands revenged themselves on unfaithful wives by lopping off their nose, a caste of Hindu potters learned how to restore them. The closely guarded art was passed only from father to son, and not until the fifteenth century did it reach Italy. Less than a century later Gasparo Tagliacozzi wrote a book on certain forms of plastic surgery, which is perhaps better described as reconstructive surgery – to use the term of its greatest exponent, Archibald McIndoe. After Tagliacozzi centuries passed before ridicule and opposition were overcome.

In 1551 another Italian pioneer, Fiorovanti, witnessed a duel in which one of the swordsmen lost his nose, which fell in sand. Fiorovanti picked it up, urinated on it to wash off the sand, sewed the nose on, rubbed balsam well in and bandaged it. He thought the nose would rot, but after eight days found that it had attached itself to the face.

Sir Charles Valadier, a noted dentist who served with the British Army during the First World War, urged the need for a plastic surgery unit behind the lines, and in the summer of 1915 he set up the first British jaw and plastic unit at Wimereux, France. He took as his assistant Harold Delf Gillies, who after a few months started a plastic unit of his own at Aldershot. At this time the Germans were also practising reconstruction, but only to get mutilated men back to the front and with little regard for how the men looked. The French, surprisingly perhaps, were also not concerned about appearance, and it was often said that a French plastic patient looked horrible when he went in and ridiculous when he came out.

Gillies was one of the first to study the aesthetics as well as the techniques of plastic surgery. After the battle of the Somme in the summer of 1916 he received 2,000 cases of jaw and facial mutilation at Aldershot, and somehow gave every man his personal attention. His pioneer work received little recognition. In January 1924 he was called to Copenhagen to treat about twenty Danish naval officers and men who had been seriously burned in an accident; the publicity made medicine aware of his brilliance.

In 1932 Gillies took as his assistant Archibald McIndoe, a distant cousin from New Zealand who had been working at the Mayo Clinic, New York. The partnership gave the ambitious McIndoe all the work he could handle and his techniques became remarkably sophisticated, but in 1938, a year before war broke out, only four men were specializing in plastic surgery in England, Rainsford Mowlem and T.P. Kilner being the other two.

In June 1938 McIndoe replaced Gillies as consultant in plastic surgery to the RAF, and soon after the war started he established himself in the Queen Victoria Hospital at East Grinstead, Sussex. Mowlem and Gillies had gone to other plastic surgery units at St Albans and Basingstoke. As with so many physicians and surgeons before him, McIndoe was worried about his status with the services. Most of his predecessors had wanted rank; McIndoe considered that the comparatively junior rank of Wing Commander which the RAF offered him would restrict his powers, so he remained a civilian, and as one was able to fight for his ends much more vigorously.

Again, like many of his predecessors, he had to fight hidebound custom, such as the routine treatment of badly burned patients by smearing their burns with tannic acid or gentian violet which McIndoe knew could cause great damage to a man badly burned about the face and hands. After a bitter argument he managed to have tannic acid prohibited as treatment for third-degree burns on the face and hands.

The air war brought to the plastic surgery hospitals many hideously mutilated young men who faced years of continual operations, as the plastic surgeons worked patiently to reconstruct faces and hands, and restore skin to ravaged bodies. Sometimes there was no possibility of repair; the surgeon would have to begin again – a new bone for the chin, new skin and flesh for the cheeks, a flap from the shaved head pulled down and filled with cartilage to form a new nose, new eyelids – painful three-year job. Burned flying men of the RAF treated by McIndoe became the famous Guinea Pigs.

Flying-Officer James Wright, DFC, after suffering dreadful burns when he crashed in Italy, had forty-six operations on his face and eight corneal graft operations. They were among the 4,000 reconstructive surgery operations McIndoe performed at East Grinstead in four years of war. In one series he carried out thirty-eight operations, carefully stitching on postage-stamp-sized grafts of skin to the fingers of a young pilot whose hands had been glued into a solid mass of fire.

McIndoe confessed to hating only two things in surgery. One was to make an ear for a man who had had his original burned away. The other was amputation: 'It's not surgery. It's butchery.'

If flying brought burns more frequently into the catalogue of service surgery it compensated for it by allowing more rapid evacuation of wounded men. Air evacuation was as important as penicillin and blood supply and it came to be used on a gigantic scale. In just one year – 1943 – the US Army alone air-evacuated 173,527 sick and wounded to base hospitals; only 11 deaths occurred in flight.[72]

But the one great asset of air evacuation is not that seriously wounded men can be evacuated in large numbers. To be flown out – ambulance helicopters were not much used in the Second World War – a man would have to be taken by road to the plane and by road from plane to hospital and his body simply would not tolerate such treatment. A man with a penetrated brain, however, would probably be air-evacuated because he needed to be watched daily for the onset of meningitis or brain abscess. But a most valuable service provided by planes was the evacuation of large numbers of sick and lightly wounded men, thus decongesting the front areas. This was especially so in some jungle campaigns where advanced surgical stations were set up next to forward air strips from which, after emergency treatment, the casualties were taken by light aircraft to corps medical centres made up of several units, such as casualty clearing stations, ophthalmic units and malaria treatment units.

Aircraft did not only take the wounded back, they took the doctors forward. In one instance, where a hospital was destroyed, eighty aircraft delivered an entirely new 200-bed hospital unit with all equipment, on one day, to an isolated American unit.

During the operation by Brigadier Wingate's Chindits, the long-range penetration group in Burma, one air evacuation was particularly interesting; seventeen wounded men were taken off by transport plane and brought out in an hour and a half over country which it would have taken ten weeks to cover on foot.

The surgeons' work in the jungle was more difficult than that of his *confrère*'s in North Africa or Western Europe. Here no well-organized chain of evacuation was possible, for neither roads nor railways nor sea lanes existed. A man had to walk out, be carried out or flown out. Since for some time in New Guinea and Papua no air strips were available many sick and wounded men survived the most remarkable bearer-portages of history, being carried along steep, muddy jungle tracks by willing and gentle though untrained native bearers. Infection was much more likely at all stages of a soldier's treatment – though DDT brought radical changes to tropical camps – and the generally oppressive atmosphere of damp jungle was hardly conducive to the degree of morale which helps patients to recover. The surgeon was just as vulnerable to this enervating atmosphere and only will-power tempered by professional pride kept some doctors going as long as they did.

Those surgeons taken prisoner by the Japanese in the jungle campaigns probably faced the most difficult challenges of all war doctors. With only their initiative to work with they took immense risks in treating patients and in *daring* to treat them.

The Japanese campaigns cost the lives of many surgeons and others of the medical services. In what was known as the siege of the Admin Box in the second Arakan campaign the Japanese butchered all but one of the staff of a dressing station, comprising three field ambulances, and the helpless wounded.[73]

There is neither room nor need to amplify the courage of surgeons and their helpers, but it was fitting that in the British service the only medical VC of the Second World War should go to an RAMC medical orderly, Lance-Corporal Eric Harden, serving a troop of Royal Marine commandos. On 23 January 1945 Harden went out under concentrated small arms fire to give treatment to wounded. He returned, slightly wounded himself and with his battledress torn with bullets, carrying a patient. Efforts to use tanks and a smoke-screen to bring in other casualties were abortive because of heavy

German anti-tank gunfire. Harden, helped by two young marines, went out a second and a third time; on the last journey, only fifty yards from his headquarters, he was shot through the head.*

At Arnhem, after the airborne landing on 15 September 1944, a field ambulance established in the town hospital was overrun on the first evening and the whole unit was taken away except the two surgeons, who began fresh surgical operations whenever the Germans tried to move them out. They managed to remain at their post for several weeks until their wounded men were fit to be taken to prisoner-of-war camps. Five hundred RAMC men dropped at Arnhem; only one officer and thirteen other ranks evaded capture.

Doctors serving on detached duty, such as with guerrillas in occupied countries, were in some ways under greater stress than those in prison camps, for the guerrilla surgeons were tense with the expectation of capture and probable torture. These men had to wash bandages perhaps as many as twelve times, before they rotted and fell to pieces; they had almost no instruments and often not even a cake of soap. The Yugoslav doctors who worked with the guerrillas in the woods and mountains were efficient when influenced by German techniques. They believed, as did most British doctors, in non-closure of all war wounds, but they used the plaster cast too freely for guerrilla conditions. These casts enabled immediate evacuation, but they produced dreadful pressure sores. Doctors carried out guillotine† operations too – the Russian method – and could not be persuaded by British doctors with the guerrillas that many limbs could easily be saved. They were obsessed with the fear of gangrene, yet frequently the British surgeons could detect no signs of it, merely local, gas-formed organisms. These Yugoslav doctors had scant sympathy for the wounded. Lindsay Rogers, a New Zealand surgeon in Yugoslavia, frequently saw wounded left lying on the table for half an hour in freezing cold while the surgical team had a conversation.[74] Massive and dangerous doses of camphor in oil were given supposedly to counteract heart failure. Dressings were not taken off carefully, but ripped off the stumps of limbs. Intravenous injections were clumsily given with needles that were too large.

Rogers had as a patient a Bosnian boy, Boris, aged eighteen, and known to all as 'the Foetus'. A bullet had hit him in the lumbar region and removed the spinous process of the vertebrae; his back muscles were gone and the large raw area gave him constant pain. He had been in a hospital the Germans had burnt, and all but Boris died; he survived by crawling into a

---

* The RAMC reached a maximum strength of 12,000 officers and 83,000 others; 2,463 were killed or died on service. Decorations: 1 VC, 3 George Medals, 49 DSOs and 3 bars, 322 MCs, 12 DCMs, 254 MMs.

† A rapid direct cut using knife and saw in which bone and soft tissues are divided at the same level without a flap being left to close the wound.

water-filled drain. The team cleaned his wound with sulphonamide powder, removed a piece of dead bone which was causing infection, and then covered the wound with grafted skin taken from all parts of his body. With the aid of a daily sedative Boris was kept at rest for a week and in a fortnight he was on his feet. Such surgery was rarely possible in the field.

Rogers one night admitted a young guerrilla blind from a penetrating brain wound just above the occiput. His skull was shaved and prepared with petrol which the team reserved for important cases. Under local anaesthetic, aided by a sedative, Rogers made an incision and dissected the flaps back to the bone, with the boy repeatedly complaining about his blindness and asking how could he live though blind. Hair and part of his cap had been driven through the oozing hole into his brain. Having no sterile water available, Rogers and his nurse washed out the debris with snow water, lifted out bone chips, enlarged the hole and at the bottom of it saw a fairly large piece of mortar shell. With great care the surgeon pruned away the bone edges until he had a hole the size of a match-box. More washing out of debris followed, then more trimming – and the metal was clearly visible. Wedged in, it had perforated the large venous sinuses, so Rogers under-ran them with fine silk taken from parachute cords. After that, with the cavity dry, he could extract the metal, which apparently had not produced any permanent brain damage. After more work another piece of cap was brought out and penicillin was dusted around the wound, probably for the first time in Slovenia. The large flaps were closed, sulphonamide powder was dusted over the muscles and the skin was closed except for a drain. In a month the patient had almost complete return of vision. Not many years before, his wound would have been considered hopeless in Yugoslavia.

The Great War of 1914–1918 had been described as 'the war to end all wars'. It wasn't. The Second World War, 1939–1945, despite its horrors, colossal casualties and wholesale destruction, also did not excise the cancer of war from mankind's soul. After 1945 military physicians and surgeons were on active service in many theatres of war. For the British, these included Palestine, Korea, Malaya, Kenya, Aden, Borneo, the Falkland Islands, the Persian Gulf, Bosnia and Northern Ireland. Over a period of more than 25 years, the British Army had more casualties in Northern Ireland than in any conflict since the Second World War.

For the Americans, there was Korea, then the drawn-out agony of Vietnam, Granada, Panama, the Persian Gulf and Bosnia. The French fought savage wars in Indo-China, Algeria and other parts of Africa. The medical services of other European countries were also tested to the limit, notably the Portuguese in Angola and Mozambique and the Dutch in Indonesia. Israeli military medical staff became some of the most experienced in the world, following their nation's wars of 1948, 1956, 1967, 1973, 1982 and the unending war against Palestinian terrorists and fanatical Islamic raiders from across the Lebanese border.

Techniques changed and improved, new drugs proliferated, new remedies were sought against new weapons – the threat of biological warfare, for instance. Not one of the many surgeons and physicians with whom I discussed the question believes that it is possible to invent a new physical weapon to mutilate a serviceman's body in a new way. Any new weapon must cut, penetrate, crush, break, bruise, blind, scratch, burn, mutilate, decapitate, emasculate, blow to pieces or rot – and all this has already been done. Forget the political intention or the strategic objective, the immediate purpose of war is to kill or wound the enemy's fighting men.

Some surgeons, as they treated feet infected by rusty nails set in pieces of wood and left as booby traps in paddy-fields (Vietnam, Malaya, Cambodia and other places), have found a return to the primitive. Crude weapons can be as effective as guided missiles.

Diseases are another matter. Few armies can now count on the enemy losing large numbers of fighting men to the old campaigning scourges and pestilences – such as typhoid, cholera and malaria. But this handicap can be remedied, to misuse a word deliberately. Iraq, Iran and North Korea have developed weapons of biological warfare (BW) such as anthrax and other poisons which can kill people in minutes, even seconds – and in large numbers.

For the moment, medical science is winning, but it is in the unhappy state of fighting against itself. That is, as some medical researchers find cures or prophylactics for disease, other specialists, betraying their calling, are looking for new diseases which can be used as weapons against enemies on the battlefield, to be spread by direct contact from an exploding missile, by spray, by vapour, by placement in water supplies. For nations without the vast amounts of money needed to develop sophisticated weaponry, such as nuclear rockets and bombs, the cost-effectiveness of BW is immensely attractive. In wars to come one of the dominant figures in military medicine – in attack and defence – will be the research chemist. The ultimate weapon is not the nuclear bomb but a BW agent that will destroy an army before it can open fire.

CHAPTER TWENTY-FIVE

Psychiatrists Join the Team

Psychiatric problems can disable a fighting man as effectively as a bullet wound, and while they cannot be dealt with exhaustively here they cannot be ignored, for the increasing stress of war makes psychiatric breakdown all the more probable. In any case, psychiatrists are among the medical men at the battle front. In Ireland in 1711 the British Army had some provision for mentally disturbed soldiers, in 1820 forms of occupational therapy were introduced at Chatham and in 1866 a block of Netley Hospital was allotted to disturbed men. Not until the First World War was wastage because of neurosis and shellshock much studied, and solutions mostly had to wait until the Second World War. No nation ever before gave attention to battle neurosis. Officers blindly and dogmatically assumed that a soldier who broke down was a coward. No attempt was made to discover why he was a 'coward'.*

The point is that there is no such thing as 'getting used to combat', a truth recognized by the appointment of psychiatrists in the British and American armies to work in the forward line and, as advisers, at corps level. Had such specialists existed in the First World War much tragedy may have been averted and High Command may have come to realize that a man wears out in combat; perhaps fewer men would have been executed for 'cowardice' or desertion.

According to official statistics, from 4 August 1914 to 31 March 1920, 3,080 death sentences were passed by courts-martial on officers and men in all theatres of war. The total number executed was 346 (11 per cent) of whom 322 were executed in France and Belgium and the remainder in other

---

* As recently as 1947 a peer said, quite inaccurately, 'In the First World War desertion was punishable by death. There were very few desertions. In the Second World War capital punishment for this offence was abolished. There were scores of thousands of deserters.' (Lord Blackford, *The Times*, 5 December 1947)

The average incidence of deserters per year, per 1,000 strength, for 1914–19 was 10.26, the yearly average varying from 6.03 to 20.70; the average incidence for 1939–45 was 6.89, the yearly incidence varying from 4.48 to 10.05. The deterrent value of the death penalty was obviously very slight.

theatres. Of these 346 men, 18 were executed for 'cowardice' and 266 for desertion.†

Among those executed, 91 men were under suspended sentences, including 9 under two suspended sentences. Of these 91 men, 40 had been previously sentenced to death – in 38 cases for desertion. One soldier had been sentenced to death for desertion on two previous occasions. These men had deserted again, in spite of the 'deterrent' effect of the death penalty.[75]

The death penalty for 'cowardice' and desertion was abolished in April 1930. In 1942 the relatively high incidence of desertion in the Middle East so seriously affected the manpower situation that the commander-in-chief, General Sir Claude Auchinleck, suggested to the War Office in May reintroduction of the death penalty for desertion in the field. He noted that no less a deterrent was required from time to time, not merely in the interests of discipline but for the conduct of operations in conditions of strain and stress.

The executive committee of the Army Council agreed unanimously that, in the interests of discipline, there could be no question as to the military desirability of the death sentence for desertion in the field and 'cowardice in the face of the enemy', but it would not be possible to reintroduce the death sentence during the war, for political reasons as well as for considerations affecting security.

In November 1942 General Alexander, the new commander in the Middle East, said that the morale of the army was high and improving, and cases of desertion and 'cowardice' were comparatively few. There was no immediate need for reintroducing the death penalty for desertion. He favoured its reintroduction; but the time was then inopportune.

The incidence of desertion in the British Army in the two world wars makes an interesting comparison (see table).[76]

Commanders apparently did not appreciate that 'cowardice' and desertion and other major service crimes are the result of many factors, many of them avoidable in a competently run military force. Not only doctors, but all officers should know men's limits under stress.

For some reason it is often assumed that soldiers of the First World War were under more stress than those in the Second World War. Several psychiatrists, notably J.W. Appel, G.W. Beebe, D.W. Hilger, E.A. Strecker, K.E. Appel and R.A. Ahrenfeldt, all with much army experience, refute this idea. They say that the strain of the Second World War was, in the long run, incomparably greater than that experienced in 1914–18, because of the high degree of speed and mechanization, dive-bombing and armoured warfare,

† German and Russian figures no longer exist and French figures have never been released, but all were higher than those for the British forces. The French were probably highest of all.

simultaneous bombing of the civil population at home, service at great distance from home and many other features. Nobody, of course, minimizes the dreadful conditions under which men lived and fought in the First World War.

period	average strength of army	total number of deserters	incidence per year per 1,000
First World War			
1/10/14–30/9/15	1,949,871	40,375	20.70
1/10/15–30/9/16	2,886,978	26,520	9.19
1/10/16–30/9/17	3,621,378	21,838	6.03
1/10/17–30/9/18	3,829,834	28,372	7.41
1/10/18–30/9/19	2,586,085	20,668	7.99
Second World War			
1/10/39–30/9/40	1,538,675	6,889	4.48
1/10/40–30/9/41	2,211,547	22,248	10.05
1/10/41–30/9/42	2,455,720	20,834	8.49
1/10/42–30/9/43	2,681,697	15,824	5.90
1/10/43–30/9/44	2,729,480	16,892	6.19
1/10/44–30/9/45	2,830,831	17,663	6.24

F.C. Bartlett, who studied many cases of anxiety neurosis or combat stress among soldiers from the trenches of the First World War, found marked symptoms among men acutely affected.[77] A man would be in a state of stupor, which might involve genuine loss of consciousness. After this the patient was excited, confused, did not know where he was, often could not find his way from place to place, might complain of violent headaches and be delirious, usually raving about enemy attacks. In other cases there was no loss of consciousness, but the patient would be incapable of voluntary movement and might be confused, unusually forgetful and apparently unable to talk. Often hallucinations occurred at this stage, generally connected with enemy aggression. He would have extraordinarily vivid nightmares accompanied by fear of a peculiarly intense type. These dreams, by inducing fear of sleep, increased fatigue. Tremors and uncontrollable quivering were often present, and any degree of bright light was apt to be distressing.

Symptoms such as these were often the prelude to desertion, perhaps under fire, if officers had not had the sense and compassion to send the man out of the line. Ahrenfeldt says:

> By attention to morale, i.e. careful training, suitable employment, good leadership, adequate welfare, etc., it is . . . possible to avoid many of the precipitating factors which contribute to mental breakdown or desertion. Without attention to these fundamental prophylactic measures, in vain may the Army hold this sword of Damocles – as it were, a suspended death sentence –

over the heads of fighting men already labouring under the intense stresses of modern warfare: they will prevent neither psychiatric breakdown nor desertion and other lesions of morale. Indeed the figures indicate with great clarity the fact that the alleged 'deterrent' effect of the death penalty for desertion is no more than a delusion.

In Italy, in the middle of 1944, two American investigators, Lieutenant Colonel J.W. Appel and Captain G.W. Beebe, made an important study of campaign stress in which they found that each moment of combat imposes a strain so great that men will break down in direct relation to the intensity and duration of their exposure. 'Thus, psychiatric casualties are as inevitable as gunshot wounds. . . .'

Because the infantry is exposed to the greatest danger it also suffers the greatest loss of manpower from psychiatric disorders: Appel and Beebe found that in the North African theatre practically all men in rifle battalions of the US Fifth Army who were not otherwise disabled ultimately became psychiatric casualties. Although only 1 to 3 per cent of the combat strength was lost from this cause during any single offensive, apparently the intensity and duration of the continued campaigns surpassed the limit of endurance of the average soldier. 'Just as an average truck wears out after a certain number of miles, it appears that the doughboy wore out, either developing an acute incapacitating neurosis or else becoming hypersensitive to shellfire, so overly cautious and jittery that he was ineffective and, even more dangerously, he was demoralising to the new men. The average point at which this occurred appears to have been in the region of 200 to 240 aggregate combat days.'

The psychiatrists equated 10 combat days with 17 calendar days. The number of men still on duty after this amount of combat experience was small and their value to their units was negligible. Results in the British Middle East forces showed that 90 per cent of men breaking down in battle could be restored to a good standard of stability; in practice a constant 30 per cent returned to combat duty.

From the Sicily campaign, in 1943, onward it was noted that an increasing number of psychiatric patients being sent back from the front line were not 'weaklings' – the rather contemptuous description applied by tough officers and NCOs – who had merely broken down after a short exposure to combat, but experienced veterans, strong men with excellent combat records, often including decorations. Most of them were NCOs, either squad, section or platoon leaders. By the spring of 1944 following the bloody Volturno, Rapido and Monte Cassino actions, there were more of these old men than new men coming in as psychiatric patients.

A notorious incident involving US General George Patton occurred on 3 August 1943. What happened was an example of a leading general with psychiatric problems of his own. Everybody recognized that Patton was irrational but as he was a competent fighting general his superiors overlooked his considerable imperfections. For instance, he recommended letting an amputee die because 'he is no God-damned use to us any more.' The incident in which he was the central performer when visiting the US 15th Evacuation Hospital near Nicosia in 1943 also revealed some of the tremendous personal problems faced by the ordinary infantryman in combat.

At the Evacuation Hospital, Patton came upon a private soldier who had recently reached the admissions ward with a diagnosis of 'psycho-neurosis anxiety state; moderate/severe.' The medics who pinned this diagnostic label to the man's uniform were mistaken – he actually had chronic dysentery and malaria and was running a high fever. Neither Patton nor anybody else knew this when the general confronted the soldier and asked what was wrong with him. The sick young soldier, who no doubt had read the 'psycho' label on his chest, said faintly, 'I guess I can't take it.'

Patton flew into a rage, as he was wont to do. He abused the man, slapped his face with his gloves, grabbed him by the shoulders and threw him out of the tent. He sprawled in front of a medical orderly who picked him up and took him to a ward.

In his diary that night, Patton wrote: 'I gave him the devil, slapped his face . . . and kicked him out of the hospital. One sometimes slaps a baby to bring it to.' Next day he issued an instruction to senior subordinate commanders: 'A very small number of soldiers are going to hospital on the pretext that they are nervously incapable of combat. Such men are cowards. Those who are not willing to fight will be tried by court-martial for cowardice in the face of the enemy.'

The following week Patton visited the 93rd Evacuation Hospital – and it must be admitted that his intention was, as always, to cheer the wounded. In the admissions ward he found a soldier lying on his bunk shivering. Medical officers had diagnosed 'severe shellshock' and this happened to be correct. Patton did not 'believe' in shellshock and in his gruff, brusque manner questioned the patient. Sobbing, the man said, 'It's my nerves. I can hear the shells coming over but I can't hear them land.'

Patton glared at the medical officers accompanying him. 'What is this man talking about?' he demanded. 'What's wrong with him, if anything?' Turning to the shivering, sobbing soldier he shouted, 'You're a God-damned coward, a yellow son of a bitch!' He repeatedly slapped him very hard, threatened to have him shot and waved his pistol in the man's face. His attack ended only when the hospital commander, hurriedly summoned to the scene, stepped between the general and his victim.

These incidents, widely publicized by war correspondents, caused outrage. In the end Patton's supreme commander compelled him to apologize for his behaviour. The affair badly damaged his reputation and career.

There was one beneficial result from the appalling attacks made by Patton on his own men. The army at last recognized that soldiers could become psychiatric casualties. A School of Military Neuro-Psychology opened at

Lawson General Hospital in Atlanta. From this beginning, by the end of 1943 psychiatrists were listed on the US Army's 'establishment.'

The credit for what then happened in the US Army in efforts to rehabilitate psychiatric casualties and make them functioning soldiers again belongs largely to Captain F.R. Hanson. Trained as a neurologist and neurosurgeon, Hanson was working in Canada when war broke out and he joined the Canadian Army. Posted to the staff of a psychiatric hospital in England, he eagerly sought experience in his chosen field. As an American citizen, he transferred to the US Army when America entered the war. He wanted battle experience to understand what happened to soldiers in combat and he volunteered to accompany the Canadians in the disastrous British-Canadian attack against the strong German defences at Dieppe, August 1942. He was one of the relatively few survivors not taken prisoner and his courage, dedication and skill were noted.

He was next active in North Africa, dealing with victims of combat stress after another British disaster, Kasserine Pass, Tunisia, February 1943. The staff at the 48th Surgical Hospital were impressed by this calm, highly observant specialist. He noted that the psychiatric casualties were exactly the same in manner and appearance as the wounded men. After examining perhaps 200 cases he concluded that the fundamental critical factor in causing their condition was nothing more or less than lack of sleep. His instructions to the nurses: 'Put these men to bed. Give heavy doses of barbiturates. Awaken them only for meals and defecation. Do nothing else. Don't even talk to them. Let them sleep.'

Military hospital staff, accustomed to by-the-hour routine of making beds, during which the patients were inevitably disturbed, and of taking temperatures at regular intervals, which also disturbed the men, nevertheless obeyed this quiet and confident specialist. Under his 'treatment' 30 per cent of the men cheerfully returned to duty within 30 hours and more than 70 per cent after 48 hours.

Hanson made other 'discoveries' that ran counter to established practice. It had been routine to take men with 'mental problems' out of the line at once and truck them hundreds of miles to the Atlantic coast for beach convalescence. Hanson found that at the end of this trip most of the patients were much worse than when they left their units. Now they suffered all manner of symptoms, such as hallucinations, battle nightmares and amnesia. They were trembling violently and some could not speak. A complex disorder was taking place, Hanson discovered. Having been accepted as patients with 'mental problems,' many men, consciously or unconsciously, further developed this condition and exaggerated any small physical problems that they might have. Their neurotic symptoms became significantly worse in this safe area where they were supposed to recover. While a few men were downright malingerers, many others were genuinely distressed about leaving their buddies in the line and to suppress their feelings of guilt they subconsciously exaggerated their symptoms.

Hanson now had a team of assistants and with their experience as well as his own, he so profoundly influenced the US Army commanders in North Africa that they adopted his new policy. Psychiatric casualties would from now on be diagnosed only with the label 'exhaustion'. In fact, Hanson had borrowed this term from the British Army, as he acknowledged.

To begin with, patients could stay four or five days in hospital but Hanson and the specialists whom he had trained found that after three days their patients developed hypochondria; deliberately or subconsciously they were trying to give the staff reasons for keeping them longer in hospital. Under friendly but firm management, they had to keep to a routine, such as washing and shaving and walking to meals. They were encouraged to talk about their experiences, just as they were permitted to sleep and to bathe. More than this, the 'authority figures' – the army doctor captains, majors and colonels, reassured and comforted them. One of the most important aspects of the 'Hanson treatment' was that it took place in forward areas where air raids could still occur.

Hanson was also training doctors whose speciality was not psychiatry or psychology. 'Remember', these officers were told, 'that normality does not mean the same thing for the civilian and the combat soldier. On the battlefield the abnormal, such as insomnia, trembling and recurrent nightmares, become normal.'

Hanson, who was promoted colonel, was not the only thoughtful senior army doctor. Colonel Norman T. Kirk, commanding one of the US Army's great general hospitals, urged systematic rotation of fighting units in line with British practice. The US Army did not heed this advice. Attempts to rotate combat troops usually took the form of efforts to relieve those individual soldiers with the longest service. This was commendable in itself but it would have been much better to establish a definite tour of duty, as the US Air Force did. Such an eminent authority as Albert E. Cowdrey, who specialized in army medicine for 15 years and wrote two of the official histories of the US medical service in the Second World War, wrote, 'In general, Americans underrated the importance of unit integrity; they could have learned much from their British allies but failed to do so.'

During the Vietnam War, 1959–73, the lessons concerning post traumatic stress disorder learned during the latter years of the Second World War were put into practice. Some men were very violent and out of their minds with disorientation, but provisions for security did not exist in the neuro-psychiatric wards of the army hospitals. No able-minded men were detailed for guard duty and the wards had no locks. Also, patients were not given the electric shock treatment that was so commonplace in civilian psychiatric hospitals.

The men understood from the time they arrived at the hospital that they were expected to get better. The entire staff made this very clear. The veteran psychiatrists in charge of treatment informed all doctors new to army psychiatry and psychology during active war service what was expected of *them* and they used simple language. It was: 'Label a soldier as mentally ill, support that illness, show him that is what interests you about him and he will be ill and stay ill.' (A recollection of Dr Ronald Glasser in his book *365 Days*, concerning his service during the Vietnam War.)

Soldier patients were not given opportunities to dwell on symptoms. The psychiatrists never allowed the patients to forget that they were still in the army; they wore their uniforms, they were given duties commensurate with their health and they obeyed orders.

There are documented cases of soldiers who said they could not move their legs, yet the doctors knew nothing was clinically wrong with their legs. They were told that meals were not served in bed and that the mess hall was a short distance along the corridor. When a soldier claimed that he could not possibly walk, a psychiatrist said, 'OK, so you can crawl. Go anyway you like.' This was said in tones of expectation, not as an order. Few patients lasted a day without food before they crawled. They moved in this way to the mess hall to embarrass the staff but nobody took any notice, beyond giving the crawler a friendly nod.

After a few days nearly all such 'paralysed' patients walked for their meals and given a little more time they walked for every other purpose, even to see the doctor in his office.

In Vietnam, the psychiatric patients returned to duty; similarly 100 per cent of the combat exhaustion cases, 90 per cent of the character-behaviour, 98 per cent of the alcoholic and drug patients, 56 per cent of the psychosis, 85 per cent of the psychoneurosis cases and many others went back. On their personal records was the diagnosis 'acute situation reaction.' This was brilliant use of language for it replaced totally the old comments on soldiers' records, such as neurosis, psychosis, chronic exhaustion and alcoholic dependency, among other terms that frightened the soldier so categorized.

The officers of his unit, who convinced themselves that they had problems ahead, now read 'acute situation reaction' and nodded approvingly – here was a label they could empathize with. They had all been in situations where they had 'reacted acutely'.

In the British Army notices were posted in all gun units in Malta, when the bombing was at its height in March 1942, that anxiety neurosis was the term employed by the medical profession to commercialize fear and that if a soldier was a man he would not permit his self-respect to admit an anxiety neurosis or to show fear.

Appel and Beebe knew that battle stress was a very real thing and not merely an excuse for 'cowardice'. They made an exhaustive survey among regimental surgeons and experienced combat leaders, particularly the infantry company commanders, since they had the most direct contact with the troops. The doctors and officers agreed that an infantryman became ineffective somewhere between 200 and 240 days of fighting. Some officers said that some men reached the limit of effectiveness after 140 days. But even then he was wearing out, for the peak of a soldier's combat usefulness was reached within 90 days. No infantry action could be regarded as 'light', but hard-fought actions, such as the battle for Monte Cassino and the fighting on the Rapido River – which some American military writers consider the toughest action US troops have fought – accelerated the wearing-out process, the front-line officers said.

The two psychiatrists observed that individuals developing psychiatric disorders after fewer than 200 combat days could be successfully returned to full fighting duty. This was done many times because of the high standard of front-line treatment. But the man who was really worn out could not again be used as a combat soldier short of six months out of action.

The effective combat life of the average infantryman appears to depend largely on how continuously he is used in combat. The British estimated that their riflemen in Italy would last about 400 regimental combat days, about twice as long as US riflemen in the heavily used US divisions in Italy. They attributed this difference to their policy of pulling infantrymen out of the line at the end of twelve days or less for a rest of four days. The American soldier in Italy was usually kept in the line without relief for twenty to thirty days, frequently for thirty to forty and occasionally for eighty days.

In the army which liberated Europe, for the first time in British military history the possibility of psychiatric casualties in large numbers had been anticipated and to some extent prepared for by the provision of an adequately equipped general hospital within ten miles of the front line. This was the 32nd General (Psychiatric) Hospital which opened thirty days after D-Day, 6 June 1944. In fact within ten days of D-Day between 10 and 20 per cent of battle casualties were psychiatric cases of 'exhaustion'. Between 6 June 1944 and 9 May 1945 there were 13,255 such cases – 16 per cent of all battle casualties.

The importance of preventive psychiatry in the army (and by association in the other services) was shown in July 1948 by the publication of an enlightened Army Council instruction that mental health had now been included in the scope of hygiene and it was intended that psychiatric specialists, working closely with hygiene officers, should give the necessary training to officers and selected NCOs of all arms in the application of the new methods of promoting mental health in a soldier's way of life. All nations now recognize that the serviceman's mind and emotions are as important as his body, a recognition apparent in the process of admission to the armed forces and in the subsequent selection of officers and men for certain duties. In future wars psychiatrists and psychologists will be even more prominent in the front line or its equivalent, i.e. in an atomic submarine, at the base of intercontinental aircraft or missiles. Like the chemist's, the psychiatrist's work is assuming an ever-increasing importance.

In the German service in 1944 psychologists co-operated with doctors in producing a lengthy guide for British and American soldiers serving in Italy who might be induced to simulate illness to avoid duty. Printed in small type on a long strip and folded into a card cover, the instructions, which looked like book-matches, were dropped by aircraft or planted by retreating soldiers. The medical advice, though sometimes dangerous, is more competent than the psychology which bred the idea.

Would-be malingerers were advised to make the impression that they hated to be ill, to decide on one kind of sickness and stick to it, not to tell the doctor too much and not to exaggerate their symptoms. Key Italian words were given for malingering aids. The illnesses or disabilities which could be simulated include:

Inflammation of the foot. Soak a ball of cotton the size of a pea in turpentine and keep it overnight between the 3rd and 4th toe. . . . Before reporting to the doctor wash your foot very thoroughly so that the smell of turpentine cannot be noted. . . .

Dysentery. Take a laxative. . . . When it has begun to work report to your doctor with the following complaints: Tell him you had a severe attack of dysentery some months ago in Africa. . . . Since that time you notice that heavy foods such as pork and beans . . . produce violent pains and diarrhoea. When the doctor examines you show painful response to pressure on the right side immediately below the ribs. . . .

A harmless inflammation of the eyes. Refrain from cleaning your teeth or rinsing your mouth for a few days. The white substance which gathers on your teeth, introduce under the eyelids. [Other methods were also given.]

Temporary paralysis. Before going to bed wrap a stone, eraser or short piece of rubber tubing in gauze tissue and fasten firmly to exert pressure on spot X [accompanying sketch showed places on arm and leg]. Fasten with tight bandage and allow to remain overnight. Take bandage off in morning. Repeat for several days until there is a numb feeling in your forearm and hand. . . which will last for an increasing length of time. When sufficient paralysis has resulted report to your doctor.

Jaundice. Get hold of thirty or forty digitalis tablets. . . . Take daily four times one tablet . . . . Carry on the procedure until your pulse-rate has slowed down to 60 or less per minute. . . . Eat a lot of chocolate. Do not clean your teeth. Take one gram of picric acid. . . . The skin and whites of your eyes will become yellow. . . . Drink three raw eggs before going to bed. [Instructions for approach to the doctor follow, but the soldier was not told that taking digitalis tablets in this way is very dangerous.]

Detailed instructions were given for feigning tuberculosis. 'To make your case convincing you must mix some tuberculosis germs into the sputum. This is difficult, but every man carries an excellent substitute with him. If you have failed to wash the foreskin of your penis for two or three days a yellow substance called smegma is deposited underneath. This contains a group of harmless bacteria . . . in appearance and staining qualities they behave exactly like the tuberculosis germs. Of this smegma you must mix a very small quantity with the sputum in your mouth. . . .'

Similarly, soldiers were instructed how to fake nervous troubles by taking drugs; stomach ulcer – involving the acquisition of a pint of cow, ox, hog or sheep blood; heart disease, induced by dangerous drugs.

Few of these simulated disabilities were practicable for the average soldier who, in any case, had plenty of tricks of his own had he wanted to use them. *The Lancet*, publishing the German instructions in March 1945, observed that 'it is curious that the psychiatric side is so lightly dismissed', implying that the man who wanted to opt out of the war might find the psychiatrist easier to deceive than the physician or surgeon. It is possible that the authors of the malingerer's guide had a very high opinion of Allied psychiatrists. It would not have been an unjustifiable opinion. But if the Germans believed it would be easy to deceive an Allied doctor in the field they were wrong, very wrong, about that.

This is not to say that Services doctors had nothing to learn. During the First World War doctors had identified 'shock,' but it had never been thoroughly explained. It was such a danger to the life of a wounded man that a study in Italy late in the Second World War produced convincing evidence that shock was the primary cause of battle casualty deaths.

The symptoms of wound shock were clear enough: low blood pressure, high pulse rate, cold extremities and acute anxiety in the patient. About one in 40 wounded soldiers were in shock when they reached hospital and it was likely that morphine injected by medics in the field had adversely affected their respiration. While it was realized that shock began a process of destructive changes the reasons were not at first understood.

A difficulty was that during the First World War doctors had separated shock from haemorrhage. This error was understandable because shock was complicated and many doctors believed there had to be a reason other than loss of blood.

Nearly twenty years after the First World War ended, researchers found out that plasma was remarkably efficacious. Plasma is the fluid part of the blood after removal of red and white cells. Its benefit in wound surgery was that it filled the arteries and veins, thus preventing a dangerous drop in blood pressure until the system regenerated red cells. Plasma looked like a miracle because it could be stored for long periods and even dried. Even better, it could be given to a patient of any blood group and, unlike whole blood, it could be conveniently carried.

However, in the really savage fighting in certain theatres of war, it was found that many men, brought out of shock with plasma, were suffering relapses that ended in death. Much was discovered from these tragedies, notably that many a wounded man was in a more dangerous condition than anybody had realized. Medical people had tended to gauge blood loss by its visible flow outside the body but after many types of wounds the blood loss was internal, with the blood soaking into the surrounding flesh and tissues, even back 'behind' the wound itself.

It was dangerous even to move a wounded man, let alone anaesthetize and operate on him. American and British surgeons found that two teams were needed to treat many wounded – the surgical team and the 'shock squad.' The anti-shock medics had to keep the patient alive while the surgeons did their work.

The fundamental conclusion was that while plasma was a godsend in keeping the wounded alive to the point of arrival at treatment stations, whole blood was essential in preparing a man for surgery. This created a medical crisis in the field which the British were the first to resolve. The army had set up its own blood banks and the donors came from troops – and nurses – in the field.

The Americans copied this system and Albert Cowdrey, the pre-eminent researcher into the US medical services during the war, estimates that staff in the field hospitals contributed more blood than any other group. Mobile blood banks in trucks busily made the rounds of camps and airfields. The need was so great that much other blood was flown into the war areas from the US and Britain and transfusions were given closer and closer to the battle line.

The Red Cross network helped greatly with blood supply as it had already done with plasma. During the war the Red Cross collected more than 13 million pints of blood and processed about 10 million into plasma. Plasma and whole blood saved the lives of thousands of soldiers, sailors and airmen, largely by eliminating or radically reducing shock.

Sadly, it has to be said that when the US entered the war in December 1941, racial discrimination was so rampant that the services refused blood donations from blacks, which to the rational mind would seem ridiculous. The Army medical chiefs lamely justified the policy by reference to 'the disinclination on the part of Caucasians to have Negro blood injected into their veins'.

Albert Cowdrey says: 'Politically the exclusion was an impossibility in wartime. Blacks made their resentment felt and many Whites joined them. The Army yielded and the Red Cross [in the US] returned to an earlier practice of taking everybody's blood and segregating the plasma... [This] fundamentally made no sense, but it accurately reflected the state of American thinking about blood, race and patriotism at the time.'

CHAPTER TWENTY-SIX

The Agony of Vietnam

The Vietnam War produced casualties on a scale and of a type not seen since 1945. Medically, it was a hideous war and the appalling conditions in which it was fought produced immense challenges for the US armed forces medical services.

The war began on 8 July 1959 when the Viet Cong (Vietnamese Communists) attacked the South Vietnamese Army near Saigon. American advisors were already in position and in 1963, at the request of President Diem, the US sent 17,000 more advisors, some of whom were actively directing South Vietnamese units.

The 'Americanization' of the war by President Johnson took place by stages between August 1964 and June 1965. At the end of that year 175,000 American servicemen were in Vietnam, or Nam as they universally called it. By the end of 1967 this number had risen to 500,000. Obviously, the potential for casualties had increased dramatically.

On 30 January 1968, during the truce which marked the Tet Buddhist new year festival, the Viet Cong began a major offensive, a term which frequently appears in the medical records and reminiscences by surgeons. The Viet Congs' seven-week offensive was unsuccessful and they lost 46,000 killed and 9,000 wounded. The Americans had 4,114 killed and 19,285 wounded, while 604 were posted missing, which usually meant that they had been killed.

American military strength in Vietnam reached a peak of 549,000 at the end of 1968. Powerful American public opinion against the war brought about a reduction of US involvement. By 1971 the US strength was down to 171,000 and on 11 August 1972 the last American combat unit was withdrawn from Vietnam, although 43,000 air force personnel remained. For the US the conflict ended on 27 January 1973 when a peace treaty was signed. By that date the American forces had lost 45,941 men killed while 300,635 were wounded. Many more had suffered illnesses in various degrees of severity. In 16 years of war 150,000 South Vietnamese troops were killed and 400,000 wounded. Many of these men were treated by American medical staff, for whom the strain had been immense.

The active-service life of a medic in the field was so fraught with tension and was so exhausting that somebody in authority, as well as with common sense – a rare commodity in Vietnam – ordained that medics would spend only seven months on duty, while their fighting buddies stayed for 365 days.

While many medics were glad of this relief from strain, many others refused to leave their units. They knew how desperately their buddies depended on them in this savage war.

Back at the four base hospitals in Japan the work was endless because never before had so many casualties been so quickly moved away from the campaigning areas. The army prided itself that no man hit in Vietnam was any longer than ten minutes away from the nearest hospital. Except in a technical sense, this was not so. Once a helicopter picked up a casualty it was a ten-minute flight to the nearest surgical or evacuation facility but longer could elapse if a man was seriously wounded and the medical evacuation system (medevac) had to fly him to the nearest small hospital and from there to the closest evacuation point.

The claim of 'expert medical help within ten minutes' was bogus. Let us suppose some men are wounded in a fight or ambush in the jungle. As soon as he is able, the patrol leader or the medic on the spot radios for a Dust Off (the soldiers' term for an evacuation helicopter) to come in but in the confusion of battle he may not be able to make this call for some minutes. The Dust Off pilot will risk his life in getting in but it will be difficult to reach the pick-up patch in the jungle. The wounded men's mates will get them onto – or under – the helicopter as rapidly as possible but probably they are under fire and they have to pick their moment. Time is ticking by and the wounded men are bleeding. The medic will do his best to keep his mates alive in the mud while the Dust Off gets in. Twenty minutes or more may have elapsed. It is still an amazingly short time but it is not ten minutes – and the helicopter still needs time to fly the casualties to safety and treatment. Nevertheless, it was true that a wounded man taken off the helicopter alive would probably live.

The Dust Off pilots were among the great heroes of the war, and many rescue helicopters were shot down. The Viet Cong did not respect Red Cross markings. Many an attempt to evacuate a few men resulted in the loss of all those trying to help them. The Viet Cong fighters were cunning. Often they would try to wound a point man – the scout in front of a patrol – rather than kill him. They knew that he would scream for the medic and the Viet Cong had learned that the medic always came when called. Then they shot him dead. They calculated that by killing the medic they were in effect killing all those men who might have been saved by him.

Wounds caused by mines and booby traps caused great problems for the medical people. The Viet Cong used plastic mines containing 10 lb of explosives and 3 lb of metal fragments. They were detonated by pressure, which could be set for particular targets, from a tank weighing many tons to a single soldier's weight. Some of these mines operated on a pull-release: A soldier walking into a hidden cord could 'pull' the mine or it could be pulled by an enemy hiding nearby in the heavy foliage.

In a particular case known to Dr Ronald Glasser, who helped to deal with it in Japan, a mine explosion blew a soldier 10 ft into the air. The medic who went to his aid found that his left leg had been blown off and his right leg was shredded up to the thigh. His penis, scrotum, lower abdomen and anus were burnt. A helicopter ferried him to the 27th Surgical Hospital where surgeons removed his testicles and penis, took out his left kidney and four inches of large bowel and stitched up his liver. These also performed a colostomy and right ureterostomy.

Three days later when the man's condition had been stabilized by blood transfusion, antibiotics and other procedures he was taken to the great US Army hospital at Zama, Japan. Here his left leg was removed by a left-hip disarticulation or 'simple' separation at the hip. Surgeons also sutured his right thumb and left index finger. They wanted to close his surgical wounds but not enough skin remained, so the wounds had to be left open and they became infected, despite intensive nursing care.

During his fourth night in the ward the soldier tried to kill himself but he was too weak. His urinary output diminished and there were other problems. On day seven his temperature soared to 106 degrees and he lost consciousness. Soon after he died.

Regulations demanded that a final pathological diagnosis be made for medical files. This particular soldier's end-of-life record is one of the saddest documents in existence, although it is not unique. It also serves to show the immense efforts made to deal with his multiple wounds and to save his life. That he lived for a full seven days after his disaster in the jungle is a measure of the human will but we can only wonder if he would have wanted to live on.

Final pathological diagnosis:

1. Death, eight days after stepping on a land mine.
2. Multiple blast injuries.
   A. Traumatic amputation of lower extremities, distal right thumb, distal left index finger.
   B. Blast injury of anus and scrotum.
   C. Avulsion of testicles.
   D. Fragment wounds of abdomen.
   E. Laceration of kidney and liver, transection of left ureter.
3. Focal interstitial myocarditis and right heart failure.
   A. Left and right ventricular dilation.
   B. Marked pulmonary edema, bilateral.
   C. Marked pulmonary effusion, bilateral (3,000 cc in the left, 1,500 in the right).
   D. Congestion of lungs and liver.
4. Patchy acute pneumonitis (Klebsiella-Aerobactoer organism).
5. Gram negative septicemia.
6. Extensive acute renal tubular necrosis, bilateral.
7. Status post multiple recent surgical procedures.
   A. Hip disarticulation with debridement of stumps, bilateral.
   B. Testicular removal bilaterally.
   C. Exploration of abdomen, suturing of lacerated liver.
   D. Removal of left kidney and ureter.
   E. Multiple blood transfusions.

External examination:

The body is that of a well-developed, well-nourished, though thin, Negro male in his late teens or early twenties, showing absence of both lower extremities and extensive blast injuries on the perineum. There is a large eight-inch surgical incision running from the chest wall to the pubis. There is a previous amputation of the distal right thumb and left index finger.

Many of the wounded brought in by the Dust Offs had up to sixty pieces of metal in their abdomen or chest. The American medics referred to them as 'frag wounds', from the fragmentations of mines and grenades. 'Frag' was a more accurate description than 'shrapnel' wounds, by which the British describe such injuries. True shrapnel was rarely used after the First World War. It was found that high explosive shells and massive use of automatic machine-guns were better killers than shrapnel. Taking sixty fragments out of a man's body generally occupied a surgical team for six hours.

All kinds of things other than fragments of shell and mine were projected into the body – stones, pieces of wood, parts of the soldier's equipment, part of his filthy germ-laden clothing. The surgeons found these bits and pieces embedded in the heart, liver, muscles, lungs, eyes, sinuses, buttocks, bones, limbs and joints. Lots of hurtling frags tore into the scrotum and occasionally something was discovered in the rectum.

Frequently a decision was made to leave debris in certain parts of the body rather than cause more damage by operating to take it out. There were cases of bullets being left in the liver and even near the heart. Another professional decision was whether to stitch up a tear in the intestines or cut out the damaged part and join up the ends. All the many surgeons who confronted wounds to the colon had to create an artificial outlet for the bowel by performing a colostomy.

And always there were amputations, some of which were carried out by medics on the spot, when the remnants of a shattered limb had been left hanging by tissue and mangled flesh. Other amputations were more deliberately performed, but always reluctantly, by surgeons in the field hospitals or back at the base hospitals in Japan.

Because every soldier knew that his time in Nam would be complete in 365 days, as the period of service became shorter and shorter, so the troops were less and less inclined to take risks. They then grew to hate the keen and thrusting leader, be he corporal or captain. The attitude was, 'If he wants to get killed that's his business but he's not taking me with him.'

This led to the practice of 'fragging.' That is, a grenade would be quietly rolled into the tent of the gung-ho leader while he slept. At such close range the explosion generally killed the victim but many medics and surgeons dealt with wounds known to have been caused by fragging. This was murder or attempted murder but only a few soldiers were charged with these crimes. Naturally, no statistics for fragging exist but anecdotal evidence suggests that it was commonplace.

Serious burns were almost as commonplace during the Vietnam War as they had been in Europe during the Second World War. Many of the burn wounds were caused when helicopters were shot down; about 4,000 of them were lost throughout the conflict. Burns also occurred through faulty handling of flame-throwers and when gasoline was set alight. Sometimes detonators being carried by a soldier were hit by enemy fire and flared into uncontrollable flames.

Even experienced nursing staff found the burn wards harrowing places. The wounds of many other patients were not visible except during dressing but a man suffering from severe burns was so obviously in trouble. Burns needed careful and slow dressing and medical staff were acutely aware of each patient's distress, even when he was sedated. Often all hair, including eyebrows and lashes had been burned away. Knowing this, some of the boys wanted to look into a mirror. They would hardly be refused but staff provided mirrors with misgivings, especially when a man's lips and ears had been destroyed by fire.

Sometimes burns covered as much as 90 per cent of the body. Blistered, charred and skinless, these men would die. Before that happened they were placed in Stryker frames, in which the victim was placed between two metal arches so that he could be turned over without causing him more pain than he was already suffering. They were the invention of an American army doctor.

An associated problem with burns patients was that only their own skin could be used for grafts. Skin from other people, other than identical twins, would not 'take'. Surgeons tried it but the new skin quickly liquefied. For a man suffering, say, 60 per cent burns, where on his body was the graft to come from? Still, near miracles were performed on some burns cases.

Of all Services medical staff, those who treated burns most fervently cursed the war and the politicians who prolonged it.

Nasty wounds were caused by the punji stakes used by the Viet Cong in ambushes. The Japanese had employed them effectively in the jungles of the south-west Pacific. On either side of a track expected to be used by enemy soldiers, the Viet Cong stuck into the ground hundreds of sharpened stakes, often of bamboo. Ankle, knee, thigh or waist high, the punjis were angled towards the track and were invisible in the heavy foliage. The Viet Cong would then lie in ambush.

As the American patrol moved cautiously forward, the Viet Cong fired straight down the track, knowing that the Americans had been trained to dart into the cover of the jungle. The punji points caused nasty wounds which were often deep and disabling, and with a high risk of infection. According to the Americans, the Viet Cong smeared the points with excrement. A punji ambush had the effect of preventing the Americans from running further than a few yards off the track and with several members of the oncoming patrol out of action the Viet Cong would then bring the Americans under fire from machine-guns, mortars and grenades.

Ronald Glasser knew of several cases in which medics showed not only great bravery but extraordinary medical skill. He told the story of a nineteen-year-old medic named Pierson who was caught with his squad on a track when a huge mine exploded. Some of the men were mangled and killed outright. Another soldier was smashed but survived – with half his bottom jaw blown off and with blood gushing out of his neck and spilling into what was left of his mouth. He was writhing on the ground and Medic Pierson had first to subdue him. Then he took out his knife and grabbing the protruding piece of jawbone, forced back the soldier's head and then, as Glasser said, 'calmly cut open his throat and punched a hole into the windpipe . . . a spattering of blood and foam came out through the incision and as his breathing eased the soldier quieted.'

Taking an endotracheal tube out of his kit, Pierson slid it through the incision and deftly threaded it into the soldier's lungs, listened to hear if all was as it should be and only then did he give the man morphine.

Some medics carried sweets in their kits which they offered to men too far gone for morphine; the sweets were placebos and, when gently placed between lips with the medics' calm assurance that they would work, they did work.

For long periods the hospitals in Japan were receiving 6,000 to 8,000 cases a month; during the Tet offensive the average was 11,000 a month.

In its way, the life of a combat surgeon in Vietnam or dealing with the war's results in the hospitals in Japan, was as grim and stressful as that of the soldiers. Doctors and nurses broke down from exhaustion and from their own kind of post traumatic stress disorder.

However, at least one surgeon found a kind of consolation. He was the battalion surgeon of 101st Airborne and he told Dr Ronald Glasser, 'If there is any blessing in being there [that is, in Vietnam] it is in the shortness of things. There is no wasting away there, no philosophical concerns about medical ethics, about pulling out the plugs and turning off the machines. When they die there they die straight out, right off the choppers. It's sort of clean work. No brain tumors to worry about, no chronic renal sclerosis, no leukemics – and no goddam families to have to worry about.'

To fight the war in Vietnam cost the United States $90 million each day. With money spent on such a vast scale the government could have funded research to eliminate most of the world's diseases.

CHAPTER TWENTY-SEVEN

War in a Cold Climate

Purely from a military point of view, the Falklands War of 1982 – known as Operation Corporate – was a remarkable conflict. It was an imperial nineteenth-century type of conflict, reminiscent of scores of British campaigns in Africa, India and Asia. Also, the British fought the war without a land base at the end of an 8,000-mile sea and air supply line.

Britain's opponent was Argentina, which had claimed the islands ever since Britain occupied and colonized them in 1833. On 2 April, 500 Argentinian troops captured the capital, Port Stanley, from 79 Royal Marines. A day later the Argentinians occupied South Georgia, another British possession. On 5–6 April the British Government led by Margaret Thatcher sent a naval task force to the South Atlantic and a battle group was formed. Meanwhile the Argentinian forces in the Falklands were built up to about 15,000. Their main strength lay in the air force, operating from the mainland. Argentinian planes sank seven British ships and badly damaged six others. British air support for the sea-borne infantry amounted to 22 Harrier jump jets, operating from the carriers *Hermes* and *Invincible*.

Of particular concern was the luxury cruise liner *Canberra*, which had been transformed into a great floating troop base. Had this ship been sunk casualties would have run into many hundreds.

Medical preparations for the campaign, however well thought out in advance, were always going to be difficult until a land base could be secured. In the meantime sick and wounded were lifted by helicopter to the hospital ship *Uganda*, which had been a cruise liner, mostly for school parties. It cost the government a charter fee of about £2 million a week. The sick bays of the larger ships were also ready to accept casualties.

In effect, medical preparations for a campaign in cold climates had been made years before the Falklands War began. One of these preparations was the 'Arctic Pack', described in the cardboard box which held it as '24-hour ration pack Arctic – one man.'

Once the troops got ashore they depended for survival on the Arctic Pack. The RAMC had been closely consulted about the contents of this pack. Four menus were available, a vast improvement on the -'take it or leave it' iron rations of 1939–45. The breakfast was the same in all four, porridge and drinking chocolate. The meal differed in choice between ham, chicken, ham *and* chicken and bacon spreads for plain biscuits. The rest of the meal consisted of fruit and chocolate biscuits, chocolate caramels, nuts and raisins and dextrose sweets. The main meal, all dehydrated, offered a choice of three soups, beef, curried beef, mutton or chicken supreme granules, rice or mashed potato powder; apple or apricot flakes completed the meal. All the soldier had to do was to add water and heat his meal with his naphthalene stove. Every man carried two Arctic Packs and the troops were resupplied every two days.

It had always been realized that fighting troops' fitness depended largely on their rations but finding suitable, reasonably palatable and, importantly, regular meals, had been difficult to achieve. The Americans had served hotel-like meals to troops behind the lines but even they had fallen short of troops' expectations in the Second World War.

Easy to carry and easy to prepare, the Falklands campaign food had all that was required to provide a fighting man with the calories needed to keep him fit and as energetic as possible. Where soldiers were within reach of the ships the crews took them vast quantities of freshly baked rolls, a luxury on a battlefield where it was difficult for field kitchens to operate. Probably, few soldiers gave any thought to the medical men who had advised on rations, but the Falklands War showed that this is an important part of the work of combat doctors.

The Argentinian soldiers in the field were equally well served, at least in quality, by their own medical-dietician staff. They were given a 'CF Ration' – C for combat, F for supplementary. The food was hermetically sealed in a tin weighing five pounds and containing 20 items based on meat and macaroni, chocolate, instant cocoa, vitamin C tablets, powdered fruit juice and biscuits. Nevertheless, the Argentinians were often hungry because ration packs were in short supply.

On medical advice, the Royal Marines used the 'buddy system' as part of their survival techniques in the harsh climate where exposure and frostbite could cause serious problems. All the men were paired off and every man had been instructed by combat doctors on how to keep watch on his partner for symptoms such as drowsiness, lassitude, unusual pallor and 'strange' behaviour, all of which could indicate frostbite or imminent collapse from exposure. The sufferer would at once get 'the treatment' – such as massage of arms and legs. Cases of exposure were more frequent than reported and when a soldier was known to be suffering he was placed in a transparent plastic bag – the 'survival bag' – in just his long underwear. His body heat, unable to escape through the plastic, helped him to recover.

The great challenge to the medical services took place on 8 June. Brigadier Wilson, commanding the 5th Brigade, was moving his Scots Guards and Welsh Guards forward from the British base at San Carlos to Lively Island. From here the landing ships *Sir Galahad* and *Sir Tristram* would bring them into the narrow inlet of Port Pleasant, or Bluff Cove, where they would disembark. The landing ships, each crewed by 19 British officers and 50 Hong Kong ratings, were important and versatile craft. Each of 5,670 tons, they could carry up to 540 troops with their heavy equipment, including 20 Wessex helicopters or 16 main battle tanks or more than 30 other vehicles. Each ship also carried 30 tons of ammunition and much fuel.

The two ships anchored under an open sky and in broad daylight. The British air defences were unloaded during the morning and the crews of the batteries of missiles were hurriedly setting them up on the hillside overlooking the water. At 2 p.m. they still needed another hour to be ready for action. *Sir Tristram* had unloaded most of its troops but *Sir Galahad* was still crowded with soldiers.

Four Argentinian planes, flying at little more than masthead height, hit *Sir Tristram* with rockets and cannon-fire while heavy bombs struck *Sir Galahad.*

Flames quickly erupted, setting off ammunition. Men rushed to the ships' sides and scrambled down ropes into rubber life-rafts. Some of these were blown by the wind into patches of burning oil while others, hit by hot debris, burst into flames. When the ship's fuel tanks exploded the *Sir Galahad* was enveloped in thick black smoke, trapping many men still aboard ship. In this desperate emergency the helicopters flew straight into the smoke while their crewmen winched down on lines to pluck men from the deck of the ship.

To the soldiers already ashore, watching in shocked and mesmerized horror, Port Pleasant was a fearful sight, with lifeboats, orange inflatable rafts and landing craft ferrying ashore survivors and injured, some of whom were screaming in agony. Soldiers ran into the freezing water to take their shocked and wounded mates onto their shoulders. At the top of the beach armoured car crews strapped the men to their vehicles and drove them to the field hospital. After treatment here they were helicoptered back to the medical centre at San Carlos and within a few hours many were aboard the hospital ship *Uganda.*

On this worst day of the war for Britain, casualties were severe; 56 soldiers, mostly Welsh Guards, were killed and about 100 wounded or burned, while others had minor injuries. On *Sir Galahad* three officers and two members of the crew were killed and two officers and nine crew members were injured. Two members of the 16th Field Ambulance were killed during the disaster, Lance-Corporal Ian Farrell and Private Kenneth Pearson.

RAMC doctors, nurses and orderlies were taxed to the limit of their skill. That so many of the wounded survived was largely due to the professionalism of the medical teams. Burns so severe had not been seen in such numbers, in the British forces, since 1945. In many cases a long period of treatment, including 'plastic surgery', continued in hospitals in Britain. The Bluff Cove episode and the resulting casualties proved the wisdom of the War Staff in London of including a hospital ship in the campaign fleet. At first, the very number of burns produced problems but there was no uncertainty in the treatment. The RAMC had long realized that the inflammable fuels used in aircraft, armoured fighting vehicles and the ships were a likely cause of injuries in action and medical staff were trained to deal with them.

Following Port Pleasant, the task force moved on to lay siege to Port Stanley, held by the Argentinians. Sappers of the Royal Engineers had particular hazards to face in dealing with mines planted to slow down the British infantry. During the siege many deeds of heroism occurred, none more noteworthy than that of Royal Marine Leading Medical Assistant Steve Hayward. During an artillery barrage he brought to safety a marine whose foot had been blown off by a mine and used his own body to shield the wounded man from flying shell splinters.

The South Atlantic Task Force of 25,000 servicemen suffered 255 killed and another 600 wounded, some of them crippled for life. Yet others had been subjected to such a high degree of physical strain that they needed time to recuperate.

Cases of post traumatic stress disorder were common after the Falklands War. Welsh Guardsmen who survived the Bluff Cove disaster were particular sufferers. Counselling for PTSD had greatly developed since 1945, largely because of total acceptance by the military medical professionals that such a condition actually existed. From such a premise, armed forces psychologists and psychiatrists were able to formulate methods of treatment. Just as importantly, perhaps, senior military officers now accepted that fighting men under stress were not cowards, a view held by certain commanders during the First World War. The British Army of 1939–1945 did not have the equivalent of American General George Patton, who disgraced his rank by abusing and striking suffering soldiers, and after 1945 it was extremely unlikely that another Patton would emerge in the American forces.

CHAPTER TWENTY-EIGHT

Combat Medicine in the Gulf

Each war produces new problems and worries for surgeons and doctors in the field. In the great wars of the twentieth century the generals of the belligerent armies have used new weapons, produced for them by inventors, scientists, physicists and chemists, that have resulted in great challenges for military medical people.

For instance, in the First World War, 1914–18, poison gas attacks found medical science as unprepared to deal with its evil effects as the troops were who were the victims of the new suffocating and blistering agents. Initially, there was fear and panic both on and off the battlefield. Gangrene, though not new in 1914, became a critical and alarming problem in Flanders, also because it had not been anticipated.

During the Second World War many more fighting men were grievously burned than in any previous war, especially aircrew trapped in blazing planes and soldiers unable to escape from tanks enveloped by fire. In both wars frontline troops were hideously burned by what, in 1914–15, was called 'liquid fire.' It spewed from the nozzles of flame-throwers.

Through brilliant inventiveness, specialist surgeons found ways of treating such wounds and on the battlefield regimental medics were able to apply a reasonable degree of first aid.

The Gulf War of 1990–91 – also known as the Persian Gulf War – produced phenomena that confounded and confused the military leadership, the combat surgeons who had to deal with the problems and later the staff of military hospitals. Even government departments were involved. They were BW (biological warfare), CW (chemical warfare), NW (nuclear warfare) and 'Gulf War Syndrome'. In some ways, the dangers were more acute in anticipation than they proved to be in the field but this in no way lessened the responsibilities of the medical staff.

It is first necessary to sketch the causes of the war itself. On 2 August 1990, the dictator of Iraq, Saddam Hussein, invaded neighbouring Kuwait, pursuing a claim that Kuwait was actually part of Iraq. The United Nations objected and in support of UN Resolution 660, the United States, Britain and other nations – collectively known as the Coalition Forces – sent troops, ships and aircraft to the Persian Gulf in what was known as Operation Desert Shield.

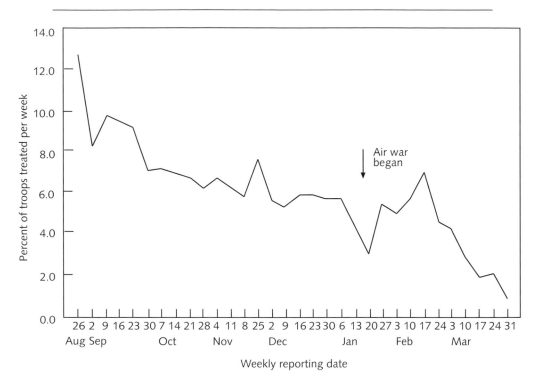

Total weekly rates of outpatient visitors among around 40,000 ground troops in Saudi Arabia during the Gulf War.

More than five months later, on 17 January 1991, Operation Desert Storm began with an air and long-range missile attack against Iraq, followed by a ground war 39 days later. Immense forces were built up. By the time hostilities ended on 27 February 1991 the US alone had 697,000 personnel in the area and Britain, the second largest contributor, had 30,000. In comparison with previous conflicts, a larger proportion of participants were women, 7 per cent of the force in the case of the US contribution and a slightly lower percentage for the British.

Operation Desert Shield and Operation Desert Storm were together a relatively brief war and the ground offensive, though violent and bloody, lasted only four days. Nevertheless, the operations left enormous medical problems in their wake.

The Allied troops had entered an extremely hot and bleak desert environment and initially they were not superior to the Iraqi Army. They were unaccustomed to the fierce heat and they carried an immense amount of equipment, more than any soldiers before had been burdened with, except perhaps, the British Marines and Paratroopers of the Falklands war.

No one could have known at the beginning of Operation Desert Shield that the Allied troops would win a quick and decisive war. A large proportion of the

British and American armies did not merely fight a 'four-day war,' the period of the most intensive hostilities; they spent months isolated in the hostile desert, under constant stress and not knowing when they would return home.

The logistic problems were immense, especially for the Americans. They had to deploy and support large numbers of troops more than 7,000 miles from the US. The British were closer to their home base and support and supply was not so difficult but like the Americans, the British troops had few amenities and lived under arduous and extreme conditions. The weather, initially so oppressively hot and humid, changed to cold and damp by the time the fighting began. Medical officers noted that few of the men and women became acclimatized because the climate of the Gulf and the surrounding deserts was unlike anything previously experienced by the troops.

Troops were crowded into warehouses, makeshift buildings and tents and privacy was minimal. Enlightened commanders have always tried to give soldiers a modicum of privacy, not only for the performance of body functions but because morale is higher when men are not living, breathing and sweating in close proximity to one another day and night. Wooden latrines were provided for sanitary needs but ablution blocks did not exist; there were only communal washing facilities. The diet consisted largely of prepacked meals, though quartermaster departments tried valiantly to supply some fruit and fresh meat.

All the British troops and most of the Americans were full-time regulars, with much training and experience behind them, so they were able to cope with the hardships. Veteran officers were heard to say, 'Thank God we aren't relying on conscripts for this war – they would never have been able to hack it.' Nevertheless, large number of reservists were with the US forces and they had greater difficulty in the trying conditions.

When hostilities finally began, the Allied troops were fully prepared and even anxious to get on with the job. They wanted to win and return home. Saudi Arabia had no leave and recreation facilities, such as most other areas of war have had during previous wars. During the Korean War most of the United Nations contingents arranged for their units to have R&R (rest and recreation) in Japan; during the Vietnam war, too, troops could go on leave to Saigon and other cities. They were squalid and diseases were rampant, including venereal infections, but at least the routine of active service was absent.

In Saudi Arabia, the principal base for the war against Iraq, any entertainment the troops enjoyed had to be taken to them. They were not permitted to visit Saudi cities. The Saudi authorities had forbidden this because they feared, no doubt with good reason, that Western troops could violate the strict Islamic way of life in Saudi Arabia.

Levels of apprehension and stress, which were very high during Operation Desert Shield, actually decreased once the war started. This was noted by all the medical teams.

The Americans, and through them their Western allies of the Coalition Forces, began Operation Desert Shield with at least one great medical advantage. The US Navy had medical research and treatment units which

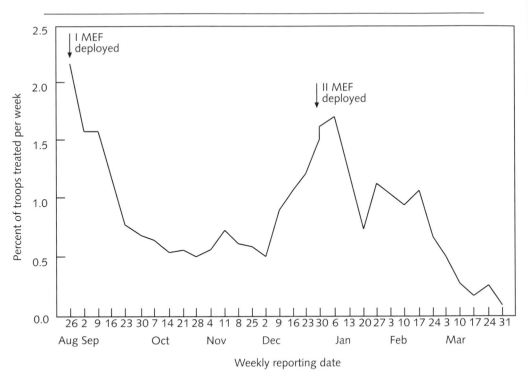

Weekly respiratory disease rates in the 40,000-strong US Marine Corps in Saudi Arabia. The two arrows indicate the points at which Marine Expeditionary Forces (MEF) were deployed.

had been operating continuously in the Middle East since 1946. They maintained their operations even during the period 1967–73 when the US and Egypt had a serious break in diplomatic relations. The base in Egypt had a long and distinguished record in training American and foreign medical personnel, even assisting local health ministries.

In all, as Desert Shield began, the USN had six overseas infectious disease research laboratories. The navy operated a sophisticated diagnostic laboratory and an active research and surveillance programme in the Middle East. With extensive experience in the region, the USN doctors knew what infectious diseases threatened the troops who were then arriving, they understood what diagnostic tests were needed in Saudi Arabia and, most importantly, they could operate effectively in the difficult political and social region. They knew 'their way around'.

Beginning in August 1990, USN preventive medicine personnel and scientists began evaluating infectious disease risks among the troops. In September, the Navy Forward Laboratory (NFL) was established in the Marine Corps Hospital in El-Jubail, Saudi Arabia. This place, taken over by the Marines, had been an unoccupied civilian hospital that had all the requirements to accommodate a modern diagnostic laboratory, as well as an unused clinical facility, running water and air conditioning. Satellite labs were established at El Mishab, El Khanjar and Kuwait city.

British and American troops were exposed to a number of diseases, including respiratory and diarrhoeal infections commonly found among troops serving overseas, as well as some tropical diseases rarely seen in the US or Western Europe. The most significant was leishmaniasis, an insect-transmitted complaint. It is not only a chronic disease but its parasites can be transmitted by blood transfusion.

American doctors diagnosed 31 cases of leishmania infection and for a time these men were not used as blood donors. In the event, no reports were made of leishmania transmission from blood donated by Desert Storm veterans.

The troops would have had no idea of the wide-ranging research and disease prevention carried out on their behalf. The medical staff sent frequent reports to the military commanders briefing them on potential dangers. For instance, they were told that two other infections found in the Middle East and which can cause chronic disease are Q-fever and brucellosis, a weakening disease caused by direct contact with infected animals or from milk, dairy products and meat from such animals.

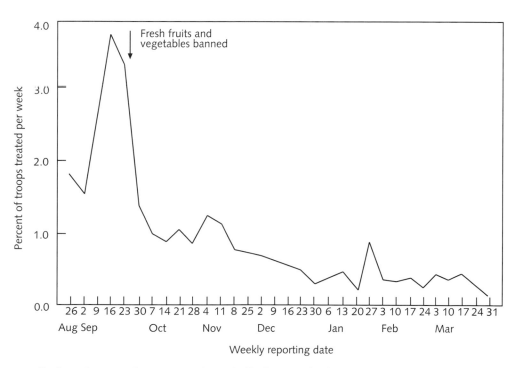

Fresh produce was shown to contain local, diarrhoea causing bacteria. A ban on the produce had a major impact on the number of US troops treated for gastroenteritis in Saudi Arabia during the Gulf War.

Close observation showed that soldiers with unexplained illnesses did not have recurrent fever or the serious complications associated with these and other infections, including pneumonia, hepatitis, osteomyelitis and meningitis.

Another report stated that known viral diseases found in the Persian Gulf – sandfly fever, Crimean-Congo haemorrhaic fever and dengue – do not cause chronic infection.

When fully operational, America's NFL served as the regional infectious diseases reference laboratory for Coalition Forces. Even countries which normally had poor relations with the US, such as Syria, called on NFL for help.

During Operation Desert Shield, the main focus of NFL was to analyse blood and stool samples from patients and to assist preventive medicine personnel in the field. In staff cars, the NFL team travelled extensively around north-eastern Saudi Arabia, evaluating patients and assessing health risks. During these travels, one of the first problems that arose concerned the numerous piles of dead animals – goats, sheep and camels – that were scattered across the desert.

The nomadic Bedouin left the dead animals in specific locations for counting and compensation by the government. Many of them had been perfectly healthy but killing them and claiming that they had died from natural causes gave the Bedouin a steady income. Some had died from natural causes. In any case, in the desert the dead animals tended to dry out rather than rot quickly.

Naturally, American and British troops who camped near these locations were worried about the risk they posed to health. The NFL teams decided the corpses were not themselves a direct health risk but they were a breeding ground for insect-transmitted disease. Military entomologists – who had never before been part of an army – sprayed the bodies with insecticide. This spraying observed by troops may explain some subsequent alarming reports of dead animals and insects, particularly among troops who arrived in Saudi Arabia in January and February 1991 at the start of the war. These newly arrived troops would not have known that dead animals had been in the desert for at least five months before hostilities began.

Acute diarrhoeal disease and common colds were the main infectious disease problems during the early stages of service in the Gulf, continuing the trend of centuries. About two-thirds of the ground troops had acute diarrhoea during both Operation Desert Shield and Operation Desert Storm. Nearly all cases were due to the infectious agents which NFL personnel had identified during earlier service periods of American troops in the Middle East. It was generally known as 'tourista,' 'the trots' or Shigella, but not a single case of typhoid fever, cholera or amoebic dysentery was identified by laboratory analysis.

There are risks at any time when troops are crowded together and rapidly deployed overseas. In Saudi Arabia, the soldiers of the US and Britain often had acute upper respiratory infections and complaints – coughs, sore throat, sneezing, runny nose. The fine blowing sand of Saudi Arabia also causes respiratory problems but they were less common among troops living in tents and open warehouses. Troops living in tightly constructed buildings had even more symptoms because in closed and crowded spaces they were more likely to pass respiratory infections to one another.

There were only seven cases of malaria, three of Q-fever, one of West Nile fever and no cases at all of brucellosis. These low figures in an area where such diseases are common says much for the effective high standards of hygiene and effective preventive medicine employed during the Gulf War.

During the Gulf War, the US Marine Corps provided one of the best examples in military history of disease prevention and surveillance. The first Marine personnel to arrive in the Gulf in August 1990 were not warriors but preventive medicine (PM) specialists. These highly trained experts were built into the Marine Table of Organization at multiple levels. They were assigned to the front line units, to the combat support elements and to the highest H/Q levels. These specialists knew precisely what illnesses might affect marines and sailors in any area, including the Persian Gulf.

Within the First Marine Division, an environmental health officer was assigned to the Division Surgeon's staff to advise on field sanitation, protection of food and water, proper immunization and the prevention of insect-borne diseases. From the beginning of Desert Shield, PM personnel were actually serving in the front lines.

For perhaps the first time, 'heat injury' was seriously considered to be one of the most significant health threats in early deployment. Also, skin conditions, a major cause of lost man hours in many previous conflicts, were under constant surveillance. Eye problems, such as 'pink eye,' can be epidemic in field conditions and corneal abrasions from blowing sand were also a risk in the desert; the PM warriors dealt with this too.

In many armies in previous wars, unexplained fevers were 'treated' simply by handing the sufferer some aspirin. The PM men and women were on the alert for such unexplained fevers because they can be the first sign of diseases, such as sandfly fever. The PM officers were also trained to notice psychiatric symptoms, which were bound to develop under stresses of active service and combat.

Each week, each unit's aid stations reviewed its sick-call log-books and determined how many marines or sailors were treated for various categories of health problems. A rate was then calculated for each category, based on how many marines or sailors were assigned to a unit. These simple calculations allowed PM personnel to determine what percentage of the unit was treated during the previous week for these problems. If the percentage was higher, the cause was investigated. The surveillance system was highly successful in keeping marines and sailors healthy during the two operations.

On average, approximately 6 per cent of ground troops were treated each week for some kind of illness or injury, this compared favourably with the rates in garrison troops at Camp Pendleton, California, where about 4 per cent of personnel per week were treated. The field rates decreased during the service period as troops adapted to conditions and PM efforts identified and controlled health threats.

Because the US military was ready for the health threats its troops encountered in the Persian Gulf War, the disease non-battle injury (DNBI) rate was lower than in previous conflicts. The good health of American troops was partly due to the comprehensive PM efforts, accurate and rapid laboratory diagnosis and the extensive health care system that was established in Saudi Arabia during Operation Desert Shield.

Besides these medical measures, several fortunate circumstances aided US and British troops.

* Deployment to barren desert locations during cooler winter months when insect activity was lowest.
* Limited contact with non-military populations.
* Very limited access to alcohol.
* The great advances made in Kuwait and Saudi Arabia during the period 1960–90 in public health and elimination of local diseases.

Wars cannot be conducted as large epidemiological studies but greater diagnostic surveillance information was collected on American troops during the Persian Gulf deployment than in previous wars. After the end of that war these data aided investigators in the search for the causes of veterans' health problems. The principal unanswered health question following the war against Iraq was the causes of the unexplained symptoms experienced by some Gulf War veterans. It is interesting that similar physical symptoms were reported by veterans during the American Civil War, 140 years earlier.

Combat casualties were fewer than anticipated. American: 389 killed, some of them accidentally, 457 wounded. Other Allied casualties: 77 killed, 830 wounded. The Iraqi loss was great – 30,000 killed, 100,000 wounded.

For the Allies, the incidence of non-battle injuries and diseases was low in comparison to other campaigns of the century, markedly lower than during the Korean, Vietnam and Falklands wars.

CHAPTER TWENTY-NINE

The Lingering Gulf War

Many nations have stocks of poison gas, napalm and anti-personnel mines and the latter, sown in their millions, have wounded many more civilians than enemy soldiers. However, few nations in history have matched the lethal depravity of Iraq in its intensive efforts to develop and use chemical and biological weapons of mass destruction. President Saddam Hussein used poison gas against his own citizens, the Kurds, proof that he would employ it against a foreign enemy. Indeed, he did just this – against the Iranians in the Iraq-Iran War of 1984–8.

The Coalition Forces were worried that Iraq would use chemical warfare and biological warfare against them during the Gulf War. Extensive preparations were made to prepare for this threat, including thorough training of medical personnel in the Western armies. Never before had specialist medical officers in the field taken a perceived threat so seriously. Tens of thousands of automatic chemical agent sensors were arrayed across the vast areas where combat was likely. These sensors were extremely sensitive in order to provide early warning.

At the beginning of the war, all US and British troops were provided with an individual CW 'warning kit' containing twenty-one 30 mg tablets of pyridostigmine bromide to help prevent the lethal effects of CW nerve agents. When the risk of chemical attack was judged to be significant, commanders instructed the troops to take one pyridostigmine tablet every eight hours. It was supposed to be a 'safe' drug but it often produced acute gastro-intestinal and urinary disturbances among Desert Storm troops.

During Operation Desert Storm the emphasis of all Service Medical personnel moved from routine infectious disease problems to the threat of biological warfare. It was well known that Saddam Hussein's scientists had developed biological weapons of mass destruction. It was obvious to all the Coalition Forces that troops had to be protected against such a threat and, first of all, there had to be methods of detecting BW agents.

The techniques used for detection were developed by international medical experts and their methods were state-of-the-art.

The most likely threat, based on the best intelligence at the time, was from the use of projectiles loaded with the bacterium clostridium botulinum, the bacteria that cause anthrax and botulism. Anthrax affects livestock and causes diseases among humans working closely with infected animals or their hides. Anthrax is an effective BW agent because, when inhaled, it causes rapid death from massive bleeding in the lungs. Botulinum toxin is a highly lethal substance which causes death, even in developed countries, when contaminated food is improperly canned or stored. Because this toxin in minute amounts causes rapid paralysis and death it is ideal for biological warfare production – and Iraqi military laboratories had stocks of it.

Despite an exhaustive, methodical and consistent search for BW agents no evidence of them was detected during Operation Desert Shield or Desert Storm, only later. The NFL staff provided commanders with accurate information about the nature of the biological threat throughout the Gulf War and their reports were considered as important as any of the military intelligence reports.

Because of frequent CW alarms during the air and ground war, troops often had to don their protective gear and take their tablets. These alarms turned out to be false and were the result of automatic detectors being triggered by 'harmless' substances, such as vehicle exhaust fumes. However, in conjunction with battlefield rumours of other units being hit by CW attacks, the troops were understandably concerned that they had been exposed to chemical warfare. On battlefields, rumours spread more rapidly than any toxic agents.

The US Department of Defense (DoD), the US Defense Science Boards Task Force on Gulf War Effects and the British Ministry of Defence (MoD) concluded that the Iraqis did not use CW/BW weapons against Coalition Forces and that there was no exposure to them of troops in Kuwait and Saudi Arabia during hostilities. No CW/BW weapons were found on the battlefield itself, only to the rear, and no intention to use CW/BW agents were uncovered during extensive and intensive interrogation of Iraqi prisoners of war.

However, there were several credible CW agent detections by Czechoslovakian chemical defence teams attached to the Saudi Arabian military. They were of extremely low, non-incapacitating levels of CW agents which did not persist for longer than a few hours. Also, the detections occurred in areas where there was no known military action or incoming Iraqi Scud missiles and where few American and British troops were located.

It is possible that the Czech findings resulted from CW agents released from Iraq production and storage facilities bombed by US and British aircraft. But CW and BW agents are highly lethal even in low concentrations and had they been released hundreds of miles inside Iraq massive fatalities would have resulted among Iraqis living near these facilities, especially as levels there would have been extremely high. Aerial photographs and intelligence reports disclosed no such disasters.

During the war there were worrying signs that something was 'wrong' with the health of some troops. The most commonly reported complaint was chronic fatigue, loss of appetite, skin rash, headache, arthralgias/ myalgias, difficulty in concentrating, irritability and forgetfulness. These symptoms were not localized to any one organ system and there was no consistent physical sign or laboratory abnormality to indicate a specific disease. The possible causes were many, exposure to dust, sand and smoke being among the more simple.

Collectively, these and many other symptoms gave rise to what soon came to be called the Gulf War Syndrome. This phenomenon demonstrated that the fighting forces need specialist medical teams long after a war ends. This had always been recognized, especially after the Second World War when veterans were treated more sympathetically and humanely than ever before. But no conflicts before that of the Persian Gulf War had left lingering medical problems on the scale of Gulf War Syndrome. The United States, Britain and other Western nations of the Coalition Forces were worried that if this syndrome were not diagnosed and treated similar problems could arise in other conflicts, leading, perhaps, to near paralysis of military effort.

There were various events in what I shall call the Lingering Gulf War that caused concern. It was essential that Saddam Hussein's munition storage depots be destroyed and one of them, that at Khamisiyah, is a worrying example. The story of what is known as 'the Operation Asp' had three parts: the efforts of the US forces to destroy Asp, the inspection of the site by the United Nations Special Commission (or UNSCOM) and the public inquiry into the events that occurred there – summed up as 'what we knew and when we knew it.'

Khamisiyah was a huge storage site, covering 30 square miles and containing about 100 ammunition bunkers and several other types of storage facilities. US forces set off two gigantic explosions in March 1991. During these operations and throughout the entire period of US occupation of Khamisiyah there were no reports of verified CW detections, nor were there reports of anybody experiencing symptoms consistent with exposure to CW.

UNSCOM later inspected Khamisiyah specifically searching for CW agents and they located three sites that had contained chemical weapons. In October 1991 UNSCOM inspectors found intact rockets containing the chemical agents sarin and cyclosarin. It was known that the Iraqis had 2,160 such rockets at Khamisiyah. Worse was to follow. The team, searching an above-ground storage site west of Khamisiyah found 6,300 intact 155 mm artillery shells filled with mustard 'gas' agent. Saddam Hussein had certainly been prepared to use CW against the Coalition Forces. 'Riot control' CS gas was also found. Many rockets were leaking, which enabled the specialists to identify chemical warfare nerve agents.

Mustard 'gas' refers to several manufactured chemicals including sulphur mustard. Mustard 'gas' does not behave as a gas under ordinary conditions and it is really a liquid. It makes the eyes burn, the eyelids swell and causes a lot of blinking. Breathing mustard 'gas' causes coughing, bronchitis and long-term respiratory problems. It was used during the Iran-Iraq War.

Sarin is a light brown liquid and is more commonly known as GB. It is toxic both as fumes and to the touch and a single milligram coming into contact with the skin is sufficient to kill. Cyclosarin, generally referred to as GF, is a nerve agent similar to sarin but more persistent.

It was not known what chemical, biological or radiological releases reached American troops in the area where the demolition explosions took place. Investigators concluded that the likely movement of vapour was to the east and northeast – away from US troops.

Letters were sent to 21,000 Gulf War veterans, to tell them of the Khamisiyah incident, to inform them of the potential for low-level exposure to CW agents and to notify them to sign up for medical examination. The US Government even established a Persian Gulf Hotline so that veterans could seek – and give – information.

Many other case incidents came to light. During February 1992 a US Marine was taking readings from a Fox chemical detector vehicle, trying to determine if enemy prisoner-of-war gear contained a chemical agent. Soon after he developed blisters. Other men who had contact with wounded Iraqi soldiers also developed an indefinable sickness, similar to that of some men who had been at Khamisiyah.

The British Ministry of Defence doctors evaluated 33 veterans predominantly complaining of fatigue, weakness, pains in muscles and joints, headache and other 'non-specific' problems.

One experimental investigation into unexplained illnesses focussed on 100 American veterans with symptoms for which there was no ready explanation. The diagnoses were diverse and included asthma, inflammatory bowel diseases and various rheumatologic, neurologic and psychiatric conditions, including post-traumatic stress disorder. In another evaluation of 42 veterans, impairments in memory and fine motor skills were found in 24 per cent and 48 per cent of patients, respectively.

Some veterans, British and American, complained of 'burning semen' during sexual intercourse. Following reports that veterans' family members had contracted unexplained illnesses from Gulf War men, services surgeons pointed out that potential infectious disease threats and likely infectious BW agents – *Bacillus anthrancis*, *Yersinia pestis* – are not transmitted by casual personal contact and are rarely if ever transmitted by sexual contact.

Two non-live vaccines, botulinum and anthrax, were postulated to be causes of unexplained illnesses which could be part of the Gulf War Syndrome. The botulinum vaccine was an unlikely factor, army doctors said, because it was given to only 8,000 troops, who were closely monitored. None reported problems with unexplained illnesses. The anthrax vaccine was given to a much larger number of men, approximately 150,000, but no association was found between this vaccine and unexplained illness.

The possibility that chronic fatigue and debility could result from the combination of vaccinations that Gulf troops were given over a short period of time, rather than any single vaccine, has been suggested. However, long-term effects have not been observed among repeatedly immunized foreign travellers. US military recruits routinely receive eight or more vaccinations during induction.

The crews of the naval vessels engaged in the Gulf operations regularly took tablets to condition their bodies against the effects of nerve gas. As a result, many sailors claimed to be suffering from tiredness, blurred vision, dizziness and flatulence. There were rumours that the medication was destroying libidos, and some men stopped taking the tablets. Ships' captains had to announce special orders, reminding their men that they were risking their lives by not following the prophylactic guidelines. Even more worrying, vaccines produced severe influenza-like symptoms for up to 48 hours.

Desert Storm troops were exposed to several potentially harmful environmental hazards, the most spectacular being the smoke from 605 oil-well fires started by the retreating Iraqi army. A concerted effort was made by services doctors to evaluate the health effects from these fires, which continued to blaze for weeks. Based on data collected between May and December 1991, the doctors, chemists and pathologists decided that the risks had been minimal because the smoke had been lofted well above ground level and there had been nearly complete combustion of most chemical substances. Significantly, the civilian fire-fighters who were highly exposed to the oil-well fires reported no symptoms of unexplained illnesses.

In addition to smoke, the doctors considered the exposure of troops to low levels of several pesticides. The vast majority of pesticides employed in the Gulf were products that had been used during numerous exercises of American and British troops in various parts of the world. Herbicides, which had definitely caused serious health problems to American and Australian troops in South-East Asia, were not used by the Coalition Forces in the desert environment. Pet flea collars, which contain potentially harmful chemicals, were used inappropriately by a small number of troops before being prohibited but they were not associated with unexplained illnesses.

American reservists, of whom there were a large number in the Gulf, were frequently classified as having unexplained illnesses. Reservists tended to be older and less physically resilient compared to active duty troops. Also, reserve personnel probably suffered increased stress because they had to leave civilian jobs and experience greater disruption of their personal lives.

It was not generally made known that some troops were exposed to a number of other potential environment hazards. They included microwaves, chemical-agent-resistant-coating (CARC) paint fumes containing the toxic isocynate, to various petroleum products like JP4 fuel used in tent heaters and on the ground to keep the sand from blowing and to other airborne allergens and irritants.

Overall, Desert Storm troops may have suffered from too much emphasis on their protection and comfort. Perhaps the combat doctors were overly concerned about their troops' welfare.

A puzzling aspect of Gulf War Syndrome is that there was no evident increase in the number of reported deaths among US Gulf War veterans to the end of 1998. While 2,000 veterans had died since the war, more than

3,000 would be expected in an age- and gender-matched US civilian population and medically screened for military service.

Whatever the doubts, fears and uncertainties about the Lingering Gulf War, one fact emerged. It was a victory for Saddam Hussein. Research, treatment and compensation for Gulf War Syndrome cost the Coalition Forces, especially the Americans, hundreds of millions of dollars. Without even actively using CW and BW agents, Saddam had the satisfaction of seeing his Western enemies confused and apprehensive about his intentions. He would expect that in the future Western leaders would be reluctant to commit ground troops to a war against him. During the decade after the Gulf War this expectation was fulfilled.

Captain Chris Craig, the senior Royal Navy officer in the Gulf, noted: 'The emotional preoccupation with chemical weapons was out of proportion with their real threat, but such is the nature of the unknown. We increased our already regular drills and were often unsettled by spurious alarms from the upper-deck chemical alarms.'

Saddam Hussein was affecting his enemies' morale without actively engaging in chemical warfare against them. We can expect the threat of using BW and CW agents to be increasingly used as a tactic of warfare, just as threats of nuclear attack were used throughout the years of the Cold War.

The United States Department of Defense appointed Bernard Rostker a retired lieutenant-general, who was also a medical doctor, as special assistant for the investigation of Gulf War illnesses. When taking up his appointment, Rostker said, 'if we can't explain what went on in the Gulf, then we will have a very poor ability to put in place military doctrine, medical policies and practical treatment of troops'.

He might equally well have said: 'We cannot afford to have medical mysteries in the armed forces – they reduce our ability to function effectively.' It seems that the work of combat surgeons is unending.

Postscript

War has produced some of medicine's greatest accomplishments, such as mass inoculation, antiseptic surgery, blood and plasma transfusions, plastic reconstruction and surgical developments, heart and lung surgery among them, that once would have seemed fantasy.

For later generations of soldiers the speed of treatment gave a much greater chance of survival, at least in the armed forces of developed countries. Casualty statistics bear this out. In the First World War the average time between injury and treatment was 10 to 18 hours and many a surgeon wrote of removing battlefield dressings to discover maggots in a wound. In Vietnam, the swiftness – and courage – of helicopter pilots on medevac duties cut the time to an average of one to two hours. In that war less than 2 per cent of wounded men who reached hospital died. Deaths from disease were infinitely fewer than during the Second World War.

But we give too little thought to the psychological impact of conflict on the wounded and most people give no thought whatever to what it does to the combat surgeon. It should be noted that in the American military all doctors are officially listed as surgeons. There is no separate classification of physician. Mankind has become ever more inventive in the destruction of his own species with resultant trauma to doctors. One regimental doctor who served in Vietnam wrote of 'mud, screams and the terrible smell of death'.

Dominique Jean-Larrey, already referred to, is said to have performed more than 200 amputations during a single day of Napoleon's doomed march on Moscow in 1812. Because of this astonishing effort, some of Larrey's patients lived. But at what cost to Larrey's peace of mind? Professional though he was, did he never hear screams in his sleep? A photograph exists of a heap of men's amputated feet and legs piled outside the door of a hospital during the American Civil War. The photographer gave it the label, 'A Morning's Work'. For the surgeons was the memory of this work difficult to live with?

I believe that it is difficult. Military physicians and surgeons become accustomed to the diseases, wounds and injuries and their treatment. That is the professional side of their work. But they are always conscious of the suffering and pain they witness and they inwardly rage against the waste of life and health, wilfully inflicted by nations and men on one another.

This is the combat surgeon's own hidden wound.

Sources

These are sources referred to by number in the text. They were published in London unless otherwise stated.

1   Blond, Georges (1966). *Verdun*. André Deutsch.
2   Mills, M. (1825). *History of Chivalry*.
3   Chevers, J. *Moral and Social Conditions of the British Soldier*; contemporary account.
4   Stevenson, Joseph, ed. (1861–4). *Letters and Papers Illustrative of the Wars of the English in France during the Reign of Henry VI*. Rolls Series.
5   Prescott, W.H. (1850). *History of the Reign of Ferdinand and Elizabeth*. 15th edn.
6   Description by Joseph Grundpeck von Burckhausen, a contemporary writer. (Geneva).
7   Grose, Francis (1801). *Military Antiquities*.
8   Monro, Donald (1765). From *Account of the Diseases most Frequent in the British Military Hospitals in Germany from January 1761 to the Return of the Troops in 1763*.
9   Hunter, John. From *Observations on the Diseases of the Army in Jamaica*.
10 Hamilton, Richard (1794). *The Duties of a Regimental Surgeon*.
11 Zimmerman, A. (1770). *Experience of Physic*. Zurich.
12 (1819). *Narrative of a Private Soldier in one of His Majesty's Regiments of Foot*. Glasgow.
13 Hamilton, see note 10.
14 Guthrie, G.J. (1827). *A Treatise on Gunshot Wounds*.
15 Longmore, Thomas Longmore was the leading English authority on ambulance transport, on which he wrote a manual, 1893. The material he amassed from many countries is now in the Muniments Room, Royal Army Medical College, London.
16 Kinkaid, John (1832). *Adventures in the Rifle Brigade*.
17 Settle, A.H. (1905). *Anecdotes of Soldiers*. Methuen.
18 Gronow, Rees Howell (1934). *Last Recollections of Captain Gronow*. Selwyn Blount.
19 Vansittart, Jane (1964). *Surgeon James' Journal*. Cassell.
20 Larrey, D.J. (1812–17). *Mémoires de Chirurgie Militaire et Campagnes du Baron*. Paris.
21 See note 20.
22 Several men who left first-hand accounts of the Russian campaign of 1812 commented on the endurance and courage of the women. Captain Franz Roeder (*The Ordeal of Captain Roeder*, Methuen, 1960) and Sergeant Bourgogne (*Memoirs of Sergeant Bourgogne*, Peter Davis, 1926) discuss it in detail.
23 Walter, R. *Lord Anson's Voyage Round in the World 1740–4*. Abbr. & ed. S.W.C. Pack, Penguin Books, 1948. His narrative is the only complete first-hand record of Anson's voyage.

24   Blane, Sir Gilbert (1785). *Observations on the Diseases of Seamen.*
25   Trotter, Thomas (1796–1803). *Medica Nautica.*
26   Lind, James (1753). *A Treatise on Scurvy.* Edinburgh.
27   Milroy, Gavin. *The Health of the Royal Navy Considered,* in a letter addressed to Rt Hon Sir John S. Pakington, MP (The Longmore Pamphlets, see note 15).
28   Southey, Robert (1807). *Espriella's Letters.*
29   Shipp, John (1843). *Memoirs of the Military Career of John Shipp.*
30   See note 10.
31   From the *United Services Journal,* 1830.
32   Cherry, F.C. (1825). *Observations on the defective state of army transport, with suggestions for improvement.*
33   Alcock, Rutherford (1838). *Notes on the Medical History and Statistics of the British Legion in Spain.*
34   Ballingall, George (1838). *Outlines of Military Surgery.* Edinburgh.
35   From an Army Medical Department memo, 20 June 1854, by Director-General Sir Andrew Smith.
36   Cattel, William. This surgeon left a vast unpublished biography from which I have extracted many details of a surgeon's life in the Crimea.
37   See note 36.
38   From a Report, 1867, on the administration of the transport and supply departments of the Army; Appendix 28.
39   *Campagne de l'Empereur Napoléon III, en Italie,* 1859. Documents officiels, 3me édit. Paris, 1865.
40   Hammond, S.P., US Surgeon-General. In the American *Medical Times.* 1862, p. 193.
41   Wilkeson, Frank (1885). *Recollections.* New York.
42   Letterman, Jo (1866). *Medical Recollections of the Army of the Potomac.* New York.
43   Longmore, See note 15.
44   Mongmore, See note 15.
45   Villiers, Frederic (1898). *Pictures of Many Wars.*
46   These figures, with others, were quoted by Surgeon-Major H. Melladew, Royal Horse Guards, in *Notes on Antiseptic Surgery in War,* 1881, a government publication.
47   Taken from *Jahresbericht,* 1880, a German translation by Surgeon-General Dr Roth of Pirogoff's report on the Russo-Turkish War. Vienna.
48   Longmore. See note 15.
49   The 1830–6 figures from the *British and Foreign Medical Quarterly Review,* April 1844, p. 313.
50   Evatt, G.H.H. (1878). *Comparative Examination of Regimental and Departmental Systems.*
51   Shipley, A.E. (1916). *The Minor Horrors of War.* Smith, Elder.
52   Corbett, A.F. (1953). *Service Through Six Reigns,* privately printed.
53   Gask, George. In a lecture to the Medical Society of London, 7 February 1921.
54   Nicholls, Lieutenant Colonel T.B. (1936 and 1940). *Organisation, Strategy and Tactics of the Army Medical Services in War.* Baillière, Tindall & Co.
55   Gask. See note 53.
56   Gibbs, Philip (1929). *Realities of War,* rev. edn. Hutchinson.
57   Sparrow, Geoffrey, & MacBean-Ross, J.N; Surgeons, RN (1918). *On Four Fronts With the Royal Naval Division.* Hodder & Stoughton.

58 Dearden, Harold (1928). *Medicine & Duty*. Written as a diary in the field, this is a surgeon's vivid but matter-of-fact account of his experiences on the Western Front.

59 Moodie, William (1930). *Crown of Honour*. Clarke. An anthology of war incidents.

60 Swindell, G.H. Manuscript. A merchant seaman who left the sea to fight in Kitchener's army, Swindell wrote a graphic diary-like account of his life in 77th Field Ambulance.

61 Gibbs. See note 56.

62 Dearden. See note 58.

63 Dolbey, Robert (1917). *A Regimental Surgeon in War and Prison*. John Murray. Taken prisoner on the Western Front, Dolbey kept a record of the rigours of prison medical work.

64 Luard, K.E., Sister (1930). *Unknown Warriors*. Chatto & Windus. Extracts from letters written home while serving in France, Sister Luard's letters are unrivalled in their graphic objectivity.

65 Anonymous (1917). *Nursing Adventures, by a FANY in France*. Hutchinson

66 Marsden, Alexandrina (1961). *Resistance Nurse*. Odhams.

67 Thurstan, Violetta (1916). *Field Hospital and Flying Column*. Putnam. An account of war nursing in Belgium and Russia.

68 Grauwin, Major (1955). *Doctor in Dien Bien Phu*. A superbly written account of the medical difficulties of the French doctors beseiged with the French army by the Vietminh.

69 Donald, Brigadier Charles (1944). *With the Eighth Army in the Field*. Monograph, BMA. I have drawn heavily from this lucid account of medical work in North Africa, Sicily, Italy. Brigadier Donald was consulting surgeon to the Eighth Army.

70 Cottrell, Anthony (1942). *R.A.M.C.* Hutchinson.

71 Pyle, Ernie (1943). *Brave Men in Action*. Henry Holt.

72 Library of Congress official information. New York.

73 Pavillard, Stanley (1960). *Bamboo Doctor*. Macmillan.

74 Rogers, Lindsay (1957). *Guerrilla Surgeon*. Collins.

75 Ahrenfeldt, R.H. (1958). *Psychiatry in the British Army in the Second World War*. Routledge & Kegan Paul.

76 Ahrenfeldt. See note 75.

77 Bartlett, F.C. (1927). *Psychology and the Soldier*. Cambridge University Press.

Among the best American authors about modern combat surgeons are Dr Albert E. Cowdrey and Dr Ronald J. Glasser.

Cowdrey is the author of *Fighting for Life: American Military Medicine in the Second World War*, The Free Press, New York, 1994. His book is the first comprehensive history of what he justifiably calls 'one of the most important yet under-appreciated weapons of the Second World War – America's extraordinary military medicine'.

Glasser wrote *365 Days*, George Braziller Inc., New York, 1971. *Newsweek*'s reviewer called this book, 'The most convincing, most moving account I have yet read about what it was like to be an American soldier in Vietnam.' I would add to this that *365 Days* – which refers to the length of time men were required to serve in Vietnam – is the most revealing account about medics and combat surgeons in Vietnam. It is essential reading about the horrors of service in Vietnam.

Apart from sources referred to specifically by reference number, I have made use of hundreds of other books, diaries and documents, in particular Peter Lovegrove's, *Not Least in the Crusade*, a short history of the RAMC, Gale & Polden, 1951. Since a full list would be tedious to read I give only my other major sources:

Barnsley, Major-General R.E. (1963). *Mars and Aesculapius*, a lecture given in the Royal Army Medical College.
Borodin, George (1944). *Red Surgeon*. Museum Press.
Caldwell, R. (1904). *Prevention of Diseases in the Army*.
Drew, Major-General W.R.M. 'Medicine's Debt to the Army and the Challenge of Tropical Medicine', from the *Journal of the RAMC*, vol. 110.
Edwards, Colonel Harold (1955). 'the Contribution of War to the Advancement of Surgery'. The Blackham Lecture.
Fergusson, William (1843). *Notes & Recollections of a Professional Life*.
Girdlestone, Dr Thomas (1787). *Essays on Hepatitis and Spasmodic Affections of India*.
Glasscheib, H.S. (1961). *The March of Medicine*. Macdonald.
Gordon, Dr C.A. (1870). *Army Surgeons and Their Works*.
Jackson, Dr Robert (1845). *Formation, Discipline and Economy of Armies*, 3rd edn.
Kraus, Felix (1861). *Das Kranken Zerstreuungs-System*. Vienna. (Concerning Solferino.)
Lande, Dr P. *Du Transport des Blessés et des Malades par Les Voies Ferrées et Navigables*.
Life Blood (1943). Official Account of the Transfusion Services, HMSO.
Makins, G.H. (1901). *Surgical Experiences in South Africa 1899–1900*. Smith Elder.
Power, Lieutenant Colonel D.O. (1915). *Wounds in War*. Oxford.
Rush, Benjamin (1789). *Medical Enquiries and Observations* (on the War of Independence). Philadelphia.
Tales of a Field Ambulance (1935). Told by the personnel. Privately printed.
Smart, William (1873). *History of the Medical Staff of the British Army Prior to the Tudors*.
Longmore pamphlets (1854–91). 8 vols. A remarkable collection of letters, documents, pamphlets. The authors include Florence Nightingale, Dunant, Paré, Larrey.
Parkes Pamphlets, 30 vols. Similar to the Longmore pamphlets but not all of military medical interest.
Various letters written by surgeons in the field to the National Society for Aid to Wounded in War and pamphlets published by the Society, especially in connection with the Russo-Turkish War, 1877. *Under the Red Crescent*, 1879, is most revealing.

Index